GUIDE TO
CANCER IMMUNOTHERAPY

Edited by
Suzanne Walker, CRNP, MSN, AOCN®, BC
Elizabeth Prechtel Dunphy, DNP, RN, CRNP, BC, AOCN®

Oncology Nursing Society
Pittsburgh, Pennsylvania

ONS Publications Department

Publisher and Director of Publications: William A. Tony, BA, CQIA
Senior Editorial Manager: Lisa M. George, BA
Assistant Editorial Manager: Amy Nicoletti, BA, JD
Acquisitions Editor: John Zaphyr, BA, MEd
Associate Staff Editors: Casey S. Kennedy, BA, Andrew Petyak, BA
Design and Production Administrator: Dany Sjoen
Editorial Assistant: Judy Holmes

Library of Congress Cataloging-in-Publication Data

Names: Walker, Suzanne (Suzanne L.), editor. | Dunphy, Elizabeth Prechtel, editor. | Oncology Nursing Society, issuing body.
Title: Guide to cancer immunotherapy / edited by Suzanne Walker, Elizabeth Prechtel Dunphy.
Description: Pittsburgh, Pennsylvania : Oncology Nursing Society, [2018] | Includes bibliographical references and index.
Identifiers: LCCN 2018018908 (print) | LCCN 2018019532 (ebook) | ISBN 9781635930191 (ebook) | ISBN 9781635930184 (pbk.) | ISBN 9781635930191 (e-book)
Subjects: | MESH: Neoplasms–therapy | Neoplasms–nursing | Immunotherapy–nursing | Oncology Nursing–methods
Classification: LCC RC266 (ebook) | LCC RC266 (print) | NLM WY 156 | DDC 616.99/40231–dc23
LC record available at https://lccn.loc.gov/2018018908

Publisher's Note

This book is published by the Oncology Nursing Society (ONS). ONS neither represents nor guarantees that the practices described herein will, if followed, ensure safe and effective patient care. The recommendations contained in this book reflect ONS's judgment regarding the state of general knowledge and practice in the field as of the date of publication. The recommendations may not be appropriate for use in all circumstances. Those who use this book should make their own determinations regarding specific safe and appropriate patient care practices, taking into account the personnel, equipment, and practices available at the hospital or other facility at which they are located. The editors and publisher cannot be held responsible for any liability incurred as a consequence from the use or application of any of the contents of this book. Figures and tables are used as examples only. They are not meant to be all-inclusive, nor do they represent endorsement of any particular institution by ONS. Mention of specific products and opinions related to those products do not indicate or imply endorsement by ONS. Websites mentioned are provided for information only; the hosts are responsible for their own content and availability. Unless otherwise indicated, dollar amounts reflect U.S. dollars.

ONS publications are originally published in English. Publishers wishing to translate ONS publications must contact ONS about licensing arrangements. ONS publications cannot be translated without obtaining written permission from ONS. (Individual tables and figures that are reprinted or adapted require additional permission from the original source.) Because translations from English may not always be accurate or precise, ONS disclaims any responsibility for inaccuracies in words or meaning that may occur as a result of the translation. Readers relying on precise information should check the original English version.

Printed in the United States of America

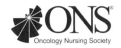

Innovation • Excellence • Advocacy

Contributors

Editors

Suzanne Walker, CRNP, MSN, AOCN®, BC
Nurse Practitioner/Coordinator for Thoracic
  Malignancies
Penn Presbyterian Medical Center
Lecturer B
Adult Oncology Specialty Minor/Post-
  Master's Certificate
University of Pennsylvania School of Nursing
Philadelphia, Pennsylvania

**Elizabeth Prechtel Dunphy, DNP, RN,
CRNP, BC, AOCN®**
Gastrointestinal Oncology Nurse Practitioner
Abramson Cancer Center at Penn
  Presbyterian Medical Center
Senior Lecturer B, Biobehavioral and Health
  Sciences Division
Adult Oncology Specialty Minor/Post-
  Master's Certificate, Advanced Practice
  Oncology Nurse
University of Pennsylvania School of Nursing
Philadelphia, Pennsylvania
Chapter 5. Bacillus Calmette-Guérin

Authors

**Kristine Deano Abueg, RN, MSN,
OCN®, CBCN®**
Oncology Clinical Trials Research Nurse
Kaiser Permanente
Roseville, California
Chapter 7. Active Immunity: Vaccine Therapy

**Kelly J. Brassil, PhD, RN, AOCNS®,
ACNS-BC**
Director, Nursing Research and Innovation
University of Texas MD Anderson Cancer
  Center
Houston, Texas
Chapter 1. History of Immunotherapy

Kevin Brigle, PhD, NP
Oncology Nurse Practitioner
Massey Cancer Center
Virginia Commonwealth University
Richmond, Virginia
Chapter 6. Oral Immunomodulatory Agents

Pamela K. Ginex, EdD, RN, OCN®
Senior Manager, Evidence-Based Practice
  and Inquiry
Oncology Nursing Society
Pittsburgh, Pennsylvania
Chapter 1. History of Immunotherapy

Brianna Hoffner, MSN, RN, AOCNP®
Lead Advanced Practice Provider, Medical
  Oncology
University of Colorado Cancer Center
Aurora, Colorado
Chapter 3. Cytokines in Immunotherapy

Lisa Kottschade, APRN, MSN, CNP
Nurse Practitioner
Associate Professor of Oncology
Mayo Clinic
Rochester, Minnesota
Chapter 9. Combination Therapies

Tracy Krause, BS, PharmD, BCOP
Oncology Clinical Pharmacist
Hospital of the University of Pennsylvania
Philadelphia, Pennsylvania
Chapter 10. Biomarkers

Susan J. McCall, MSN, ANP-BC, AOCNP®
Clinical Trials Nurse Practitioner
Memorial Sloan Kettering Cancer Center
New York, New York
*Chapter 11. Case-Based Management Strategies
and Patient Education*

**Barbara Barnes Rogers, CRNP, MN,
AOCN®, ANP-BC**
Adult Hematology-Oncology Nurse
    Practitioner
Fox Chase Cancer Center
Philadelphia, Pennsylvania
Chapter 8. Passive/Adoptive Immunotherapy

Rowena N. Schwartz, PharmD, BCOP
Associate Professor of Pharmacy Practice
    and Administrative Sciences
University of Cincinnati James L. Winkle
    College of Pharmacy
Cincinnati, Ohio
*Chapter 2. Principles of Immunology and
Immunotherapy*

Victoria Sherry, DNP, CRNP, AOCNP®
Oncology Nurse Practitioner for Thoracic
    Malignancies
Abramson Cancer Center
University of Pennsylvania Health System
    Faculty
Adult Oncology Specialty Minor/Post-
    Master's Certificate Program
University of Pennsylvania School of Nursing
Philadelphia, Pennsylvania
Chapter 4. Immune Checkpoint Inhibitors

**Susan Stonehouse-Lee, MSN, CRNP,
AOCNP®**
Oncology Nurse Practitioner
Abramson Cancer Center
University of Pennsylvania
Philadelphia, Pennsylvania
Chapter 4. Immune Checkpoint Inhibitors

Disclosure

Editors and authors of books and guidelines provided by the Oncology Nursing Society are expected to disclose to the readers any significant financial interest or other relationships with the manufacturer(s) of any commercial products.

A vested interest may be considered to exist if a contributor is affiliated with or has a financial interest in commercial organizations that may have a direct or indirect interest in the subject matter. A "financial interest" may include, but is not limited to, being a shareholder in the organization; being an employee of the commercial organization; serving on an organization's speakers bureau; or receiving research funding from the organization. An "affiliation" may be holding a position on an advisory board or some other role of benefit to the commercial organization. Vested interest statements appear in the front matter for each publication.

Contributors are expected to disclose any unlabeled or investigational use of products discussed in their content. This information is acknowledged solely for the information of the readers.

The contributors provided the following disclosure and vested interest information:
Kristine Deano Abueg, RN, MSN, OCN®, CBCN®: Greater Sacramento Chapter Oncology
    Nursing Society, honoraria
Kelly J. Brassil, PhD, RN, AOCNS®, ACNS-BC: Genentech, Inc., Premier Inc., consultant or
    advisory role; Oncology Nursing Society, honoraria; Genentech, Inc., research funding
Kevin Brigle, PhD, NP: Amgen Inc., Celgene Corp, Genentech, Inc., Takeda Oncology,
    Novartis Pharmaceuticals Corp., consultant or advisory role
Brianna Hoffner, MSN, RN, AOCNP®: Array BioPharma, AXIS Medical Education, Merck
    and Co., Inc., Terranova Medica, consultant or advisory role
Lisa Kottschade, APRN, MSN, CNP: Array BioPharma, consultant or advisory role;
    Bristol-Myers Squibb Co., research funding
Susan J. McCall, MSN, ANP-BC, AOCNP®: Seattle Genetics, Inc., consultant or advisory role;
    Creative Educational Concepts, Inc., Research To Practice, honoraria
Rowena N. Schwartz, PharmD, BCOP: Clinical Care Options, Horizon, Prime, Tesaro, Inc.,
    consultant or advisory role

Contents

Preface..ix

Acknowledgments xi

chapter one | **History of Immunotherapy**.. 1
    Introduction...1
    The First Hint Toward Immunotherapy..1
    1900s–1980s: From Coley Toxins to a Renewed Look at Immunotherapy 3
    1980s–Present: Immunotherapy Comes of Age 5
    Summary 12
    References...13

chapter two | **Principles of Immunology and Immunotherapy** 19
    Introduction...19
    The Immune System...20
    Innate and Adaptive Immune Recognition and Response 21
    Immune Tolerance 39
    Cancer and the Immune System..40
    The Cancer–Immunity Cycle 41
    The Evolution of Immunotherapy in Cancer 44
    Summary 49
    References...50

chapter three | **Cytokines in Immunotherapy**... 53
    Introduction...53
    Cytokines..53
    Chemokines...54
    Types of Cytokines 55
    Immunocytokines..60
    Cytokines and Cancer Symptoms 61
    Nursing Implications...62
    Summary 63
    References...63

chapter four | **Immune Checkpoint Inhibitors** 67
    Introduction...67
    Checkpoint Receptors..67
    Checkpoint Inhibitors 70
    Other Promising Checkpoint Inhibitors...73
    Costimulatory Receptors 74
    Combination Therapies 74
    Nursing Administration..76
    Adverse Effects 76
    Pregnancy and Lactation..88
    Summary 88
    References...89

chapter five | **Bacillus Calmette-Guérin**..**95**
    Introduction..95
    History..95
    Mechanism of Action..96
    Nursing Administration..97
    Side Effects..99
    Summary...100
    References...100

chapter six | **Oral Immunomodulatory Agents**..**103**
    Introduction..103
    History..103
    Mechanism of Action..105
    Risk Evaluation and Mitigation Strategy.....................................106
    Clinical Applications..107
    Nursing Implications...114
    Summary...114
    References...114

chapter seven | **Active Immunity: Vaccine Therapy**...................................**119**
    Introduction..119
    Development of Immunity From Vaccines......................................120
    Considerations in Vaccine Development..122
    Ex Vivo Dendritic Cell Therapy..129
    Oncolytic Viral Therapy...130
    Approved Agents..130
    Summary...134
    References...134

chapter eight | **Passive/Adoptive Immunotherapy**....................................**139**
    Introduction..139
    Tumor-Targeting Monoclonal Antibodies......................................139
    Epidermal Growth Factor Receptor–Specific Monoclonal Antibodies.....141
    HER2-Targeted Monoclonal Antibodies.......................................155
    Vascular Endothelial Growth Factor Receptor Inhibitors................161
    Platelet-Derived Growth Factor Alpha Inhibitors.........................167
    CD20-Targeted Monoclonal Antibodies.......................................168
    SLAMF7-Targeted Antibodies..176
    CD38-Targeted Monoclonal Antibodies.......................................178
    Interleukin-6–Targeted Monoclonal Antibodies............................180
    CD52-Targeted Antibodies..182
    Receptor Activator of Nuclear Factor Kappa-B Ligand...................183
    Antibody–Drug Conjugates..184
    Antibody–Radiopharmaceutical Conjugates.................................191
    Bispecific T-Cell Engager Antibodies..194
    Hypersensitivity Reactions..196
    Adoptive Cell Transfer..197
    Chimeric Antigen Receptor T Cells..198
    Summary...201
    References...201

chapter nine | **Combination Therapies**...**215**
    Introduction..215
    Chemoimmunotherapy..215
    Radioimmunotherapy...219
    Combination Immunotherapy..221

Summary 223
References..224

chapter ten | **Biomarkers** 227
Introduction..227
History...228
Development..229
Clinical Uses..230
Benefits..236
Challenges..237
Future Directions..238
Nursing Implications 238
Summary 239
References..239

chapter eleven | **Case-Based Management Strategies and Patient Education** 241
Introduction..241
Immune-Related Adverse Events From Checkpoint Inhibitors...................241
Case-Based Management of Toxicities Related to Therapy 247
Immune-Related Adverse Events From Other Agents.................................277
Special Populations 284
Pseudoprogression 286
Adherence to Oral Therapy..288
Financial Considerations...289
Summary 292
References..293

Index 303

Preface

Major advances in immunotherapy over the past few years have revolutionized cancer care. These breakthroughs have also brought forth shifts in the delivery of treatments as well as the management of their toxicities. Oncology nurses are at the forefront of prevention and management of immune-mediated toxicities and leaders in patient education in this rapidly evolving field. The Oncology Nursing Society recognized the need to develop an in-depth immunotherapy book for oncology nurses and healthcare professionals. As editors, we were honored to be selected as the leaders of this first-time endeavor. One of the major challenges of producing an immunotherapy book is the continual development of new agents and classes of agents. This book not only provides its readers with an overview of these agents, but also establishes a solid foundation for understanding the complexities of the immune system and how it can be harnessed to fight cancer.

We were thrilled to attract a variety of chapter authors who are experts in their field and leaders in cancer care. The opening chapters showcase this expertise with a fundamental look at the history of immunotherapy, the principles of immunology, and cancer and the immune system. These are followed by chapters on immunotherapy and immunomodulatory agents, including nonspecific immune system modulators, immune checkpoint inhibitors, bacillus Calmette-Guérin, and oral immunomodulators. Additional chapters detail active immunization (vaccines), passive/adoptive immunotherapy, combination therapies, and biomarkers. The book closes with a focus on nursing implications using a case-based discussion.

Although immunotherapy has proved to be effective for a variety of cancers, many types of malignancies have yet to see success with this new and evolving class of agents. Additionally, the management and exploration of short- and long-term toxicities remain underexplored areas. As the scientific understanding of the complex interaction between cancer and the immune system continues to grow, oncology healthcare providers will be called upon to assume an increasingly important role in the management of patients receiving immunotherapy treatments. This comprehensive and contemporary overview of immunotherapy will hopefully serve as a valuable reference for clinical practice.

Acknowledgments

The editors thank all the amazing authors who have dedicated a significant amount of time to crafting their respective chapters. Thank you to the ONS Publications Department staff for mentoring us through this process.

Thank you to my husband, kids, dog, and cat for supporting me through this project while I worked full time and simultaneously pursued a nursing PhD degree, and thank you to my parents for always believing in me.

—Suzanne Walker

Thank you for all of your support, Jake, Gen, and Mom, as well as my mentor, Nevena Damjanov.

—Elizabeth Prechtel Dunphy

History of Immunotherapy

Kelly J. Brassil, PhD, RN, AOCNS®, ACNS-BC
Pamela K. Ginex, EdD, RN, OCN®

Introduction

The promise of immunotherapy as a cancer treatment relies on using the entire immune system—its cells, molecules, and rules of engagement—to fight a cancer. Like chemotherapy and radiation, the two historical pillars of cancer treatment, immunotherapy has a long history of highs and lows. As immunotherapy research progresses at a rapid pace, it is important to understand the beginnings of this promising therapy and its significant milestones, both accomplishments and challenges, from a historical perspective. This chapter will reflect on the history of immunotherapy and establish a foundation for subsequent chapters, which will delve further into the diverse immunotherapeutic approaches for cancer.

The First Hint Toward Immunotherapy

Immunotherapy as it is known today arose from the spirit of inquiry of pioneering scientists and, as is the case with many scientific discoveries, chance. Before the immune system and its functionality were fully understood, the first sparks of inquiry were ignited near the end of the 19th century, when a young woman presented with a unique disease state in New York City. The narrative of this woman, Bessie Dashiell, is further elucidated in *A Commotion in the Blood: Life, Death, and the Immune System* (Hall, 1997), a key text that narrates the extraordinary events that precipitated the use of the immune system to fight cancer.

In the summer of 1890, 17-year-old Dashiell was experiencing nagging pain from a wound in her hand, an injury she believed occurred when traveling across country by train. When Dashiell's wound worsened, she was referred to Dr. William Coley, a young surgeon in New York City. On first appearance, Coley observed that Dashiell's right hand did not have the typical presentation of an infection. On closer examination, which included opening the wound, Coley found a small amount of pus and tissue that seemed "abnormally hard and more of a grayish color than normal" (Hall, 1997, p. 25). As Dashiell's pain and symptoms increased, Coley reopened the wound to find "grayish granulations" (Hall, 1997, p. 25) and a bone that appeared normal. It seemed to Coley that this was something other than an infection, and he became increasingly concerned that Dashiell had a sarcoma. A biopsy of the tissue confirmed his suspicion, revealing round cell sarcoma. The best available therapy at the time was amputation, which came with a survival rate of 1 out of 10 patients. In November 1890, two days after the biopsy results, Coley performed an amputation of Dashiell's right arm below the elbow (Hall, 1997). Following the amputation, however, Dashiell's disease spread rapidly, and tumors appeared throughout her body. Her symptoms were managed with the best supportive care available at that time, but in January 1891, with Coley at her bedside, Dashiell died of her disease at the age of 18 (Hall, 1997).

Dashiell's dramatic suffering, accelerated decline, and death at such a young age had a profound effect on two people very close to her. John D. Rockefeller Jr., an American financier and philanthropist, considered Dashiell his adopted sister (Hall, 1997). Her death was a great shock to him, and he focused much of his philanthropic work after her death on health care and cancer research. Specifically, he supported Coley's work and made significant donations to what is now known as Rockefeller University and the Memorial Sloan Kettering Cancer Center (Hall, 1997).

Coley was so affected by Dashiell's death that he referred to her case nearly 50 years later in his last scientific paper, stating that it had left a "deep impression" on him (Hall, 1997, p. 29). His determination to prevent the same fate in others led Coley through a scientific journey that began with a retrospective chart review to gain a baseline understanding of sarcoma treatments and outcomes. He identified and reviewed 90 cases of sarcoma over the previous 15 years. One particular case stood out that involved a man in his thirties with round cell sarcoma, the same malignancy as Dashiell. The patient had four tumors on his neck and face and needed multiple surgeries, the last so extensive that it required skin grafts, which ultimately failed. Following his last operation, the patient developed erysipelas, a common infection at the time believed to be caused by *Streptococcus pyogenes* (Hall, 1997). The patient experienced two occurrences of this infection, but remarkably, his disease disappeared, and his large wound healed.

Coley was so intrigued by this case that he started his own epidemiologic investigation, searching for the patient among New York City's tenement buildings. Surprisingly, he found the patient alive and well years after his cancer diagnosis. Coley concluded that if an accidental infection could lead to complete regression of this patient's sarcoma, it seemed fair to assume that the same could occur when an infection was artificially produced (Hall, 1997).

Through research, Coley found a history of manipulating the immune system, either deliberately or accidentally, to treat illness. One paper identified 14 cases of patients with a malignant disease who also came down with erysipelas. Five of the cases were sarcoma, three of which were either fully or permanently cured (Hall, 1997). Based on his experience and the literature, Coley made the decision to inoculate the next patient with inoperable sarcoma presented to him.

In May 1891, just months after Dashiell's death, Coley was introduced to a patient with an inoperable sarcoma of the neck and a large tonsil tumor. The patient was unable to talk or eat solids and could barely swallow liquids. He had previous surgeries on his neck tumor, which left an open wound that would not heal. Coley injected cultures of erysipelas into the patient and his wound. The injections occurred in the patient's apartment, as hospitals were reluctant to host the experiment because of the infection risk to other patients and staff. The inoculations did not work at first, forcing Coley to test different preparations for months; however, he eventually induced a full infection. As a result, the patient had a complete disappearance of his neck tumor and a decrease in the size of his tonsil tumor. The patient lived for eight more years before dying of a local recurrence (Hall, 1997).

Coley experimented with the use of infections to treat cancer for the rest of his career. He eventually progressed from using live bacteria to using heat-killed bacteria, a treatment that became known as Coley toxins (Tontonoz, 2015). Coley was investigating this phenomenon at a time when little was known about the immune system or how it worked. No one, including Coley, had an explanation as to how exactly the toxins worked. Other investigators attempted to use Coley toxins to treat patients, but none were as successful (Hall, 1997). Coley was developing this therapy at a time when radiation was introduced as a treatment option. Unlike Coley toxins, which worked sporadically with an unknown mechanism of action, radiation therapy was successful in most patients (Tontonoz, 2015). This led most cancer specialists to dismiss Coley toxins as a treatment option. Coley continued his research but was never able to see his toxins become a standard treatment for cancer.

1900s–1980s: From Coley Toxins to a Renewed Look at Immunotherapy

Despite the development of radiation therapy and chemotherapy as standard treatments for cancer, scientists remained intrigued by the underlying mechanisms of Coley toxins that led to responses in some patients (Balkwill, 2009). In the 1930s and 1940s, animal studies showed that bacteria caused tumor necrosis and that serum from endotoxin-treated tumors could be reintroduced to tumors (O'Malley, Achinstein, & Shear, 1962). The serum caused the tumors to necrose, leading investigators to state that it contained a "tumor necrotizing factor" (O'Malley et al., 1962). Later research discovered that tumor destruction was caused by host cells in response to the endotoxin and *not* by the endotoxin itself, leading to the modified term *tumor necrosis factor* (TNF) (Carswell et al., 1975). TNF was initially thought to be an important new treatment for patients with cancer, and research on the subject progressed rapidly. Unfortunately, systemic TNF administration was found to be associated with unacceptable severe toxicity and side effects, including fever, headache, rigor, hypotension, and pulmonary edema (Balkwill, 2009; Morice, Blick, Ali, & Gutterman, 1987). Research also emerged that TNF may stimulate tumor growth (Leibovich et al., 1987). Because of these associations, its use in cancer treatment has been severely limited.

Around the time that Coley was working on his theory of infection and cancer regression, two Frenchmen—Albert Calmette, a bacteriologist, and Camille Guérin, a veterinarian—were on a lifelong quest to develop a vaccine against tuberculosis (TB) (Herr & Morales, 2008). Calmette and Guérin isolated a virulent strain of *Mycobacterium bovis* (closely related to the human strain of TB) and worked years to make *tubercle bacillus* nonvirulent and genetically stable. The unique strain they developed was named bacillus Calmette-Guérin, or BCG, after the two scientists (Herr & Morales, 2008). In the early 1920s, Calmette and Guérin administered an oral form of the vaccine to children in Paris, none of whom developed TB. In 1929, researchers at Johns Hopkins noted a lower incidence of cancer in patients with TB, and later research found antitumor effects against several malignant cell lines after immunization with BCG (Alcorn, Burton, & Topping, 2015).

Unfortunately, a tragedy put the promise of BCG as a cancer therapy on hold. From 1929 to 1933, a laboratory error led to the continued vaccination of 251 German babies with a preparation of BCG that was contaminated with a virulent strain of TB. A total of 173 babies developed TB, and 72 died in what became known as the Lübeck disaster (Herr & Morales, 2008). Because of this tragedy, enthusiasm for BCG as a cancer therapy dampened for more than three decades.

In the 1950s, Dr. Lloyd Old conducted studies that provided the first direct evidence that BCG had antitumor effects (Herr & Morales, 2008; Old, Clarke, & Benacerraf, 1959). BCG was further studied clinically by international investigators as a treatment for leukemia and melanoma, as well as for lung, prostate, bladder, colon, and kidney cancer; however, the early promise of BCG as an effective treatment was unfulfilled, and it was soon replaced by other treatment options for most cancer types (Herr & Morales, 2008). Alvaro Morales, a urologist from Canada, indicated a notable exception when he published the first use of intravesicular BCG against superficial bladder cancer in 1976 (Morales, Eidinger, & Bruce, 1976). The schedule and dosing for BCG in this study were scientifically based, and preliminary results persuaded the National Cancer Institute to fund randomized controlled trials to test the effectiveness of a BCG regimen in superficial bladder cancers (Camacho, Pinsky, Kerr, Whitmore, & Oettgen, 1980; Lamm et al., 1980). These trials found that BCG was markedly effective in reducing the frequency of tumor recurrence compared to a control group treated with surgery alone (Herr & Morales, 2008). In 1990, with data from more than 2,500 cases worldwide, the U.S. Food and Drug Administration (FDA) approved the use of BCG in patients with superficial bladder cancer. Today, BCG remains the standard treatment for high-grade noninvasive bladder cancer (Herr & Morales, 2008). In 1999, Taniguchi et al. noted that BCG induces both a local and systemic immune response associated with the elimination or reduction of cells linked to non-muscle invasive bladder cancer.

1980s–Present: Immunotherapy Comes of Age

Immunotherapy research over the past 40 years has resulted in synchronous advancements in both bench and translational science. Timelines related to immunotherapy have been published and include notable scientific and treatment advances (see Bachireddy, Burkhardt, Rajasagi, & Wu, 2015; Cancer Research Institute, n.d.; Pardoll, 2011; Parish, 2003). Additional institution-specific timelines are also available (see Johns Hopkins Medicine, n.d.; Memorial Sloan Kettering Cancer Center, n.d.).

1980s: Conflicting Scientific Evidence Highlights a Decade of Immunotherapeutic Uncertainty

As research emerged on the role of the immune system as a mediator to cancer, opinions and attitudes toward cancer immunotherapy changed. In the 1970s, scientific evidence contradicting the capacity for immune-driven mediation of tumors resulted in the perception of cancer immunotherapy as an ineffectual treatment approach (Parish, 2003; Stutman, 1975, 1979a, 1979b). Specifically, studies demonstrated that T-cell–deficient mice and syngeneic wild-type mice had a similar incidence of tumor occurrence, negating the implication of

T-cell–facilitated immunosurveillance in preventing tumors (Parish, 2003). Immunotherapy research regained traction in the 1980s, when a study demonstrating the capacity of autoreactive T cells to escape thymic deletion and a study discussing the potential of tumor-associated antigens to mediate immunosurveillance contradicted previous findings (Parish, 2003). Among these new findings was the identification of cancer antigens in melanoma, which suggested the possibility of targeted immune therapies (Houghton, Eisinger, Albino, Cairncross, & Old, 1982; Houghton, Thomson, Gross, Oettgen, & Old, 1984; Livingston et al., 1985). In addition, the first studies suggesting T cells could be used to attack tumors, specifically malignant melanoma, were conducted (Knuth, Danowski, Oettgen, & Old, 1984), leading to the identification of cytotoxic T-lymphocyte antigen 4 (CTLA-4) (Brunet et al., 1987). This discovery would become the foundation for the development of checkpoint inhibitors.

Perhaps most profound was further research involving interleukin-2 (IL-2), which was first discovered in 1976 (Morgan, Ruscetti, & Gallo, 1976). In 1984, IL-2 was identified as an immunologic-based treatment in the management of a 33-year-old woman with metastatic melanoma. The patient demonstrated complete tumor necrosis and no evidence of disease following recombinant IL-2 administration (Rosenberg, 2014). This result was further validated in a study by the National Cancer Institute, in which escalating doses of IL-2 in patients with metastatic melanoma and renal cell cancer demonstrated tumor regression in those who had previously failed standard-of-care treatment (e.g., chemotherapy, surgery, radiation) (Rosenberg et al., 1985). In 1992, based on the durability of response seen in multiple trials, FDA approved high-dose IL-2 for the treatment of patients with metastatic renal cell cancer (Rosenberg, 2007). A series of studies of high-dose IL-2 in melanoma had an overall response rate of 16% and led to the approval of high-dose IL-2 for advanced melanoma in 1998 (Amin & White, 2013). IL-2 was also explored as a contributor to adoptive cell therapy in the stimulation of human tumor-infiltrating lymphocytes (Rosenberg, Spiess, & Lafreniere, 1986). The positive responses seen with IL-2 demonstrated to scientists and clinicians that immunologic manipulation was possible and could lead to the regression of cancers. This established IL-2 as a foundation of modern immunotherapy.

1990s: The Reemergence of Immunosurveillance Drives a Decade of Progressive Discoveries in Bench Science

The discovery of immunogenicity in IL-2 led to a rapid progression of the science in the 1990s. This decade contributed to many of the recent immunotherapeutic breakthroughs, including the scientific establishment of immunosurveillance through several bench studies. Key clinical questions addressed the lack of costimulatory molecules for tumors cells (necessary for the initiation of immune response) and the potential for a T-cell tolerance that would prevent tumor-specific immunity (Allison & Krummel, 1995; Parish, 2003; Schwartz, 1992). Further exploration examined tumor immunosurveillance with natural killer (NK) cells, NK T cells, and gammadelta T cells (Girardi et al., 2001; Lanier, 2001; Smyth, Godfrey, & Trapani, 2001; Smyth, Thia, Street, Cretney, et al., 2000). The identification of a modulator, namely dendritic cell maturation in response to microbial and proinflammatory mediators, provided insight into the relationship between innate and adaptive immune responses (Cella, Engering, Pinet, Pieters, & Lanzavecchia, 1997; Pierre et al., 1997). This led to the use of dendritic cells in cancer vaccines to facilitate tumor-specific T-cell immunity, which demonstrated induction of antitumor immune responses across diverse tumor types (Brossart, Wirths, Brugger, & Kanz, 2001; Brugger et al., 2001; Mukherji et al., 1995; Parish, 2003; Steinman & Dhodapkar, 2001). Type 1 interferons were also explored because of their relationship with NK cells, cytotoxic T lymphocytes, and macrophages, which signal and engage an immune response that can be directed toward tumor cells, specifically targeting the Janus kinase (JAK) inhibitors and signal transducer and activator of transcription (STAT) pathways (Constantinescu et al., 1994; Lee & Margolin, 2011). Further, Janus kinase 3, or JAK-3, was discovered to be coupled to the IL-2 receptor in human peripheral blood T cells and NK cells (Johnston et al., 1994). The discovery of NY-ESO-1 (Chen et al., 1997), a cancer/testis antigen associated with advanced melanomas, contributed to a rapid progression in diverse immunotherapeutic treatments, as this antigen can be targeted for vaccine-induced tumor response (Gnjatic et al., 2006). The GVAX vaccine (Dranoff et al., 1993), first developed in 1989, proceeded with promising clinical trials for pancreatic and non-small cell lung cancers in the 2000s ("Cell Genesys," 2002; Nemunaitis, 2003, 2005). Monoclonal antibodies also emerged as a treatment option for patients with solid tumors (Minasian et al., 1994). In 1997, rituximab (Rituxan®) was the first monoclonal antibody approved for treatment of malignancies, specifically non-Hodgkin lymphoma (Ribatti, 2014). The use of interferon alfa was explored in clinical trials throughout the decade as treatment for melanoma, though results were mixed (Lee & Margolin, 2011). Although the use of interferon alfa as an adjuvant agent produced results in relapse-free survival, significant improvements in overall survival were observed in only 4 out of 14 studies (Eggermont, 2001; Mocellin, Pasquali, Rossi, & Nitti, 2010). Interferon alfa-2b (Intron A®) was first approved for hairy cell leukemia in 1986, with subsequent approvals as adjuvant therapy for malignant melanoma in 1995 and treatment of follicular lymphoma in 1997 (Ningrum, 2014).

2000s: Discoveries at the Bench Translate to Immunotherapeutic Advances at the Bedside

The 21st century witnessed dramatic discoveries at the bench and rapid acceleration of clinical trials, resulting in new and emerging immunotherapeutic treatment options. Several new classes of agents were either introduced in clinical trials or received FDA approval during this period (see Table 1-1). Immunotherapeutic approaches include cytokines, monoclonal antibodies, checkpoint inhibitors, vaccines, and adoptive cell transfer.

Cytokines (Interferons)

The theory of cancer immunosurveillance was revisited based on laboratory data demonstrating increased susceptibility to B-cell lymphomas in mice lacking interferon gamma, interferon gamma receptors, or interferon gamma–producing cells (Shankaran et al., 2001; Smyth, Thia, Street, Cretney, et al., 2000; Smyth, Thia, Street, MacGregor, et al., 2000). This was further evidence of the presence of immunosurveillance and further justification for the exploration of targeted and immunotherapeutic approaches to cancer treatment. The neoadjuvant effects of interferon alfa-2b were revealed as the result of an indirect immunomodulatory mechanism in a trial of patients with stage IIIB melanoma (Moschos et al., 2006). This led to FDA approval of peginterferon alfa-2b (PegIntron®) for metastatic melanoma in 2011.

Monoclonal Antibodies

Although monoclonal antibodies have been present since the FDA approval of muromonab-CD3 in 1986, the emergence of trastuzumab (Herceptin®) and rituximab in the 1990s revolutionized cancer treatment. As of the time of this writing, 30 monoclonal antibodies are approved for a diversity of treatment indications (Buss, Henderson, McFarlane, Shenton, & de Haan, 2012). Most notably in cancer care, tositumomab (Bexxar®) was approved for the treatment of non-Hodgkin lymphoma in 2003. This was followed in 2004 by bevacizumab (Avastin®) and cetuximab (Erbitux®) for the treatment of metastatic colorectal cancer. In 2010, brentuximab (Adcetris®), a targeted agent, was approved for treatment of relapsed/refractory classical Hodgkin lymphoma and systemic anaplastic large-cell lymphoma. Obinutuzumab (Gazyva®) was approved for the treatment of chronic lymphocytic leukemia in 2013 and follicular lymphoma in 2016. In 2014, blinatumomab (Blincyto®) was approved for the treatment of relapsed/refractory B-cell acute lymphoblastic leukemia (ALL).

TABLE 1-1   Timeline of Immunotherapeutic Agents Approved by the U.S. Food and Drug Administration

Agent	Indications
Checkpoint Inhibitors	
Atezolizumab (Tecentriq®)	Bladder cancer (2017), lung cancer (2017)
Axicabtagene ciloleucel (Yescarta®)	B-cell non-Hodgkin lymphoma (2017)
Ipilimumab (Yervoy®)	Metastatic melanoma (2011)
Ipilimumab (Yervoy) + nivolumab (Opdivo®)	Advanced melanoma (2015)
Nivolumab (Opdivo)	Bladder cancer (2017), follicular lymphoma (2016), head and neck cancer (2016), kidney cancer (2015), lung cancer (2015), melanoma (2014)
Pembrolizumab (Keytruda®)	Adult and pediatric lymphoma (2017), head and neck cancer (2016), lung cancer (2016, 2015)
Tisagenlecleucel (Kymriah®)	Pediatric and young adult acute lymphoblastic leukemia (2017)
Cytokine Therapies	
Interferon alfa-2b (Intron A®)	Follicular lymphoma (1997), malignant melanoma (1995), hairy cell leukemia (1986)
Interleukin-2 (aldesleukin; Proleukin®)	Metastatic melanoma (1998), metastatic kidney cancer (1992)
Peginterferon alfa-2b (Sylatron®)	Melanoma (2011)
Monoclonal Antibodies	
Alemtuzumab (Campath-1H®)	Chronic lymphocytic leukemia (2001)
Basiliximab (Simulect®)	Prophylaxis for transplant rejection (1998)
Bevacizumab (Avastin®)	Metastatic colorectal cancer (2004)
Blinatumomab (Blincyto®)	B-cell acute lymphoblastic leukemia (2014)
Cetuximab (Erbitux®)	Metastatic colorectal cancer (2004)
Daclizumab (Zenapax®)	Prophylaxis for transplant rejection (1997)
Daratumumab (Darzalex®)	Expanded access for myeloma (2016), multiple myeloma (2015)
Elotuzumab (Empliciti™)	Multiple myeloma (2015)

(Continued on next page)

TABLE 1-1   Timeline of Immunotherapeutic Agents Approved by the U.S. Food and Drug Administration *(Continued)*

Agent	Indications
Monoclonal Antibodies *(cont.)*	
Gemtuzumab (Mylotarg®)	Leukemia (2000)
Ibritumomab tiuxetan (Zevalin®)	Non-Hodgkin lymphoma (2002)
Muromonab-CD3 (Orthoclone OKT3®)	Prophylaxis for transplant rejection (1986)
Obinutuzumab (Gazyva®)	Follicular lymphoma (2016), chronic lymphocytic leukemia (2013)
Ofatumumab (Arzerra®)	Leukemia (2016), chronic lymphocytic leukemia (2010)
Olaratumab (Lartruvo®)	Sarcoma (2016)
Panitumumab (Vectibix®)	Metastatic colorectal cancer (2006)
Pertuzumab (Perjeta®)	HER2-positive breast cancer (2012)
Ramucirumab (Cyramza®)	Stomach cancer (2014)
Rituximab (Rituxan®)	Non-Hodgkin lymphoma (1997)
Tositumomab (Bexxar®)	Non-Hodgkin lymphoma (2003)
Trastuzumab (Herceptin®)	HER2-positive breast cancer (2006), metastatic breast cancer (1998)
Oncolytic Viral Therapies	
Human papillomavirus vaccine (Cervarix®)	Human papillomavirus linked to cervical cancer (2009)
Oncophage (Vitespen®)	Kidney cancer (2008)
Quadrivalent human papillomavirus recombinant vaccine (Gardasil®)	Human papillomavirus linked to cervical cancer (2006)
Sipuleucel-T (Provenge®)	Prostate cancer (2010)
Talimogene laherparepvec (Imlygic®)	Melanoma (2015)
Targeted Therapies	
Brentuximab vedotin (Adcetris®)	Hodgkin and anaplastic large-cell lymphoma (2011)
Vemurafenib (Zelboraf®)	Advanced melanoma (2011)

Note. Based on information from National Cancer Institute, 2018.

Checkpoint Inhibitors

The discovery of cellular checkpoints contributed to the introduction of checkpoint inhibitors. A CTLA-4–specific antibody is identified as an immune checkpoint inhibitor associated with clinical regression in melanoma and immune-mediated toxicities (Egen, Kuhns, & Allison, 2002). In 2002, the first clinical trials of monoclonal antibodies to induce CTLA-4 blockade were conducted in renal and prostate cancers (Fong & Small, 2008; Small et al., 2007; Yang et al., 2007). This led to FDA approval of ipilimumab (Yervoy®) in 2011 for the treatment of melanoma (Hodi et al., 2010; Pennock, Waterfield, & Wolchok, 2012; Wolchok et al., 2010).

Programmed cell death protein 1 (PD-1), previously identified as being directly involved in cell death (Agata et al., 1996), was identified as an immune checkpoint in bench studies (Nishimura, Nose, Hiai, Minato, & Honjo, 1999). These studies included identification of PD-1's two ligands, programmed cell death-ligand 1 (PD-L1) and programmed cell death-ligand 2 (PD-L2) (Tseng et al., 2001).

In 2010 alone, nivolumab (Opdivo®) was tested in early clinical trials (Brahmer et al., 2010); ipilimumab demonstrated survival advantage for patients with advanced melanoma (Friedlander & Hodi, 2010; Hodi et al., 2010); and exploration of the PD-1 checkpoint blockade demonstrated tumor regression in melanoma and in renal, lung, and colon cancers (Brahmer et al., 2010). Nivolumab (BMS-936558) demonstrated dramatic results across cancer types in a phase 1 trial (Topalian et al., 2012). In 2013, it was approved for relapsed/refractory classical Hodgkin lymphoma after stem cell transplantation and brentuximab.

Pembrolizumab (Keytruda®) was granted accelerated approval in 2014 for advanced or unresectable melanoma. It was the first PD-1 inhibitor cleared in the United States. In 2015, the first combination therapy for melanoma, ipilimumab plus nivolumab, was FDA approved (Wolchok et al., 2013). In the same year, nivolumab alone was FDA approved for advanced renal cell carcinoma (George et al., 2016; Motzer et al., 2015). Nivolumab and ipilimumab used in combination produced a 60% response rate in patients with melanoma (Larkin, Hodi, & Wolchok, 2015). These agents continue to be explored individually and in combination for diverse diagnoses.

Vaccines

The development and testing of a vaccine to prevent human papillomavirus (HPV)–associated cancers demonstrated a durable response in women with HPV 16–positive vulvar intraepithelial neoplasia, resulting in the first FDA-approved HPV vaccination (Gardasil®) in 2006 (Kenter et al., 2009). In 2014, granulocyte macrophage–colony-stimulating factor–secreting allogeneic pancreatic tumor cells (GVAX Pancreas) and the CRS-207 cancer vaccine demonstrated survival benefit for patients with pancreatic cancer in a phase 2 multicenter trial (Le et al., 2015). In 2015, talimogene laherparepvec (Imlygic®) was FDA approved for intralesional injection in patients with melanoma (Johnson, Puzanov, & Kelley, 2015). Research has also explored the role of viral therapies in patients with brain tumors (Martin, 2017).

Adoptive Cell Therapy

In the early 2000s, T cells were further explored for therapeutic purposes, including the use of adoptive T-cell therapies to produce tumor regression in melanoma (Dudley et al., 2002; Yee et al., 2002) and for the development of chimeric antigen receptor (CAR) T cells (Sadelain, Brentjens, & Rivière, 2013). This exploration also included attention to the expanding role of IL-2 with high-dose chemotherapy to facilitate adoptive cell transfer, which contributes to objective cancer response and proliferation of transferred cells (Dudley et al., 2002; Rosenberg, 2014). Genetically engineered T cells were used to induce clinical responses in patients with B-cell lymphomas (Till et al., 2008), and genetically modified T cells were observed to produce durable response in patients with chronic lymphocytic leukemia (Kalos et al., 2011; Porter, Levine, Kalos, Bagg, & June, 2011). In 2013, clinical trials of CAR T-cell therapies produced dramatic results, attaining a complete response in patients with B-cell ALL (Brentjens et al., 2013), an 89% response rate in children and adults with ALL (Grupp et al., 2013; Maude et al., 2014), and a 92% response rate in patients with aggressive non-Hodgkin lymphoma (Kochenderfer et al., 2015). In 2017, tisagenlecleucel (Kymriah®), a CAR T-cell therapy, was approved for pediatric and young adult ALL, becoming the first FDA-approved treatment of its kind.

Summary

Immunotherapy is well established as both a field for rich scientific discovery and an opportunity for accelerated cancer treatments. Clinical trials have contributed to rapid exploration of safety, efficacy, and survival outcomes for several key immunotherapeutic agents. The robust advances of immunotherapy over the past two decades will only be further accelerated by the National Cancer Moonshot Initiative, which prioritizes collaborative approaches to developing, testing, and evaluating immunotherapeutic agents (Singer, Jacks, & Jaffee, 2016). The Cancer Moonshot emphasizes the importance of symptom management, a robust area for nursing contribution (Ginex, Brassil, & Ely, 2017). Future immunotherapy research may focus on exploration of combination therapies (Bernier, 2016; Jiang & Zhou, 2015), the use of existing agents with new disease presentations, the late effects and long-term sequelae of newly approved therapies, and the evaluation of the cost and sustainability of these therapies off protocol. A focus on the *types* of patients that respond to immunotherapeutic agents will be imperative to expanding the potential benefits of these treatment types to a broader population.

As this science advances, so too will questions concerning how immunotherapy physiologically and psychologically affects patients. Nurses have had an integral role in the clinical care of patients receiving these agents and are well positioned to address these concerns through research, clinical practice, and education.

References

Agata, Y., Kawasaki, A., Nishimura, H., Ishida, Y., Tsubat, T., Yagita, H., & Honjo, T. (1996). Expression of the PD-1 antigen on the surface of stimulated mouse T and B lymphocytes. *International Immunology, 8*, 765–772. https://doi.org/10.1093/intimm/8.5.765

Alcorn, J., Burton, R., & Topping, A. (2015). BCG treatment for bladder cancer, from past to present use. *International Journal of Urological Nursing, 9*, 177–186. https://doi.org/10.1111/ijun.12064

Allison, J.P., & Krummel, M.F. (1995). The yin and yang of T cell costimulation. *Science, 270*, 932–933. https://doi.org/10.1126/science.270.5238.932

Amin, A., & White, R.L., Jr. (2013). High-dose interleukin-2: Is it still indicated for melanoma and RCC in an era of targeted therapies? *Oncology, 27*, 680–691.

Bachireddy, P., Burkhardt, U.E., Rajasagi, M., & Wu, C.J. (2015). Haematological malignancies: At the forefront of immunotherapeutic innovation. *Nature Reviews Cancer, 15*, 201–215. https://doi.org/10.1038/nrc3907

Balkwill, F. (2009). Tumour necrosis factor and cancer. *Nature Reviews Cancer, 9*, 361–371. https://doi.org/10.1038/nrc2628

Bernier, J. (2016). Immuno-oncology: Allying forces of radio- and immuno-therapy to enhance cancer cell killing. *Critical Reviews in Oncology/Hematology, 108*, 97–108. https://doi.org/10.1016/j.critrevonc.2016.11.001

Brahmer, J.R., Drake, C.G., Wollner, I., Powderly, J.D., Picus, J., Sharfman, W.H., ... Topalian, S.L. (2010). Phase I study of single-agent anti-programmed death-1 (MDX-1106) in refractory solid tumors: Safety, clinical activity, pharmacodynamics, and immunologic correlates. *Journal of Clinical Oncology, 28*, 3167–3175. https://doi.org/10.1200/JCO.2009.26.7609

Brentjens, R.J., Davila, M.L., Riviere, I., Park, J., Wang, X., Cowell, L.G., ... Sadelain, M. (2013). CD19-targeted T cells rapidly induce molecular remissions in adults with chemotherapy-refractory acute lymphoblastic leukemia. *Science Translational Medicine, 5*, 177ra138. https://doi.org/10.1126/scitranslmed.3005930

Brossart, P., Wirths, S., Brugger, W., & Kanz, L. (2001). Dendritic cells in cancer vaccines. *Experimental Hematology, 29*, 1247–1255. https://doi.org/10.1016/S0301-472X(01)00730-5

Brugger, W., Schneider, A., Schammann, T., Dill, P., Grünebach, F., Bühring, H.-J., ... Brossart, P. (2001). Dendritic cell-based vaccines in patients with hematological malignancies. *Annals of the New York Academy of Sciences, 938*, 359–363. https://doi.org/10.1111/j.1749-6632.2001.tb03603.x

Brunet, J.-F., Denizot, F., Luciani, M.-F., Roux-Dosseto, M., Suzan, M., Mattei, M.-G., & Golstein, P. (1987). A new member of the immunoglobulin superfamily—CTLA-4. *Nature, 328*, 267–270. https://doi.org/10.1038/328267a0

Buss, N.A.P.S., Henderson, S.J., McFarlane, M., Shenton, J.M., & de Haan, L. (2012). Monoclonal antibody therapeutics: History and future. *Current Opinion in Pharmacology, 12*, 615–622. https://doi.org/10.1016/j.coph.2012.08.001

Camacho, F., Pinsky, C., Kerr, D., Whitmore, W., & Oettgen, H. (1980). Treatment of superficial bladder cancer with intravesical BCG. *Proceedings of the American Association for Cancer Research, 21,* 359.

Cancer Research Institute. (n.d.). Timeline of progress. Retrieved from https://www.cancerresearch.org/cri-impact/timeline-of-progress

Carswell, E.A., Old, L.J., Kassel, R.L., Green, S., Fiore, N., & Williamson, B. (1975). An endotoxin-induced serum factor that causes necrosis of tumors. *Proceedings of the National Academy of Sciences of the United States of America, 72,* 3666–3670. https://doi.org/10.1073/pnas.72.9.3666

Cella, M., Engering, A., Pinet, V., Pieters, J., & Lanzavecchia, A. (1997). Inflammatory stimuli induce accumulation of MHC class II complexes on dendritic cells. *Nature, 388,* 782–787. https://doi.org/10.1038/42030

Cell Genesys reports long-term survival data in phase II trial of GVAX. (2002). *Expert Review of Anticancer Therapy, 2,* 245–246.

Chen, Y.-T., Boyer, A.D., Viars, C.S., Tsang, S., Old, L.J., & Arden, K.C. (1997). Genomic cloning and localization of CTAG, a gene encoding an autoimmunogenic cancer-testis antigen NY-ESO-1 to human chromosome Xq28. *Cytogenetics and Cell Genetics, 79,* 237–240. https://doi.org/10.1159/000134734

Constantinescu, S.N., Croze, E., Wang, C., Murti, A., Basu, L., Mullersman, J.E., & Pfeffer, L.M. (1994). Role of interferon alpha/beta receptor chain 1 in the structure and transmembrane signaling of the interferon alpha/beta receptor complex. *Proceedings of the National Academy of Sciences of the United States of America, 91,* 9602–9606. https://doi.org/10.1073/pnas.91.20.9602

Dranoff, G., Jaffee, E., Lazenby, A., Golumbek, P., Levitsky, H., Brose, K., ... Mulligan, R.C. (1993). Vaccination with irradiated tumor cells engineered to secrete murine granulocyte-macrophage colony-stimulating factor stimulates potent, specific, and long-lasting anti-tumor immunity. *Proceedings of the National Academy of Sciences of the United States of America, 90,* 3539–3543. https://doi.org/10.1073/pnas.90.8.3539

Dudley, M.E., Wunderlich, J.R., Robbins, P.F., Yang, J.C., Hwu, P., Schwartzentruber, D.J., ... Rosenberg, S.A. (2002). Cancer regression and autoimmunity in patients after clonal repopulation with antitumor lymphocytes. *Science, 298,* 850–854. https://doi.org/10.1126/science.1076514

Egen, J.G., Kuhns, M.S., & Allison, J.P. (2002). CTLA-4: New insights into its biological function and use in tumor immunotherapy. *Nature Immunology, 3,* 611–618. https://doi.org/10.1038/ni0702-611

Eggermont, A.M.M. (2001). The role of interferon-alpha in malignant melanoma remains to be defined. *European Journal of Cancer, 37,* 2147–2153. https://doi.org/10.1016/S0959-8049(01)00272-6

Fong, L., & Small, E.J. (2008). Anti-cytotoxic T-lymphocyte antigen-4 antibody: The first in an emerging class of immunomodulatory antibodies for cancer treatment. *Journal of Clinical Oncology, 26,* 5275–5283. https://doi.org/10.1200/JCO.2008.17.8954

Friedlander, P., & Hodi, F.S. (2010). Advances in targeted therapy for melanoma. *Clinical Advances in Hematology and Oncology, 8,* 619–627.

George, S., Motzer, R.J., Hammers, H.J., Redman, B.G., Kuzel, T.M., Tykodi, S.S., ... Rini, B.I. (2016). Safety and efficacy of nivolumab in patients with metastatic renal cell carcinoma treated beyond progression: A subgroup analysis of a randomized clinical trial. *JAMA Oncology, 2,* 1179–1186. https://doi.org/10.1001/jamaoncol.2016.0775

Ginex, P.K., Brassil, K., & Ely, B. (2017). Immunotherapy: Exploring the state of the science. *Clinical Journal of Oncology Nursing, 21*(Suppl. 2), 9–12. https://doi.org/10.1188/17.CJON.S2.9-12

Girardi, M., Oppenheim, D.E., Steele, C.R., Lewis, J.M., Glusac, E., Filler, R., ... Hayday, A.C. (2001). Regulation of cutaneous malignancy by gamma delta T cells. *Science, 294,* 605–609. https://doi.org/10.1126/science.1063916

Gnjatic, S., Nishikawa, H., Jungbluth, A.A., Güre, A.O., Ritter, G., Jäger, E., ... Old, L.J. (2006). NY-ESO-1: Review of an immunogenic tumor antigen. In G.F. Vande Woude &

G. Klein (Eds.), *Advances in Cancer Research: Vol. 95* (pp. 1–30). https://doi.org/10.1016/S0065-230X(06)95001-5

Grupp, S.A., Kalos, M., Barrett, D., Aplenc, R., Porter, D.L., Rheingold, S.R., … June, C.H. (2013). Chimeric antigen receptor–modified T cells for acute lymphoid leukemia. *New England Journal of Medicine, 368,* 1509–1518. https://doi.org/10.1056/NEJMoa1215134

Hall, S.H. (1997). *A commotion in the blood: Life, death, and the immune system.* New York, NY: Henry Holt and Company.

Herr, H.W., & Morales, A. (2008). History of bacillus Calmette-Guérin and bladder cancer: An immunotherapy success story. *Journal of Urology, 179,* 53–56. https://doi.org/10.1016/j.juro.2007.08.122

Hodi, F.S., O'Day, S.J., McDermott, D.F., Weber, R.W., Sosman, J.A., Haanen, J.B., … Urba, W.J. (2010). Improved survival with ipilimumab in patients with metastatic melanoma. *New England Journal of Medicine, 363,* 711–723. https://doi.org/10.1056/NEJMoa1003466

Houghton, A.N., Eisinger, M., Albino, A.P., Cairncross, J.G., & Old, L.J. (1982). Surface antigens of melanocytes and melanomas. Markers of melanocyte differentiation and melanoma subsets. *Journal of Experimental Medicine, 156,* 1755–1766. https://doi.org/10.1084/jem.156.6.1755

Houghton, A.N., Thomson, T.M., Gross, D., Oettgen, H.F., & Old, L.J. (1984). Surface antigens of melanoma and melanocytes. Specificity of induction of Ia antigens by human gamma-interferon. *Journal of Experimental Medicine, 160,* 255–269. https://doi.org/10.1084/jem.160.1.255

Jiang, T., & Zhou, C. (2015). The past, present and future of immunotherapy against tumor. *Translational Lung Cancer Research, 4,* 253–264. http://doi.org/10.3978/j.issn.2218-6751.2015.01.06

Johns Hopkins Medicine. (n.d.). Immunotherapy research timeline. Retrieved from http://www.hopkinsmedicine.org/kimmel_cancer_center/centers/bloomberg_kimmel_institute_for_cancer_immunotherapy/about_bki/immunotherapy-research-timeline.html

Johnson, D.B., Puzanov, I., & Kelley, M.C. (2015). Talimogene laherparepvec (T-VEC) for the treatment of advanced melanoma. *Immunotherapy, 7,* 611–619. https://doi.org/10.2217/imt.15.35

Johnston, J.A., Kawamura, M., Kirken, R.A., Chen, Y.-Q., Blake, T.B., Shibuya, K., … O'Shea, J.J. (1994). Phosphorylation and activation of the Jak-3 Janus kinase in response to interleukin-2. *Nature, 370,* 151–153. https://doi.org/10.1038/370151a0

Kalos, M., Levine, B.L., Porter, D.L., Katz, S., Grupp, S.A., Bagg, A., & June, C.H. (2011). T cells with chimeric antigen receptors have potent antitumor effects and can establish memory in patients with advanced leukemia. *Science Translational Medicine, 3,* 95ra73. https://doi.org/10.1126/scitranslmed.3002842

Kenter, G.G., Welters, M.J.P., Valentijn, A.R.P.M., Lowik, M.J.G., Berends-van der Meer, D.M.A., Vloon, A.P.G., … Melief, C.J.M. (2009). Vaccination against HPV-16 oncoproteins for vulvar intraepithelial neoplasia. *New England Journal of Medicine, 361,* 1838–1847. https://doi.org/10.1056/NEJMoa0810097

Knuth, A., Danowski, B., Oettgen, H.F., & Old, L.J. (1984). T-cell-mediated cytotoxicity against autologous malignant melanoma: Analysis with interleukin 2-dependent T-cell cultures. *Proceedings of the National Academy of Sciences of the United States of America, 81,* 3511–3515. https://doi.org/10.1073/pnas.81.11.3511

Kochenderfer, J.N., Dudley, M.E., Kassim, S.H., Somerville, R.P.T., Carpenter, R.O., Stetler-Stevenson, M., … Rosenberg, S.A. (2015). Chemotherapy-refractory diffuse large B-cell lymphoma and indolent B-cell malignancies can be effectively treated with autologous T cells expressing an anti-CD19 chimeric antigen receptor. *Journal of Clinical Oncology, 33,* 540–549. https://doi.org/10.1200/JCO.2014.56.2025

Lamm, D.L., Thor, D.E., Harris, S.C., Reyna, J.A., Stogdill, V.D., & Radwin, H.M. (1980). Bacillus Calmette-Guérin immunotherapy of superficial bladder cancer. *Journal of Urology, 124,* 38–42. https://doi.org/10.1016/S0022-5347(17)55282-9

Lanier, L.L. (2001). A renaissance for the tumor immunosurveillance hypothesis. *Nature Medicine, 7,* 1178–1180. https://doi.org/10.1038/nm1101-1178

Larkin, J., Hodi, F.S., & Wolchok, J.D. (2015). Combined nivolumab and ipilimumab or monotherapy in untreated melanoma. *New England Journal of Medicine, 373*, 1270–1271. https://doi.org/10.1056/NEJMc1509660

Le, D.T., Wang-Gillam, A., Picozzi, V., Greten, T.F., Crocenzi, T., Springett, G., ... Jaffee, E.M. (2015). Safety and survival with GVAX Pancreas Prime and Listeria monocytogenes-expressing mesothelin (CRS-207) boost vaccines for metastatic pancreatic cancer. *Journal of Clinical Oncology, 33*, 1325–1333. https://doi.org/10.1200/JCO.2014.57.4244

Lee, S., & Margolin, K. (2011). Cytokines in cancer immunotherapy. *Cancers, 3*, 3856–3893. https://doi.org/10.3390/cancers3043856

Leibovich, S.J., Polverini, P.J., Shepard, H.M., Wiseman, D.M., Shively, V., & Nuseir, N. (1987). Macrophage-induced angiogenesis is mediated by tumour necrosis factor-alpha. *Nature, 329*, 630–632. https://doi.org/10.1038/329630a0

Livingston, P.O., Albino, A.P., Chung, T.J.C., Real, F.X., Houghton, A.N., Oettgen, H.F., & Old, L.J. (1985). Serological response of melanoma patients to vaccines prepared from VSV lysates of autologous and allogeneic cultured melanoma cells. *Cancer, 55*, 713–720. https://doi.org/10.1002/1097-0142(19850215)55:4<713::AID-CNCR2820550407>3.0.CO;2-D

Martin, C. (2017). Oncolytic viruses: Treatment and implications for patients with gliomas. *Clinical Journal of Oncology Nursing, 21*(Suppl. 2), 60–64. https://doi.org/10.1188/17.CJON.S2.60-64

Maude, S.L., Frey, N., Shaw, P.A., Aplenc, R., Barrett, D.M., Bunin, N.J., ... Grupp, S.A. (2014). Chimeric antigen receptor T cells for sustained remissions in leukemia. *New England Journal of Medicine, 371*, 1507–1517. https://doi.org/10.1056/NEJMoa1407222

Memorial Sloan Kettering Cancer Center. (n.d.). MSK immunotherapy—Timeline of progress. Retrieved from https://www.mskcc.org/timeline/immunotherapy-msk

Minasian, L.M., Szatrowski, T.P., Rosenblum, M., Steffens, T., Morrison, M.E., Chapman, P.B., ... Houghton, A.N. (1994). Hemorrhagic tumor necrosis during a pilot trial of tumor necrosis factor-alpha and anti-GD3 ganglioside monoclonal antibody in patients with metastatic melanoma. *Blood, 83*, 56–64.

Mocellin, S., Pasquali, S., Rossi, C.R., & Nitti, D. (2010). Interferon alpha adjuvant therapy in patients with high-risk melanoma: A systematic review and meta-analysis. *Journal of the National Cancer Institute, 102*, 493–501. https://doi.org/10.1093/jnci/djq009

Morales, A., Eidinger, D., & Bruce, A.W. (1976). Intracavitary Bacillus Calmette-Guérin in the treatment of superficial bladder tumors. *Journal of Urology, 116*, 180–182. https://doi.org/10.1016/S0022-5347(17)58737-6

Morgan, D.A., Ruscetti, F.W., & Gallo, R. (1976). Selective in vitro growth of T lymphocytes from normal human bone marrows. *Science, 193*, 1007–1008. https://doi.org/10.1126/science.181845

Morice, R.C., Blick, M.B., Ali, M.K., & Gutterman, J.U. (1987). Pulmonary toxicity of recombinant tumor necrosis factor. *Proceedings of the American Society of Clinical Oncology, 6*, 29.

Moschos, S.J., Edington, H.D., Land, S.R., Rao, U.N., Jukic, D., Shipe-Spotloe, J., & Kirkwood, J.M. (2006). Neoadjuvant treatment of regional stage IIIB melanoma with high dose interferon alfa-2b induces objective tumor regression in association with modulation of tumor infiltrating host cellular immune responses. *Journal of Clinical Oncology, 24*, 3164–3171. https://doi.org/10.1200/JCO.2005.05.2498

Motzer, R.J., Rini, B.I., McDermott, D.F., Redman, B.G., Kuzel, T.M., Harrison, M.R., ... Hammers, H.J. (2015). Nivolumab for metastatic renal cell carcinoma: Results of a randomized phase II trial. *Journal of Clinical Oncology, 33*, 1430–1437. https://doi.org/10.1200/JCO.2014.59.0703

Mukherji, B., Chakraborty, N.G., Yamasaki, S., Okino, T., Yamase, H., Sporn, J.R., ... Meehan, J. (1995). Induction of antigen-specific cytolytic T cells in situ in human melanoma by immunization with synthetic peptide-pulsed autologous antigen presenting cells. *Proceedings of the National Academy of Sciences of the United States of America, 92*, 8078–8082. https://doi.org/10.1073/pnas.92.17.8078

National Cancer Institute. (2018, April 3). A to Z list of cancer drugs. Retrieved from https://www.cancer.gov/about-cancer/treatment/drugs

Nemunaitis, J. (2003). GVAX (GMCSF gene modified tumor vaccine) in advanced stage non small cell lung cancer. *Journal of Controlled Release, 91*, 225–231. https://doi.org/10.1016/S0168-3659(03)00210-4

Nemunaitis, J. (2005). Vaccines in cancer: GVAX®, a GM-CSF gene vaccine. *Expert Review of Vaccines, 4*, 259–274. https://doi.org/10.1586/14760584.4.3.259

Ningrum, R.A. (2014). Human interferon alpha-2b: A therapeutic protein for cancer treatment. *Scientifica, 2014*, 970315. https://doi.org/10.1155/2014/970315

Nishimura, H., Nose, M., Hiai, H., Minato, N., & Honjo, T. (1999). Development of lupus-like autoimmune diseases by disruption of the PD-1 gene encoding an ITIM motif-carrying immunoreceptor. *Immunity, 11*, 141–151. https://doi.org/10.1016/S1074-7613(00)80089-8

Old, L.J., Clarke, D.A., & Benacerraf, B. (1959). Effect of Bacillus Calmette-Guerin infection on transplanted tumours in the mouse. *Nature, 184*, 291–292.

O'Malley, W.E., Achinstein, B., & Shear, M.J. (1962). Action of bacterial polysaccharide on tumors. II. Damage of sarcoma 37 by serum of mice treated with Serratia marcescens polysaccharide, and induced tolerance. *Journal of the National Cancer Institute, 29*, 1169–1175.

Pardoll, D. (2011). Timeline: A decade of advances in immunotherapy. *Nature Medicine, 17*, 296. https://doi.org/10.1038/nm0311-296

Parish, C.R. (2003). Cancer immunotherapy: The past, the present and the future. *Immunology and Cell Biology, 81*, 106–113. https://doi.org/10.1046/j.0818-9641.2003.01151.x

Pennock, G.K., Waterfield, W., & Wolchok, J.D. (2012). Patient responses to ipilimumab, a novel immunopotentiator for metastatic melanoma: How different are these from conventional treatment responses? *American Journal of Clinical Oncology, 35*, 606–611. https://doi.org/10.1097/COC.0b013e318209cda9

Pierre, P., Turley, S.J., Gatti, E., Hull, M., Meltzer, J., Mirza, A., … Mellman, I. (1997). Developmental regulation of MHC class II transport in mouse dendritic cells. *Nature, 388*, 787–792. https://doi.org/10.1038/42039

Porter, D.L., Levine, B.L., Kalos, M., Bagg, A., & June, C.H. (2011). Chimeric antigen receptor–modified T cells in chronic lymphoid leukemia. *New England Journal of Medicine, 365*, 725–733. https://doi.org/10.1056/NEJMoa1103849

Ribatti, D. (2014). From the discovery of monoclonal antibodies to their therapeutic application: An historical reappraisal. *Immunology Letters, 161*, 96–99. https://doi.org/10.1016/j.imlet.2014.05.010

Rosenberg, S.A. (2007). Interleukin-2 for patients with renal cancer. *Nature Clinical Practice Oncology, 4*, 497. https://doi.org/10.1038/ncponc0926

Rosenberg, S.A. (2014). IL-2: The first effective immunotherapy for human cancer. *Journal of Immunology, 192*, 5451–5458. https://doi.org/10.4049/jimmunol.1490019

Rosenberg, S.A., Lotze, M.T., Muul, L.M., Leitman, S., Chang, A.E., Ettinghausen, S.E., … Reichert, C.M. (1985). Observations on the systemic administration of autologous lymphokine-activated killer cells and recombinant interleukin-2 to patients with metastatic cancer. *New England Journal of Medicine, 313*, 1485–1492. https://doi.org/10.1056/NEJM198512053132327

Rosenberg, S.A., Spiess, P., & Lafreniere, R. (1986). A new approach to the adoptive immunotherapy of cancer with tumor-infiltrating lymphocytes. *Science, 233*, 1318–1321. https://doi.org/10.1126/science.3489291

Sadelain, M., Brentjens, R., & Rivière, I. (2013). The basic principles of chimeric antigen receptor design. *Cancer Discovery, 3*, 388–398. https://doi.org/10.1158/2159-8290.CD-12-0548

Schwartz, R.H. (1992). Costimulation of T lymphocytes: The role of CD28, CTLA-4, and B7/BB1 in interleukin-2 production and immunotherapy. *Cell, 71*, 1065–1068. https://doi.org/10.1016/S0092-8674(05)80055-8

Shankaran, V., Ikeda, H., Bruce, A.T., White, J.M., Swanson, P.E., Old, L.J., & Schreiber, R.D. (2001). IFNγ and lymphocytes prevent primary tumour development and shape tumour immunogenicity. *Nature, 410*, 1107–1111. https://doi.org/10.1038/35074122

Singer, D.S., Jacks, T., & Jaffee, E. (2016). A U.S. "Cancer Moonshot" to accelerate cancer research. *Science, 353*, 1105–1106. https://doi.org/10.1126/science.aai7862

Small, E.J., Sacks, N., Nemunaitis, J., Urba, W.J., Dula, E., Centeno, A.S., ... Simons, J.W. (2007). Granulocyte macrophage colony-stimulating factor. Secreting allogeneic cellular immunotherapy for hormone-refractory prostate cancer. *Clinical Cancer Research, 13,* 3883–3891. https://doi.org/10.1158/1078-0432.CCR-06-2937

Smyth, M.J., Godfrey, D.I., & Trapani, J.A. (2001). A fresh look at tumor immunosurveillance and immunotherapy. *Nature Immunology, 2,* 293–299. https://doi.org/10.1038/86297

Smyth, M.J., Thia, K.Y.T., Street, S.E.A., Cretney, E., Trapani, J.A., Taniguchi, M., ... Godfrey, D.I. (2000). Differential tumor surveillance by natural killer (Nk) and Nkt cells. *Journal of Experimental Medicine, 191,* 661–668. https://doi.org/10.1084/jem.191.4.661

Smyth, M.J., Thia, K.Y.T., Street, S.E.A., MacGregor, D., Godfrey, D.I., & Trapani, J.A. (2000). Perforin-mediated cytotoxicity is critical for surveillance of spontaneous lymphoma. *Journal of Experimental Medicine, 192,* 755–760. https://doi.org/10.1084/jem.192.5.755

Steinman, R.M., & Dhodapkar, M. (2001). Active immunization against cancer with dendritic cells: The near future. *International Journal of Cancer, 94,* 459–473. https://doi.org/10.1002/ijc.1503

Stutman, O. (1975). Immunodepression and malignancy. In G. Klein, S. Weinhouse, & A. Haddow (Eds.), *Advances in Cancer Research: Vol. 22* (pp. 261–422). https://doi.org/10.1016/S0065-230X(08)60179-7

Stutman, O. (1979a). Chemical carcinogenesis in nude mice: Comparison between nude mice from homozygous matings and heterozygous matings and effect of age and carcinogen dose. *Journal of the National Cancer Institute, 62,* 353–358.

Stutman, O. (1979b). Spontaneous tumors in nude mice: Effect of the viable yellow gene. *Experimental Cell Biology, 47,* 129–135. https://doi.org/10.1159/000162929

Taniguchi, K., Koga, S., Nishikido, M., Yamashita, S., Sakuragi, T., Kanetake, H., & Saito, Y. (1999). Systemic immune response after intravesical instillation of bacille Calmette-Guérin (BCG) for superficial bladder cancer. *Clinical and Experimental Immunology, 115,* 131–135. https://doi.org/10.1046/j.1365-2249.1999.00756.x

Till, B.G., Jensen, M.C., Wang, J., Chen, E.Y., Wood, B.L., Greisman, H.A., ... Press, O.W. (2008). Adoptive immunotherapy for indolent non-Hodgkin lymphoma and mantle cell lymphoma using genetically modified autologous CD20-specific T cells. *Blood, 112,* 2261–2271. https://doi.org/10.1182/blood-2007-12-128843

Tontonoz, M. (2015). Immunotherapy: Revolutionizing cancer treatment since 1891. Retrieved from https://www.mskcc.org/blog/immunotherapy-revolutionizing-cancer -treatment-1891

Topalian, S.L., Hodi, F.S., Brahmer, J.R., Gettinger, S.N., Smith, D.C., McDermott, D.F., ... Sznol, M. (2012). Safety, activity, and immune correlates of anti–PD-1 antibody in cancer. *New England Journal of Medicine, 366,* 2443–2454. https://doi.org/10.1056 /NEJMoa1200690

Tseng, S.-Y., Otsuji, M., Gorski, K., Huang, X., Slansky, J.E., Pai, S.I., ... Tsuchiya, H. (2001). B7-Dc, a new dendritic cell molecule with potent costimulatory properties for T cells. *Journal of Experimental Medicine, 193,* 839–846. https://doi.org/10.1084/jem.193.7.839

Wolchok, J.D., Kluger, H., Callahan, M.K., Postow, M.A., Rizvi, N.A., Lesokhin, A.M., ... Sznol, M. (2013). Nivolumab plus ipilimumab in advanced melanoma. *New England Journal of Medicine, 369,* 122–133. https://doi.org/10.1056/NEJMoa1302369

Wolchok, J.D., Weber, J.S., Hamid, O., Lebbé, C., Maio, M., Schadendorf, D., ... O'Day, S.J. (2010). Ipilimumab efficacy and safety in patients with advanced melanoma: A retrospective analysis of HLA subtype from four trials. *Cancer Immunology, 10,* 9.

Yang, J.C., Hughes, M., Kammula, U., Royal, R., Sherry, R.M., Topalian, S.L., ... Rosenberg, S.A. (2007). Ipilimumab (anti-CTLA4 antibody) causes regression of metastatic renal cell cancer associated with enteritis and hypophysitis. *Journal of Immunotherapy, 30,* 825–830. https://doi.org/10.1097/CJI.0b013e318156e47e

Yee, C., Thompson, J.A., Byrd, D., Riddell, S.R., Roche, P., Celis, E., & Greenberg, P.D. (2002). Adoptive T cell therapy using antigen-specific CD8+ T cell clones for the treatment of patients with metastatic melanoma: In vivo persistence, migration, and antitumor effect of transferred T cells. *Proceedings of the National Academy of Sciences of the United States of America, 99,* 16168–16173. https://doi.org/10.1073/pnas.242600099

Principles of Immunology and Immunotherapy

Rowena N. Schwartz, PharmD, BCOP

Introduction

One of the most exciting and rapidly evolving advances in cancer treatment is the use of immunotherapy, or the augmentation of the immune system's ability to fight cancer. This therapy is being used alone or in combination with more traditional therapies for the treatment of a growing number of cancers. Advancements in immunotherapy parallel the progress seen with immunology, the understanding of the biology of the immune response, and drug development. This complex interaction between the immune system and cancer continues to be deciphered, and both clinical successes and the limitations of immunotherapy in practice drive the development of new approaches and strategies (Chen & Mellman, 2013).

Historically, the understanding of immunity has focused on the body's strategies to mount a response to infectious diseases. The immune system is a complex network of cells, tissues, and organs that function together to defend the body against foreign invaders, such as bacteria, viruses, parasites, or fungi. It exists to protect individuals from infection and to recognize and respond to other deviations from normal physiologic homeostasis (Dunn & Okada, 2015). *Immunity* is the ability of the body to respond to foreign substances, including microbes and noninfectious molecules. The complex network that mediates the immune response to infection is as important as the immune response to cancer. An area of great interest regarding immunotherapy is the role of the immune system during the formation of cancer, or tumorigenesis, and during cancer progression. Investigation into the complex and interrelated cellular and molecular mechanisms that influence and regulate the immune response has led to the development, evaluation, and clinical application of novel strategies for immunotherapy in cancer treatment.

Therapies that stimulate the immune system, or immunostimulatory therapies, include approaches that range from cytokines (e.g., interferons [IFNs], interleukins [ILs]) that stimulate immune response, to monoclonal antibodies that target the regulators of immune response (e.g., checkpoint inhibitors). The goal of immunostimulatory therapy is to enhance the immune response to cancer cells. Further evaluation will help determine how to best sequence and combine immunostimulatory therapies with other cancer treatments (e.g., radiation therapy, chemotherapy).

Immunology and immunopharmacology are rapidly evolving fields. As such, it is crucial to keep abreast of the new literature on the science of immunity and the transformation of care. New immune targets for drug therapy are being identified, and therapies directed at these targets are being developed, evaluated, marketed, and integrated into the standard of care for many cancers. This chapter will provide a foundational review of the current understanding of the immune system. This knowledge is essential, as the immunotherapy approach is very different from more familiar therapies.

The Immune System

The human immune system is a highly efficient and complex network of antigen-specific and antigen-nonspecific tissue barriers, specialized cells, and soluble factors that help the body distinguish "self" from "nonself." Exposure to a pathogen, or nonself, triggers a rapid nonspecific response that attempts to isolate the invader (innate immune response). This subsequently initiates the antigen-specific arm of the immune system (adaptive immune response).

Immunity also can be described as the balanced state of having adequate biologic defenses to fight infection, disease, and other unwanted biologic invasions. A key function of the immune system is to eradicate microbial pathogens and prevent infection. Unsurprisingly, the literature has largely focused on the role of immunity in infection. However, immunity and immunology play important roles in many diseases, including cancer.

An antigen is a molecule capable of triggering an immune response. It can be a microbe, such as a virus; a tissue from another person (e.g., organ transplantation); or part of the body's own tissues (e.g., autoimmune disease). In the latter scenario, the body mistakes self for nonself, and the immune system attacks a specific organ or tissue (e.g., rheumatoid arthritis, type 1 diabetes mellitus) or has a more generalized response (e.g., systemic lupus erythematosus).

Cancer ultimately occurs when mutations of a cancer cell trigger the oncogenic process. These mutations can be from known (e.g., smoking) or unknown factors and may cause the development of neoantigens, or new proteins or peptide sequences. Neoantigens are recognizable by the immune system. This recognition and the subsequent downstream effects of the immune response are important to the understanding of immunity's relationship with cancer (Chen & Mellman, 2017).

Innate and Adaptive Immune Recognition and Response

The function of the immune system is to identify and destroy foreign cells and substances in the body. Host defenses are often categorized as either innate immunity, which provides immediate protection to the host, or adaptive immunity, which develops more slowly (see Figure 2-1). Innate immunity does not adapt following pathogen invasion because of a lack of immunologic memory. In contrast, adaptive immune response is enhanced with each successive encounter with a specific pathogen.

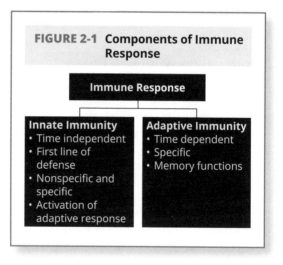

FIGURE 2-1 Components of Immune Response

Immune Response

Innate Immunity	Adaptive Immunity
• Time independent • First line of defense • Nonspecific and specific • Activation of adaptive response	• Time dependent • Specific • Memory functions

Innate Immunity

The innate immune response includes two key reactions: an acute inflammatory response and the activation of antiviral defense mechanisms. Inflammation is central to innate immunity and involves the recruitment of immune cells and plasma proteins to the invasion site; however, this can result in tissue damage or pathogen exposure (Shalapour & Karin, 2015). Acute-phase proteins (e.g., C-reactive proteins) are a heterogeneous group of plasma proteins that can be a marker for inflammation in some clinical situations (Markanday, 2015). Cytokines and other soluble products generated by immune cells increase the permeability of blood vessels and result in subsequent accumulation of complement and leukocytes into the tissues to promote repair. Phagocytic cells of the innate immune system are recruited to the infection site and activated through the engagement of surface receptors. Neutrophils and monocytes migrate to sites of extravascular infection or tissue damage in response to chemoattractant, a substance produced by tissue cells reacting to infection or injury. Chemoattractant provokes the movement of a cell, or chemotaxis. Neutrophils and macrophages ingest microbes, which may result in microbe death via enzymes and nitric oxide. Neutrophils can also destroy microbes through the release of substances into the extracellular environment.

Familiar clinical hallmarks of inflammation include redness (rubor), heat (calor), pain (dolor), and swelling (tumor). In clinical practice, signs of inflammation are used as an indication of infection or as a parameter to assess the response of an infection to treatment. As many of these signs are mediated by the presence of white blood cells, they may be absent in leukopenic individuals with an infection.

Chronic inflammation may contribute to the pathogenesis of some diseases, including cancer (Coates, FitzGerald, Helliwell, & Paul, 2016; Harris & Drake, 2013; Hong et al., 2017). The impact of inflammation with the use of immunostimulatory agents in cancer treatments is not known at this time.

Components of Innate Immunity

Many components of innate immunity are also important in adaptive immunity. These components are discussed in this section. Cellular components of innate immunity are also summarized in Table 2-1.

Neutrophils

Neutrophils, or polymorphonuclear leukocytes, are circulating phagocytes that are recruited to infection sites. They ingest microbes for intracellular killing (Amulic, Cazalet, Hayes, Metzler, & Zychlinsky, 2012). In response to an infection, colony-stimulating factor (CSF), or white blood cell growth factor, rapidly stimulates neutrophil production from bone marrow, resulting in an increase in neutrophil number and the release of immature neutrophils (bands) into the blood. CSF triggers hematopoietic stem cells, resulting in proliferation and maturation of neutrophil precursors. Neutrophils are frequently the initial immune cells involved in the response to bacterial and fungal infections and are the dominant cells during acute inflammation. Neutrophils also play a major role in cancer immunity when recruited to the tumor microenvironment (TME). These tumor-associated neutrophils are thought to be involved in the development and proliferation of tumor cells (Hurt, Schulick, Edil, El Kasmi, & Barnett, 2017).

TABLE 2-1 Cells of the Innate Immune Response

Cell	Description
Basophils	Originate from the common myeloid progenitor cells in the bone marrow and released into the circulation as mature cells Travel to sites of inflammation and infection in response to locally released cytokines and chemokines Believed to promote neoplastic angiogenesis
Dendritic cells	Antigen-presenting cells that reside in most tissues of the body Link the innate immune system to adaptive immune response Ensure triggering of antigen-presenting machinery Classified as migratory or lymphoid tissue-resident
Eosinophils	Traditionally associated with the host defense against certain parasites and fungi with allergic conditions Express chemokine, cytokine, immunoglobulin, Toll-like recognition, and histamine receptors When the receptors are engaged, a variety of cytotoxic proteins are released from cytoplasmic secretory granules; also found in the tumor-infiltrating area Express major histocompatibility complex class II and costimulatory molecules, whereby they function as antigen-presenting cells and initiate antigen-specific immune responses by T cells
Hematopoietic stem cells	All cells of the immune system originate from the pluripotent hematopoietic stem cells in the bone marrow. Divide to produce the common lymphoid progenitor cells and common myeloid progenitor cells Common lymphoid progenitor cells give rise to B lymphocytes, T lymphocytes, and natural killer cells. Common myeloid progenitor cells give rise to the cells of the innate immune system (e.g., leukocytes, mast cells, dendritic cells, erythrocytes, megakaryocytes).
Mast cells	Derived in the bone marrow and present in skin and mucosal epithelium Have cytoplasmic granules that contain vasoactive substances, such as histamine, that can cause vasodilatation and increase capillary permeability and proteolytic enzymes Synthesize and secrete prostaglandins and cytokines, such as tumor necrosis factor Can be activated by microbial products binding to Toll-like receptors as part of innate immunity or by special antibody-dependent mechanisms
Monocytes	Derived from the common myeloid progenitor cells Migrate into the tissues, where they differentiate rapidly and mature into distinct macrophages depending on the tissue of activation

(Continued on next page)

TABLE 2-1   Cells of the Innate Immune Response *(Continued)*

Cell	Description
Natural killer cells	Do not express antigen-specific surface receptors Express activating and inhibitory cell surface receptors Identify and eliminate cells that do not produce self-major histo-compatibility complex class I molecules Effector function triggered by activating cell surface receptors and dependent on cellular cross talk Induce cytotoxicity and promote cytokine production when activated
Neutrophils	Circulate in the blood as dormant cells and are recruited to infection sites by specific cytokines and cell adhesion molecules When activated, upregulate the production of cytokines and chemokines critical for chemotaxis and recruitment of additional neutrophils, macrophages, and T lymphocytes

Note. Based on information from Abbas et al., 2016; Delves & Roitt, 2000a, 2000b; Stephen & Hajjar, 2017.

Monocytes

Monocytes are circulating phagocytes that ingest microbes in blood and tissue. During inflammation, monocytes enter extravascular tissues and differentiate into macrophages. In cancer immunity, monocytes are attracted to the TME by tumor-derived cytokines. Once in the TME, monocytes differentiate into tissue-resident macrophages. Tumor-associated macrophages are influenced by the cytokine profile of the TME and are key regulators of tumor vascularization, lymphangiogenesis, metastasis, and immunosuppression (Fukuda, Kobayashi, & Watabe, 2012).

Macrophages

Macrophages are phagocytes found in tissues. Specialized types of macrophages are found in organs, including the lungs, kidneys, brain, and liver. Macrophages engulf and destroy invading microorganisms and release cytokines and chemokines to recruit other cells to the inflammation site. They are important in innate immune response and are effector cells in both the cell-mediated and humoral arms of adaptive immunity. Macrophages induce expression of costimulatory molecules on antigen-presenting cells (APCs) to initiate adaptive immune response and dispose of destroyed pathogens. Monocytes and macrophages are two stages of the same cellular lineage, the mononuclear phagocyte system.

Dendritic Cells

The gatekeepers of the immune system, dendritic cells (DCs), are APCs that link the innate immune system to adaptive immune response. DCs are concentrated in the secondary lymphoid tissues (e.g., spleen, lymph nodes, mucosal tissue associated with lymphoid tissue), where they continually inspect the TME, interpret clues, and coordinate immune response. The microarchitecture of secondary lymphoid tissue facilitates the interaction between DCs and the cellular components of adaptive immunity (Merad, Sathe, Helft, Miller, & Mortha, 2013).

The epithelia and T-cell–rich areas of secondary lymphoid tissue contain a network of the two major DC populations: classical and plasmacytoid. These populations differ in surface markers, location, receptor expression, cytokine production, and function. Plasmacytoid DCs are morphologically like plasma cells. When stimulated, DCs produce cytokines such as IL-1 and tumor necrosis factor (TNF) to initiate inflammation. Immature DCs also take up antigens through pinocytosis, a process when the antigen is internalized and ultimately degraded. Cytokine production and the signaling initiated through receptor binding ultimately stimulate an adaptive immune response (Mildner & Jung, 2014).

When activated, immature DCs stop taking up antigens and lose their adhesiveness to epithelial tissues. These DCs then travel to secondary lymphoid tissue, which is rich in T cells. During this migration, the DCs mature and have increased expression of major histocompatibility complex (MHC) molecules, the membrane proteins that display peptide antigens for recognition by T lymphocytes. Mature DCs become APCs and can stimulate T cells with the appropriate costimulatory signals. The binding of ligands to costimulatory molecules on T cells leads to T-cell activation. Based on the type of pathogen and the other maturation signals received, activated T cells are educated to proliferate and differentiate and become potent effector cytotoxic T cells or helper cells.

Pattern Recognition Receptors

Macrophages and DCs can express pattern recognition receptors (PRRs) to identify conserved structures found during tissue damage and cell death (Dunn & Okada, 2015). PRRs are germline-encoded host sensors expressed on many types of cell surfaces, including phagocytes, neutrophils, and DCs. They are also called *primitive pattern recognition receptors* because they evolved earlier than other parts of the immune system. Toll-like receptors (TLRs), expressed on the plasma membranes and endosomes of many cells, are PRRs that recognize different microbial products and signal the immune process through cytokine selection.

PRRs are identical in all cells and used by the innate immune system against microbes and damaged cells. Cells with PRRs bind to microbial unique molecular sequences called pathogen-associated molecular patterns (PAMPs). Once activated, PRRs initiate the production of various cytokines from DCs. These cytokine profiles are important in determining different immune responses. PRR recognition of conserved molecular components on the cell surface of receptors on the pathogen (PAMPS) is crucial to innate immunity (Takeuchi & Akira, 2010). PRRs also recognize damage-associated molecular patterns, which are related to the components of the cell released during cell damage or death.

Innate Lymphoid Cells

Innate lymphoid cells (ILCs) are lymphocyte-like cells that function like T lymphocytes but do not express T-cell antigen receptors (Mattner & Wirtz, 2017). They appear to provide early defense against infections and facilitate T-cell response. ILCs respond rapidly and are functionally analogous to diverse T-cell subsets. These cells may be a potential target for cancer therapy, as they are an innate immune cell population endowed with potent immunomodulatory properties.

Natural Killer Cells

Natural killer (NK) cells are cytotoxic lymphocytes of the innate immune system that specialize in early defense against virus-infected and transformed cells (Muntasell et al., 2017). NK cells originate from the common lymphoid progenitor cells in the bone marrow and are in peripheral tissues. NK cells do *not* express antigen-specific surface receptors, but they *do* express many activating and inhibitory cell surface receptors. Subsets of NK cells are classified based on the expression of cell surface molecules (e.g., CD16, CD56).

A primary function of NK cells is to identify and eliminate cells that do not produce self-MHC molecules. NK-cell–mediated cytotoxicity is similar in many ways to T-cell cytotoxicity; however, NK cells do not require antigen presentation. Activation of the effector function of NK cells occurs once cell surface receptors are engaged by PAMPs. This helps to identify infected nonself cells and stressed self-cells and successively initiates the effector function of NK cells. NK-cell–mediated cytotoxicity may occur before initiation of adaptive immune response (Vivier, Tomasello, Baratin, Walzer, & Ugolini, 2008).

NK-cell activation is dependent on cross talk with the cells (e.g., DCs, neutrophils, macrophages, mast cells) and cytokines (e.g., IL-2, IL-12) involved in immune response. DCs prime NK cells through direct contact or secretion of cytokines. NK cells recognize infected and stressed cells and respond by killing these cells and secreting cytokines such as IFN gamma (IFN-γ) and TNF. The production of these cytokines increases the activity of other immune cells. For example, IFN-γ activates macrophages to become more effective at killing phagocytosed microbes. Cytokines, such as ILs and IFNs secreted by other cells (e.g., DCs, macrophages), can enhance NK cells, showcasing an example of cooperative functioning (Abbas, Lichtman, & Pillai, 2016).

NK cells also exhibit some characteristics of T cells and can mount a rapid immune response on secondary exposure. The immune memory function of NK cells lasts for months after initial exposure and is antigen specific and transferable. Interest is growing in the manipulation or transfer of NK cells as a form of immunotherapy (Granzin et al., 2017).

Soluble Factors of Innate Immunity: Complement and Cytokines

Complement and its proteins, cytokines and chemokines, are important components of innate immune response. Complement provides clearance for apoptotic, or dying, cells (Kolev, Towner, & Donev, 2011). The complement cascade, a network of more than 35 soluble circulating and membrane-bound proteins, plays a vital role in maintaining host defenses during the early stages of microbial invasion. Initially, complement proteins circulate in the blood in an inactive form. When the first protein in the complement series is activated, the complement cascade begins.

The complement system is activated through either innate or adaptive immunity via three main pathways: classical, lectin, and alternative. The classical pathway is triggered by antibodies that bind to antigens or microbes via the humoral arm of adaptive immunity (Liszewski & Atkinson, 2015). The lectin pathway is activated when a carbohydrate-binding plasma protein binds to surface glycoproteins of microbes (innate immunity). The alternative pathway is initiated when complement proteins are activated on microbial surfaces (innate immunity).

Complement activation in innate immune response involves the binding of circulating mediators to invading microbial cells and the enhancing of antigen-nonspecific cell activity by chemotaxis and/or by facilitating phagocytosis via macrophages or neutrophils. Complement opsonizes microbes for phagocytosis, stimulating inflammation and cell lysis. The complement system also works to "complement" the action of antibodies (humoral immunity).

Complement-dependent cytotoxicity is the process in which pathogens are killed by damaging their membranes without the involvement of antibodies or the cells of the immune system. Therapeutic monoclonal antibodies for cancer treatment, such as rituximab, are believed to use this as a mechanism to exert an antitumor effect (Kolev et al., 2011).

Cytokines, or "cell movers," are a large family of low-molecular-weight soluble proteins with diverse biologic functions that mediate immune and inflammatory reactions and coordinate communication between cells. They are secreted in response to stimuli by many of the cells that participate in the immune response. Most cytokines act on the cells that produce them or on adjacent cells. Distinct cytokines may have overlapping effects that provide a level of redundancy (Butterfield, Kaufman, & Marincola, 2017).

Interleukins, a type of cytokine, were named as such because they were believed to coordinate communication "between leukocytes." ILs include many proteins with a wide range of functions. The physiologic role of the IL family extends far beyond leukocytes and is important in the coordination of communication between many cells of the immune system. ILs, IFNs, chemokines, mesenchymal growth factors, adipokines, and TNF make up the functional classes of cytokines. TNF, IL-1, and chemokines (chemoattractant cytokines) are involved in the recruitment of neutrophils and monocytes to infection sites (Delves & Roitt, 2000a) (see Table 2-2).

To review, cytokines are secreted by cells involved in innate immune response and facilitate the mediation of cellular reactions in innate immunity. Cytokines involved in innate immunity stimulate inflammation, activate NK cells and macrophages, and prevent viral infections (e.g., type 1 IFNs). DCs, macrophages, mast cells, and ILCs respond to microbes by producing cytokines that stimulate inflammation and activate NK cells to produce IFN-γ, which plays a key role in the activation of macrophages.

Adaptive Immunity: Humoral and Cell-Mediated Immunity

Adaptive immunity, also called specific or acquired immunity, is initiated by the recognition of antigens by antigen receptors on lymphocytes. The term *acquired immunity* comes from the understanding that pathogen-specific receptors are "acquired" over a lifetime and that antigen exposure "adapts" the body for future challenges with that antigen. Lymphocytes, the worker cells of adaptive immunity, are coordinated by signals from the cells and proteins (e.g., cytokines, complement) of both innate and adaptive immunity. See Table 2-3 for information on the cells of the adaptive immune system.

The hallmark of adaptive immunity is the specificity of immune response to antigens. Antigen recognition during presentation results in the clonal expansion of antigen-specific lymphocytes that facilitate the removal of the recognized antigen. Unlike the rapid immune response seen with innate immunity, a delay occurs before naïve T and B cells can exert effector functions in adaptive immunity. Immunologic memory can develop through memory T and B cells in adaptive immunity, which is unlike the general, nonspecific responses seen in innate immunity (Delves & Roitt, 2000a).

TABLE 2-2   Key Cytokines of Innate Immunity

Cytokine	Main Source
Chemokines	Macrophages, T cells, mast cells
Interferon alfa (type I)	Dendritic cells, macrophages
Interferon beta (type I)	Fibroblasts
Interferon gamma	Natural killer cells, T lymphocytes
Interleukin-1	Macrophages, dendritic cells, endothelial cells, mast cells
Interleukin-6	Macrophages, endothelial cells, T cells
Interleukin-10	Macrophages, dendritic cells, T cells
Interleukin-12	Dendritic cells, macrophages
Interleukin-15	Macrophages
Interleukin-18	Macrophages
Transforming growth factor beta	Many sources
Tumor necrosis factor	Macrophages, T cells, mast cells

Note. Based on information from Abbas et al., 2016; Butterfield et al., 2017.

The two arms, or subsystems, of adaptive immune response are humoral and cell-mediated immunity. Humoral immunity is predominantly mediated by B lymphocytes, or B cells. B lymphocytes can recognize a variety of substances as nonself, including both extracellular macromolecules and small chemicals. Cell-mediated immunity is mediated by T lymphocytes, or T cells. T cells recognize peptide fragments when antigens are presented as small antigenic determinants on MHC molecules. The antigen receptor of most T cells only recognizes peptides as antigens when they are presented by specialized molecules. Most T-lymphocyte antigen receptors can only recognize peptide fragments of protein antigens, while B lymphocytes can recognize nonprotein substances.

Humoral Immunity

Humoral immunity neutralizes and eliminates extracellular microbes and microbial toxins mediated through B-cell recognition. It is the principal defense mechanism against microbes with capsules rich in polysaccharides and lipids, as T cells are not able to respond to these nonprotein antigens. Humoral immunity is initiated when an

TABLE 2-3   Cells of the Adaptive Immune System

Cell	Description
B lymphocytes	B cell from lymphoid progenitor cells Precursors include pre/pro-B cells, early pro-B cells, late pro-B cells, and pre-B cells. All precursors do not have surface immunoglobulin. Activated B cells differentiate into plasma cells that produce high-affinity secreted antibody. Each B cell produces a single kind of antibody.
T lymphocytes	Progenitor cells migrate from bone marrow to thymus to undergo differentiation and proliferation. In absence of antigenic stimuli, naïve T cells enter the bloodstream to travel to peripheral lymphoid tissue. Activation by antigens causes clonal expansion and differentiation into helper T and cytotoxic T cells.
Helper T cells (CD4+)	Helper T cells secrete cytokines and chemokines that help coordinate the immune response. Helper T cells can differentiate into the following: • Type 1 T helper cells (Th1)—aid in cellular immunity through activation of CD8+ T cells • Type 2 T helper cells (Th2)—aid in humoral immunity by activation of B cells • T helper 17 (Th17) • Induced regulatory T cells (iTregs) • T follicular helper cells (Tfh) • Type 9 T helper cells (Th9)
Cytotoxic T cells (CD8+)	T lymphocytes that express CD8. These cells kill target cells upon recognizing complexes of antigen and major histocompatibility complex (MHC) on the target cell membranes. Activated by antigen presentation on MHC class I molecules or through helper T cells
Regulatory T cells (Tregs; CD4+)	Specialized T cells that suppress function of other T cells Classified as natural Tregs or inducible Tregs Decreasing Treg activity can enhance innate and adaptive immune response.

Note. Based on information from Abbas et al., 2016.

antigen is recognized by a specific membrane antibody on the B lymphocyte. The B-cell receptor (BCR), a transmembrane receptor protein located on the outer surface of the B lymphocyte, binds to the antigen, resulting in proliferation and differentiation of the B lymphocyte. This generates a population of antibody-secreting plasma B cells and memory B cells. BCR is required for antibody production, and defects in BCR signal transduction may lead to immunodeficiency and B-cell malignancy.

B cells develop from hematopoietic stem cells that originate in the bone marrow. Hematopoietic stem cells differentiate into multipotent progenitor cells and then to common lymphoid progenitor cells. B-cell precursors that develop from common lymphoid progenitor cells include pre/pro-B cells, early pro-B cells, late pro-B cells, and pre-B cells.

B cells undergo selection to ensure proper development. Immature B cells migrate to the spleen as transitional cells. Further development of B cells is influenced by growth factors, cytokines, and chemokines. B cells that develop the earliest are called B1 cells. These cells express CD5 (an adhesion and signaling cell surface molecule), are reactive to different antigens, and have relatively low affinity. Within the spleen, B1 cells transition to B2 cells. Depending on signaling, these B2 cells further differentiate to follicular B cells or marginal zone B cells. Once differentiated, they are considered naïve B cells. Immature B cells express BCR class immunoglobulin (Ig) H, but once transition to B2 cells occurs, this expression changes to IgM or IgD (Abbas et al., 2016).

B-cell activation occurs in lymph nodes and other lymphoid organs, such as the spleen, and is initiated when the B cell binds to an antigen via the BCR (Cooper, 2015). This causes the proliferation of antigen-specific B cells, resulting in the expansion of antigen-specific clones (or clonal expansion) and subsequent differentiation into plasma cells. Plasma cells are effector cells of humoral immunity. They are long-lived, nonproliferating cells that actively secrete antibodies. Every plasma cell descended from a given B cell manufactures identical antibodies. Antibodies from plasma cells are produced in both lymphoid tissues and bone marrow; however, they ultimately enter the circulation to travel to the infection site.

Antigen binding to naïve B lymphocytes initiates a process of B-cell proliferation, IgM secretion. This prepares the B cell for interaction with helper T cells. Antigens that activate B cells without T cells are T-independent antigens. This response tends to be rapid. Antigens that activate B cells with the help of T cells are T-dependent antigens (e.g., foreign proteins). Memory B cells, which share the same BCR as their parent B cells, circulate through the body and initiate a stronger and more rapid antibody response if they can detect the antigen that activated their parent B cell. Regulatory B cells are immunosuppressive B cells that play a role in the modulation of the inflammatory responses that occur during autoimmune disease (Cooper, 2015).

B cells, known for their ability to produce antibodies, also can release cytokines as part of the immune response. Antibodies are glycoprotein products of plasma cells. The core antibody, or Ig structure, includes a domain or region with a unique role in immune response. Each antibody comprises two identical heavy chains and two identical light chains that are united by disulfide bonds (see Figure 2-2).

The amino terminus, or N-terminus, of both chains possesses a variable region or domain that binds antigens to

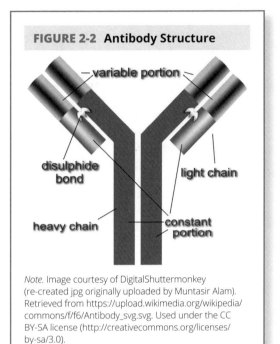

FIGURE 2-2 Antibody Structure

Note. Image courtesy of DigitalShuttermonkey (re-created jpg originally uploaded by Muntasir Alam). Retrieved from https://upload.wikimedia.org/wikipedia/commons/f/f6/Antibody_svg.svg. Used under the CC BY-SA license (http://creativecommons.org/licenses/by-sa/3.0).

antibody. The fragment antigen-binding (Fab) region refers to the proteolytic fragment required for antigen recognition, or the region of the antibody that binds to an antigen. Within these variable regions are areas called hypervariable regions, or complementarity-determining regions, which form the antigen-binding sites.

The carboxy-terminus, or C-terminus, of both chains possesses a domain that forms the constant regions, which define the class and subclass of the antibody. The fragment crystallizable (Fc) region contains most of the constant region of the heavy chains and tends to crystallize in solution (Delves & Roitt, 2000b). This region is responsible for interacting with cells of the immune system and for the biologic activity and effector functions of the antibody.

The amino acid sequence of the constant region of heavy chains specifies the classes or isotypes of Igs (e.g., IgA, IgD, IgE, IgG, IgM), four subclasses of IgG, and two subclasses of IgA. These classes and subclasses have the following functions (Abbas et al., 2016):

- IgA is found in mucosal tissue, such as in the respiratory and gastrointestinal tracts, and in secretions, such as saliva and tears. It guards the entrances of the body.
- IgD remains attached to B cells. It functions primarily as an antigen receptor on B cells and stimulates the production of basophils and mast cells.

• IgE is important for protection against parasites and is involved in allergic reactions. With activation, it triggers the release of histamine from mast cells and basophils.

• IgG provides the foundation of antibody-based immunity and expedites the uptake of microbes by other cells of the immune system. It can cross the placenta and provide passive immunity to the fetus. IgG is an isotype used for many of the approved monoclonal antibodies developed for drug therapy in cancer and other specialties.

• IgM is expressed on the surface of B cells. It is released early in humoral immunity, prior to the production of IgG.

The T-cell–dependent response of humoral immunity to protein antigens is initiated by the binding of protein to specific Ig receptors of naïve B cells in lymphoid follicles. This helps prepare the B cell for interaction with helper T cells.

Cell-Mediated Immunity

Cell-mediated immunity is the arm of adaptive immunity regulated by T lymphocytes. It is initiated by the capture and subsequent display of protein antigens by the naïve T cells specific to these antigens. T cells can be distinguished from other lymphocytes by the presence of a T-cell receptor (TCR) on the cell surface. T cells originate from the hematopoietic stem cells in the bone marrow. The "T" in T cells refers to the thymus because they mature in the thymus (or tonsils) from thymocytes. Lymphoid progenitor cells differentiate into T-cell precursors, or thymocytes, in the thymus. Very early T-cell precursors do not express the cell surface molecules CD4+ or CD8+; however, they will express both at some point during development. Once released from the thymus, mature T cells express either CD4+ or CD8+. As individuals age, T-cell production from the thymus slows; therefore, clonal expansion of existing naïve T cells is believed to be a primary source of T cells for older adults (Robey & Fowlkes, 1994).

Antigens, such as microbes, that enter the body through epithelia are captured by DCs and transported through the lymphatic system. Once captured, they are displayed by APCs to naïve T lymphocytes. The TCR engages with the antigen presented by MHC molecules on an APC. Naïve T cells are activated through exposure to antigenic determinants by antigen-presenting DCs or APCs. DCs are the principal inducers of T-cell–dependent immune responses, although macrophages are also important APCs.

MHC molecules on APCs display antigens to T lymphocytes. The two classes of MHC molecules, class I and class II, are expressed on different types of cells and are recognized by a different type of T cell.

MHC class I molecules are expressed on all nucleated cells. They display peptides from intracellular pathogens and present shorter peptides (antigens) to cytotoxic T cells (CD8+). Once activated by APC binding, cytotoxic T cells may later recognize cells that express the same antigen, resulting in cell-mediated cytotoxicity. MHC class II expression is restricted to macrophages, DCs, and some epithelial and endothelial cells that function as APCs. These molecules display peptides from extracellular pathogens and present longer peptides to helper T cells (CD4+). MHC molecules are highly polymorphic (have multiple forms). An antigen that may be recognized by one individual may not be recognized by another with a distinct set of MHC alleles.

T-cell activation is a complex process. As investigations into the complex process of T-cell activation continue, new and important aspects are being uncovered, such as the importance of antigen presentation. It is now recognized that T-cell activation requires both the engagement of the TCR and the costimulation of the T cell by stimulatory checkpoints to signal a cell-mediated immune response. It should be noted that a negative or inhibitory checkpoint signal can impair T-cell response (Greenwald, Freeman, & Sharpe, 2005).

Costimulatory signaling is initiated through the binding of ligands to stimulatory receptors on T cells, resulting in the formation of effector T cells that can either destroy the foreign substance or attract other immune cells to the site. T-cell response is regulated through a balance of costimulatory and inhibitory signals that serve as immune checkpoints. Costimulatory receptors include CD28, ICOS (inducible costimulatory molecule), 4-1BB (D137), and OX40 (CD134). Coinhibitory receptors include cytotoxic T-lymphocyte antigen 4 (CTLA-4), TIM-3, and programmed cell death protein 1 (PD-1) (see Table 2-4).

T-cell recognition, followed by costimulation, galvanizes T-cell proliferation, leading to the production of effector molecules that control the pathogen or foreign protein. Activation includes secretion of cytokines, increased expression of cytokines, and proliferation of antigen-specific activated T cells (clonal expansion). Activated T lymphocytes ultimately differentiate into effector cells that eradicate the foreign pathogen. Some antigen-activated T cells develop into long-lived memory T cells. These cells are functionally inactive but survive after the pathogen is eradicated, putting them in the position to respond with repeated exposure to the same pathogen.

An adequate adaptive immune response takes days to develop after initial exposure because of the time required for lymphocyte selection, clonal expansion, and subsequent lymphocyte differentiation. T lymphocytes recognize an antigen through membrane-bound TCRs. Each mature T lymphocyte (and its progeny cell) expresses a unique TCR repertoire. A mature T cell expresses thousands of TCRs, each identical in specificity for the same antigen.

TABLE 2-4   Inhibitory Checkpoints for T Cells

Coinhibitory Checkpoint	Receptor	Ligand	Drug Targeting
CTLA-4	Activated CD8+ T cells Regulatory T cells	CD80 CD86	Ipilimumab
LAG-3	B cells Natural killer cells T cells	MHC II molecule	–
PD-1	Activated CD8+ T cells Dendritic cells Macrophages Natural killer cells Regulatory T cells	PD-L1 PD-L2	PD-1 • Nivolumab • Pembrolizumab PD-L1 • Atezolizumab • Avelumab • Durvalumab
TIGIT	Natural killer cells T cells	CD112 CD113 CD155 Nectins	–
TIM-3	B cells Dendritic cells Macrophages Natural killer cells T cells	Galectin-9 phosphatidylserine	–
VISTA	CD11b myeloid cells Dendritic cells T cells	VISTA-immunoglobulin fusion protein	–

CD—cluster of differentiation; CTLA-4—cytotoxic T-lymphocyte antigen 4; LAG-3—lymphocyte-activation gene 3; MHC—major histocompatibility complex; PD-1—programmed cell death protein 1; PD-L1—programmed cell death-ligand 1; PD-L2—programmed cell death-ligand 2; TIM-3—T cell membrane protein 3
Note. Based on information from Sharma & Allison, 2015.

Once the T cell is engaged, a series of signals, including transcription factors such as NF-AT, NF-κB, and AP-1, initiates the activation of signaling cascades. NF-AT, or nuclear factor of activated T cells, is a family now known to have an important role in immunity. NF-κB, nuclear factor kappa-light-chain-enhancer of activated B cells, controls the transcription of DNA, cytokine production, and cell survival. This family also plays a role in the immune response to infection. NF-κB dysregulation has been linked to cancer and inflammation (Panday et al., 2016). AP-1, activator protein 1, regulates gene expression in response to signals from both immune cells and infection. The mammalian target of rapamycin (mTOR) pathway also plays a role in T-cell activation and function and is emerging as an important druggable target for some cancers (Harris & Drake, 2013).

T-cell activation leads to the expansion of T cells, called clonal expansion, and the further differentiation of naïve T cells to helper T cells (CD4+) and cytotoxic effector T cells (CD8+). Helper T cells can differentiate into one of several subtypes, including Th1 (type 1 T helper), Th2, Th3, Th17, Th9, or Tfh (T follicular helper cells), depending on the environment of the immune response. These helper T cells secrete cytokines and chemokines that regulate the immune response and appear to be important in autoimmunity and disease. The understanding of these subtypes and their role in disease continues to evolve.

T-cell activation is influenced by various cytokines throughout the activation process. Different cytokine profiles appear to impact transcription factors, ultimately influencing the function of T cells. For example, some cytokines exert their immunologic effects by modulating the function of signal transducer and activator of transcription (STAT) proteins during T-cell activation. STAT proteins are a family of transcription factors that help coordinate cellular proliferation, apoptosis, differentiation, and immunity. These proteins are activated by membrane receptor–associated Janus kinases (JAKs). Dysregulation in JAK-STAT pathways has been associated with cancer immunosuppression (Villarino, Kanno, & O'Shea, 2017). STAT proteins are a potential actionable drug target for disease, and inhibitors for STAT are currently in clinical trials for cancer and a variety of inflammatory diseases.

A unique feature of adaptive immunity is its ability to confer immunologic memory, allowing for a more rapid and enhanced T- and B-cell response on reexposure to antigens or pathogens (Saied, Pillarisetty, & Katz, 2014). Once activated, some T cells become long-lived memory cells that facilitate the immune response when an antigen is reencountered. Central memory cells have a high proliferative rate once restimulated. Tissue-resident memory cells are associated with organ-specific distribution (Abbas et al., 2016). Therefore, during a secondary response, memory B and T lymphocytes can respond more quickly to previously encountered antigens. On repeated exposures to the same immunogen, memory lymphocytes orchestrate an even faster and more efficient response.

Components of Adaptive Immunity

Adaptive immune response requires coordination between immune cells, glycoproteins, and cytokines. The receptors on these cells (e.g.,

PD-1, CTLA-4) and their ligands are considered crucial elements to this response.

Antibodies

Antibodies, or Igs, are glycoproteins produced by B lymphocytes and that bind antigens. Every individual has millions of different antibodies. Secreted antibodies are the foundation of humoral immune response, and effector function includes the neutralizing of antigens.

T Cells

Helper T cells (CD4+) recruit and activate phagocytes to kill and ingest microbes. CD4+ cells can differentiate into effector cells that produce different cytokines. These cells express TCR with an affinity for MHC class II molecules found on the surfaces of APCs. Effector cells recognize antigens that have been ingested by macrophages and produce cytokines such as IFN-γ, which helps to activate macrophages (Abbas et al., 2016).

Cytotoxic T lymphocytes (CD8+) kill cells that harbor microbes and cancer cells, mainly by inducing apoptosis. Most cytotoxic T lymphocytes express TCRs that recognize a specific antigen and express CD8+, which has high affinity for MHC molecules (Abbas et al., 2016).

Some T cells are intrinsically more likely to become memory T cells. These cells can be classified into subsets, including effector memory T cells and central memory T cells. Effector memory T cells display effector functions of the immune response, while central memory T cells are important in stimulating other cells of the immune system (e.g., DCs).

Regulatory T cells (Tregs) help maintain immune homeostasis and are important in the prevention of autoimmunity and chronic inflammatory disease. They are characterized by the expression of the transcription factor FOXP3 (Forkhead box protein 3). Two primary populations of Tregs include tTregs (develop in the thymus) and pTregs (develop in the periphery) (Abbas et al., 2016). Tregs appear to facilitate CTLA-4–mediated suppression of immune responses, secrete immunosuppressive cytokines, and consume stimulatory cytokines such as IL-2. Depletion of Tregs may enhance antitumor immunity (see Table 2-5).

Coinhibitors

The term *checkpoint* describes a time or place when a process is stopped for evaluation, such as a road checkpoint, where traffic is stopped for inspection. The immune system also has checkpoints. Recognition of these checkpoints and their role in the regulation of T cells has resulted in one of the most rapidly progressing areas in drug development for cancer treatment (Sharma & Allison, 2015; Velcheti & Schalper, 2016) (see Table 2-4).

TABLE 2-5   Cytokines Produced by Helper T Cells (CD4+)

Cytokine	Cellular Sources	Action
Interferon gamma	CD4+ T cells CD8+ T cells Natural killer cells	Activation of macrophages
Interleukin-2	Activated T cells	T-cell proliferation Regulatory T-cell survival
Interleukin-4	CD4+ T cells Mast cells	B cell to immunoglobulin E
Interleukin-5	CD4+ T cells Innate lymphoid cells Mast cells	Activation of eosinophils
Interleukin-17	CD4+ T cells	Inflammation
Interleukin-22	CD4+ T cells Innate lymphoid cells Natural killer cells	Maintenance of epithelial barrier function

Note. Based on information from Abbas et al., 2016.

CTLA-4, or CD152, is a protein receptor expressed mainly on Tregs and activated T cells. It may also be expressed on other immune cells. CTLA-4 acts as a negative regulatory receptor of T cells during the priming phase of antigen presentation, functioning as an immune checkpoint. CLTA-4 is structurally homologous to the costimulatory receptor CD28. It is induced after activation of naïve T cells and exerts an inhibitory effect on T-cell activation, as well as the induction phase of T-cell response. CTLA-4 is expressed when T cells are activated through antigen presentation by APCs and when costimulation begins. Tregs express high levels of CTLA-4 to block the activation of cytotoxic T cells. Ipilimumab, a monoclonal antibody used in the treatment of melanoma, targets and inhibits CTLA-4, resulting in T-cell activation (Ott, Hodi, & Robert, 2013).

PD-1, or CD279, is a coinhibitory cell surface receptor highly expressed on activated T cells, B lymphocytes, and NK cells. PD-1 expression is induced by TCR-antigen engagement and through the activity of several cytokines. It has two known ligands: programmed cell death-ligand 1 (PD-L1) and programmed cell death-ligand 2 (PD-L2), which are expressed on a variety of cells, including APCs and tumor cells. PD-1 has different functions than CTLA-4, although there may be some overlap. PD-1 inhibits chronic antigen receptor stimulation and appears to have a greater inhibitory effect on the effector phase of T cells. Nivolumab and pembrolizumab are monoclonal antibodies that target PD-1. The monoclonal antibodies atezolizumab, avelumab, and durvalumab target PD-L1. Through inhibition of PD-1 and ligand binding, these checkpoint inhibitors allow T-cell activation (Hamanishi et al., 2016). Additional checkpoint inhibitors are listed in Table 2-4.

Cytokines

TNF is a cytokine involved in a variety of physiologic processes that control inflammation, antitumor responses, and immune homeostasis. It is a product of effector T cells and is important in modulating T-cell activity. TNF can promote the proliferation and activation of naïve and effector T cells. In addition, it can induce apoptosis of activated effector T cells, influencing the amount of T cells available during the immune response. It also affects Tregs and appears to play a role in some autoimmune diseases (Mehta, Gracias, & Croft, 2016). The TNF superfamily of receptors and ligands is critical in coordinating signals between immune cells during both innate and adaptive immune response (Ward-Kavanagh, Lin, Šedý, & Ware, 2016).

IL-2 is a protein that activates leukocytes responsible for immunity. Its effects are mediated through binding to IL-2 receptors expressed on lymphocytes. Once called T-cell growth factor, IL-2 stimulates the proliferation and survival of T cells. It is important for Tregs and plays a role in controlling immune responses (Abbas et al., 2016). IL-2 also promotes differentiation of T cells into effector and memory T cells. Aldesleukin, an IL-2 manufactured via recombinant DNA technology, is approved by the U.S. Food and Drug Administration for the treatment of advanced melanoma and renal cell cancer.

Cytokine function is the result, in part, of the activation of transcription factors. For example, the STAT family is critical to the signaling that happens between cells of the immune system. The JAK-STAT pathway is now known to operate downstream of many cytokines and growth factors and is believed to be a central communication mechanism for the immune system (Villarino et al., 2017).

Immune Tolerance

Immune tolerance occurs when the immune system does not respond to a stimulus that has the capacity to elicit an immune response. It is an active phenomenon in that an antigen is recognized, but there is not an effective immune response (Bluestone, Bour-Jordan, Cheng, & Anderson, 2015).

Central tolerance is an immune tolerance that occurs within the generative lymphoid tissue of the immune system, such as the bone marrow or thymus. This corresponds with either the death of self-reactive immature T cells or the generation of CD4+ Tregs. It also can occur when bone marrow does not produce B cells. Central tolerance ensures the elimination of T and B cells that initiate an immune response to host tissue.

Peripheral tolerance occurs when mature T cells in peripheral tissues recognize self-antigen but are hindered by immune response inactivation. The term *anergy* describes this functional inactivation, which may be caused by suppression of Tregs or when antigen recognition occurs without adequate costimulation.

With self-tolerance, an individual (or host) is tolerant to their own antigens. When self-tolerance does not occur, an individual's immune system may identify a self-antigen as foreign and elicit a response. Some microbes and cancers can invoke self-tolerance and are able to avoid detection and subsequent immune response.

Autoimmune diseases result from the failure of immune tolerance or self-tolerance. Autoimmunity may occur secondary to the presence of inherited susceptibility genes, environment, and infections. Infection pathogens are believed to lead to autoimmunity through a variety of mechanisms, such as through inflammation caused by infection, which leads to nonspecific activation of autoimmune cells and molecular mimicry, or when a pathogen mimics self-antigen (Ercolini & Miller, 2009). Abatacept and belatcept are CTLA-4/CD28 cosignaling pathway blockades used for the treatment of autoimmune diseases (Crepeau & Ford, 2017).

Cancer and the Immune System

A complex interplay exists between the immune system and cancer (Antonia, Larkin, & Ascierto, 2014; Chen & Mellman, 2017). The immune system could play a key role in cancer protection *only* if cancer can be recognized as foreign. This protection potential has been the focus of decades of research. Recent advances in immunology have provided an avenue to enhance the immune response to cancer. An intricate balance exists between the immune system's ability to recognize cancer (immune recognition) and eradicate tumors and the ability of cancer to escape from the immune system and promote cancer progression. Cancer immunoediting, the balance of protection provided from the immune system against cancer and the evasion of cancer from the immune response, is a process by which adaptive and innate immunity can control tumor growth and shape immunogenicity. Cancer immunoediting has been described in three phases: cancer immunosurveillance (elimination), equilibrium, and escape (Dunn, Old, & Schreiber, 2004; Mittal, Gubin, Schreiber, & Smyth, 2014).

Cancer immunosurveillance, or the elimination phase, is when the immune system can detect cancer cells as different from noncancer cells, ultimately preventing cancer formation in the body. Cancer cells are identified and destroyed through both adaptive and innate immunity. The key element of this phase is the immune system's ability to recognize subtle differences between cancer and noncancer cells. This recognition causes the release of inflammatory signals, which are important to the recruitment of immune cells to the cancer site, and results in cancer cell death. Cancer immunosurveillance may be suboptimal in individuals that have a compromised immune response (e.g., immunosuppressive therapy), which may explain the increased incidence of malignancies in these individuals (Mittal et al., 2014).

The equilibrium phase begins when balance shifts between prevention of tumor growth and immunogenicity of cancer cells. During equilibrium, the immune system is unable to eliminate all cancer cells but can prevent further cancer growth. A continuous interaction exists between immune cells and the tumor cells that escaped immunosurveillance.

In the escape phase, the immune system is not able to eliminate and control the growth of the tumor because the cancer has evolved under the selective pressure of the immune system. Cancer cells with the ability to evade and/or suppress the immune response can proliferate and spread. Cancers can avoid recognition and elimination by the immune system in many ways, including by disrupting antigen presentation mechanisms for T cells, suppressing T-cell activation, inhibiting T-cell function, and suppressing the recruitment of immune cells to the cancer site (Antonia et al., 2014). The immune response may become less and less effective as the cancer progresses (Disis, 2014).

The Cancer–Immunity Cycle

Mutations during the oncogenic process can lead to the generation of new protein or peptide sequences, or neoantigens. These mutations facilitate the differentiation of cancer cells from noncancer cells by the immune system. The mutational burden of cancer is also believed to be important in its immune recognition (Chen & Mellman, 2017). Ultimately, the degree or type of mutation may determine the potential success of immune-directed treatment.

The cancer–immunity cycle describes the immune response that results from the killing of cancer cells (see Figure 2-3) (Chen & Mellman, 2013). The creation of neoantigens begins the oncogenesis process. Neo-

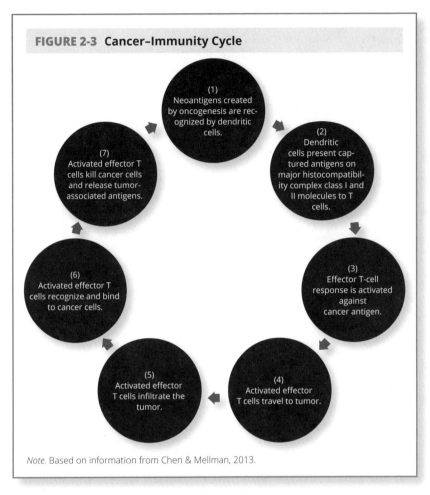

FIGURE 2-3 Cancer–Immunity Cycle

(1) Neoantigens created by oncogenesis are recognized by dendritic cells.

(2) Dendritic cells present captured antigens on major histocompatibility complex class I and II molecules to T cells.

(3) Effector T-cell response is activated against cancer antigen.

(4) Activated effector T cells travel to tumor.

(5) Activated effector T cells infiltrate the tumor.

(6) Activated effector T cells recognize and bind to cancer cells.

(7) Activated effector T cells kill cancer cells and release tumor-associated antigens.

Note. Based on information from Chen & Mellman, 2013.

antigens associated with cancer cells are detected by DCs and presented on MHC molecules to T cells. Effector T cells are primed and activated against the cancer-specific antigens. Activated T cells then travel to the tumor, infiltrate the TME, and ultimately kill the cancer. This immune response results in the release of additional tumor-associated antigens that can reinitiate this process (Chen & Mellman, 2013). An important part of the cancer–immunity cycle is the costimulation of T cells. If T cells are inhibited, immune response is suppressed, and the immune system does not effectively kill the cancer.

Some mechanisms can limit a robust antitumor immune response to cancer. Immunity may be influenced by numerous factors that ultimately determine the strength and timing of the immune response, including host factors, the cancer itself, and the TME. The immune response to cancer is dependent on T lymphocytes that recognize cancer-associated antigens. Tumor antigens may be undetectable by the immune system; therefore, the cancer cell does not interact with DCs or may not be perceived by T cells as foreign. The tumor may also activate mechanisms that enable cancer cells to actively escape detection; however, oncogenesis genomic mutations can occur that may make the cancer more likely to be recognized as foreign.

The importance of cancer cell recognition has led to further investigation into the tumor genome as a driver for cancer immunity, including both the type and degree of mutational burden. For example, the cancer-associated neoantigens that occur secondary to viral etiology, such as the human papillomavirus 16 associated with head and neck and cervical cancers, may be identified differently by the immune system compared to neoantigens caused by other mutations. This suggests the potential for different responses to immunotherapy strategies based on the recognition of an antigen type (Varelas & Kukuruzinska, 2014).

T cells and their function are key to the immune response to cancer. T cells that target tumor neoantigens from cancer mutations are a primary focus for research, as their role in response to cancer therapy appears critical (Tran, Robbins, & Rosenberg, 2017). Focus on the T cell in the development of immunotherapy has led to new strategies for cancer therapies, including T-cell expansion, activation and subsequent response, and increase at the tumor proximity. The trafficking of T cells into tumor and the TME, including T-cell migration through tumor stroma, can potentially optimize responses with immunotherapy.

A cancer may avoid or minimize immune response via activation of regulatory pathways that suppress the function of immune cells. The tumors ability to suppress immune response through negative regulatory pathways, or immune checkpoints, enables the tumor to escape from host immunity (Chen & Mellman, 2017). Immunosuppressive cosignals mediated by PD-1 and PD-L1 in the TME play an important role in this escape from host immunity. The presence of immunosuppressive factors within the TME suppress the effects of T cells and other cells involved in the immune response (Hamanishi et al., 2016).

The regulation of T-cell metabolism is another potential target for immunotherapy. The energy-demanding processes of T-cell activation and clonal expansion require nutrient uptake and cellular metabolism. Nutrient metabolism and utilization may affect T-cell function and are potential targets for immunotherapy (Chang & Pearce, 2016).

The TME plays an important role in cancer immunity. It is a complex cellular environment that includes blood vessels, immune cells, signaling molecules, the extracellular matrix, and proinflammatory cytokines, which are important for T-cell activation and expansion. In addition to the presence of T cells, B cells in the TME affect T-cell production and function. The immune response for cancer requires the presence of effector cells at the cancer site. The exclusion of relevant immune cells from the TME may play a key role in the failure of some immunotherapies. Inflammation may also contribute to the function of the immune system on cancer in the TME (Byrne, Vonderheide, Jaffee, & Armstrong, 2015). The dynamic relationship between cancer and the TME is an area of great interest, and evaluation of the TME may help determine the clinical benefit for immunotherapy in some situations (Gajewski et al., 2013).

Myeloid cells, including DCs and macrophages, can also drive antitumor immune response. NK cells can recognize cancer cells and promote elimination. The important role of NK cells in both detecting and eliminating cancer has generated interest in capitalizing on this effect in clinical practice. Initial approaches focused on boosting the number of NK cells and harvesting them for anticancer therapy. Currently, chimeric antigen receptor–engineered NK cells are generating high interest as a cancer treatment (Bollino & Webb, 2017).

Beyond the cells and cytokines found in the TME, other factors are likely to play a role in the immune response. The continuous metabolism of glucose to lactate by cancer cells results in a TME rich in lactic acid, a substance thought to be related to tumor progression because of its role in immune evasion and inhibition of T-cell function (Brand et al., 2016).

The role of inflammation, historically viewed as a benefit of the immune response, is being examined in many diseases, including cancer (Harris & Drake, 2013). Tumor-related chronic inflammation shapes local and systemic immunity to promote tumor development and an immunosuppressive TME, whereas acute inflammation can enhance antitumor immunity by promoting DC maturation and function and effector T-cell priming (Shalapour & Karin, 2015).

Much of the success of immunotherapy in recent years is directed at optimizing T-cell–mediated immune response. A barrier to success with T-cell–directed therapy is tumor development caused by T-cell exclusion (Aguilera & Giaccia, 2017). The innate pathways that contribute to T-cell exclusion in cancer include β-catenin (catenin beta-1), STAT3, NF-κB, PTEN (phosphatase and tensin homolog), and the UFO/AXL receptor tyrosine kinase. These provide additional targets for future anticancer strategies.

The Evolution of Immunotherapy in Cancer

The fundamental goal of cancer immunotherapy is to boost and restore the ability of the immune system to detect and destroy cancer cells through mechanisms that shift toward immune protection. *Immu-*

TABLE 2-6 Terminology

Term	Definition
Acute-phase proteins	Proteins synthesized in response to inflammatory cytokines as part of the inflammatory response (e.g., C-reactive, fibrinogen)
Adaptive immunity (acquired or specific immunity)	Immune response mediated by B and T lymphocytes and characterized by specificity to distinct macromolecule and memory
Adoptive transfer	Transfer of cells after in vitro activation and/or expansion, such as with regulatory T cells for cancer treatment
Antibody-dependent cellular cytotoxicity (ADCC)	Process by which natural killer cells are targeted to immunoglobulin G–coated cells, resulting in cell lysis; a mechanism for therapeutic monoclonal antibodies to cause cancer cell death
Antigen	Molecule that binds to an antibody or T-cell receptor
Antigen-presenting cell (APC)	Cell that displays a protein antigen in association with major histocompatibility complex molecules (peptide-MHC complex) on its surface; may activate antigen-specific T cells and other T lymphocytes
B-cell receptor (BCR)	Cell surface antigen receptor on B lymphocytes; a multiprotein complex on B lymphocytes that recognizes antigen and transduces activating signals into the cell
B lymphocytes (B cells)	Develop in the bone marrow and found in lymphoid follicles in lymphoid tissues, bone marrow, and the circulation; can produce antibody molecules and mediate immune the humoral responses
Cell-mediated immunity	Form of adaptive immunity mediated by T lymphocytes
Checkpoint inhibition	Evolving therapeutic strategy to increase host immune response against tumors by blocking inhibitory signals for T lymphocytes. Inhibitory signals, or checkpoint signals, include cytotoxic T-lymphocyte antigen 4 (CTLA-4) and programmed cell death protein 1 (PD-1).
Chemokines	Family of low-molecular-weight cytokines that stimulate cell movement
Cluster of differentiation (CD) molecules	Cell surface molecules expressed on cells of the immune system (see www.hcdm.org)

(Continued on next page)

TABLE 2-6   Terminology *(Continued)*

Term	Definition
Complement	Serum and cell surface proteins of the immune system that generate effectors of innate and adaptive immune response. The three complement pathways are classical, alternative, and lectin.
Cytokines	Large family of soluble proteins that are produced and secreted by cells and coordinate inflammatory and immune responses
Genome	Genetic material of an organism that includes both genes and noncoding sequences of DNA (or RNA in RNA viruses) and the generic material of mitochondria
Germ line	Genetic material carried by ova and sperm that contains genes transmitted by parents to offspring
Immune tolerance	Unresponsiveness of the immune system to substances that can elicit an immune response (self-antigens)
Immunity	Ability to respond to a foreign substance, including microbes and noninfectious substances; the protection against disease mediated by cells, tissues, and soluble proteins
Immunogen	Substance, such as an antigen, that can provoke immune system recognition and response. Not all antigens are immunogens.
Immunoglobulin (Ig)	A type of antibody; Y-shaped proteins that contain two identical L chains and two identical H chains. Each L and H chain are divided into a variable and constant region. Based on the amino acid sequence in the constant region of the H chains Ig are classified into IgM, IgD, IgG, IgE and IgA with different biologic functions.
Inflammation	Complex reaction to infection or cell injury that involves accumulation of plasma proteins and leukocytes; an immune response that helps to control infections and promote tissue repair but may also result in tissue damage
Innate immunity	Provides rapid response against infection and reacts in essentially the same way to repeated infections
Major histocompatibility complex (MHC)	A set of cell surface proteins essential for the acquired immune system to recognize foreign molecules. The main function of MHC molecules is to bind to antigens derived from pathogens and display them on the cell surface for recognition by the appropriate T cells.

(Continued on next page)

TABLE 2-6   Terminology *(Continued)*

Term	Definition
Monoclonal antibody (mAb)	Antibody specific to one antigen. Once a naïve B cell is activated, it differentiates into a clone of plasma cells that produces antibodies that have the same antigen-binding sites as the activated B-cell receptor.
Neoantigen	Newly expressed protein on a cancer cell that may be a result of an oncovirus or other mutations
Opsonization	Process in which particles, such as bacterial, are marked by a substance to assure identification for macrophages
Pathogen-associated molecular patterns (PAMPs)	Molecular component associated with groups of pathogens recognized by cells of the innate immune system; recognized by Toll-like receptors and other pattern recognition receptors
Pattern recognition receptors (PRRs)	Receptors on the monocyte (phagocytes) (e.g., Toll-like receptors)
Phagocytosis	Process by which a target cell is engulfed and enzymatically destroyed. Neutrophils, macrophages, and dendritic cells are phagocytic cells.
Polyclonal antibody	Antibodies secreted by different B-cell clones that bind with different epitopes on the same antigen
T-cell receptor (TCR)	Antigen receptor on helper T cells (CD4+) and cytotoxic T cells (CD8+) that recognizes complexes of antigen bound to major histocompatibility complex molecules on the surface of an antigen-presenting cell
Toll-like receptor (TLR)	Pattern recognition receptor on monocytes. Has a specific ligand that can activate it; once activated, can activate various signaling pathways. These pathways can induce cytokines and chemokines to activate both innate and adaptive immune responses.

Note. Based on information from Abbas et al., 2016.

notherapy, a term used for therapeutic modalities that lead to manipulation of the immune system, is not a new concept or clinical practice in cancer treatment. Other terminology for immunotherapy can be found in Table 2-6. Use of the bacillus Calmette-Guérin vaccine for the treatment of bladder cancer dates to the 1970s. IFN and IL use for the treatment of melanoma and renal cell cancer was established in the 1980s and is still used in select patients. Historically, the potential of cancer immunotherapy has been limited by modest therapy responses and challenging side effects in some patients (e.g., capillary leak syndrome with high-dose aldesleukin). Recent advances have provided opportunities to capitalize on new therapeutic approaches that optimize the cancer immune response. Some strategies have resulted in the development of immunotherapies that have wide-ranging application in many cancers (e.g., checkpoint inhibition with PD-1 and PD-L1). Other strategies have focused on select tumor types (e.g., chimeric antigen receptor T cells) but have the potential expand to other cancers. Available immunotherapy approaches for cancer range from nonspecific immunostimulation to the production of exquisitely specific, genetically modified T cells (Saied et al., 2014).

At this time in cancer care, immunotherapy strategies have undergone extensive development and clinical testing. The number and types of immunotherapy drugs used in cancer treatment are expanding, and the applications for these agents have evolved through clinical trials that have demonstrated activity in a variety of cancers and treatment settings. This evolution will continue as the understanding of the immune system and cancer biology improves.

A key approach to immunotherapy is to enhance the adaptive immune response. Adaptive immunity is enticing, as long-term memory against cancer cells may improve and yield more durable responses. Early approaches to immunotherapy focused on tumor-specific T cells and used tumor vaccines and cytokines, such as recombinant IL-2. Recently, immunotherapy efforts have focused on a variety of strategies to increase the broad immune response, such as improving the presentation of tumor antigens to the immune system; increasing triggers to adaptive immunity, innate immune activation, and inflammation in the TME (Disis, 2014); and regulating immune regulatory mechanisms with the use of monoclonal antibodies targeted at checkpoint receptors.

The loss or downregulation of antigen presentation has been identified as a major immune escape mechanism for cancer (de Charette, Marabelle, & Houot, 2016). One strategy to address this downregulation is to look at MHC expression on tumor cells, as restoring or enhancing antigen presentation by tumor cells may enhance tumor immunogenicity. Immune checkpoint inhibitors appear to overcome the mechanisms that tumors use to suppress the antitumor immune response (Disis, 2014). Potential strategies for overcoming tumor immune evasion mechanisms include reversing the inhibition of adaptive immunity by blocking T-cell checkpoint pathways, switching on adaptive immunity by promoting T-cell costimulatory receptor signaling with agonist antibodies, improving the function of innate immune cells, and activating the immune system through potentiating immune cell effector function (Antonia et al., 2014).

Advances in the understanding of the molecular mechanisms of T-cell activation and inhibition and immune homeostasis have resulted in the rational development of immunologically targeted therapies for cancer. For example, Tregs, responsible for maintaining immune homeostasis and preventing autoimmunity, have been shown to infiltrate human tumors and may limit antitumor immunity (Liu, Workman, & Vignali, 2016). T-cell metabolism is also of interest, as it has been shown that the immune response is an energetically demanding process. The regulation of nutrient uptake and its use in T cells has been shown as critical to T-cell differentiation and function. Strategies to enhance nutrient uptake and cellular metabolism are a potential target for immunotherapy (Buck, O'Sullivan, & Pearce, 2015; Patel & Powell, 2017).

Immunotherapies can be categorized as passive or active based on the mechanism of the agent, although this classification does not properly reflect the complexity of the drug-host-tumor interaction. Some strategies specifically target defined tumor-associated antigens, and others are relatively nonspecific and boost natural or therapy-elicited anticancer immune responses. Examples of passive immunity include tumor-targeting monoclonal antibodies and adoptive cell transfer (chimeric antigen receptor T cells). Active immunotherapy includes anticancer vaccines, immunostimulatory cytokines, and checkpoint inhibitor monoclonal antibodies.

With the emergence of new immunotherapy strategies for the management of cancer, many important questions. For one, what is the optimal place in therapy for the still-evolving field of immunotherapy? The answer may differ depending on the cancer. An ultimate answer may be found with a better understanding of immunotherapy's place in early (e.g., adjuvant therapy) and advanced disease (e.g., locally advanced and metastatic disease); a clearer picture of the optimal sequence of therapies (e.g., neoadjuvant therapy); and further research into the role of combination immunotherapy with other established drug and nondrug therapies. An equally important question is how to find the individuals most likely to respond to this therapy, realizing that the answer may change throughout the disease course.

Summary

Exciting advances in immunotherapy are providing additional treatment options for many individuals affected by cancer. With this evolution comes significant responsibilities for the clinician, including the need to learn about new therapies, how these therapies fit into care, and how to optimize care for each patient receiving immunotherapy. Side effect and toxicity mitigation and management, quality-of-life issues, and practical ways to optimize therapy should be discussed. As many of these strategies are new to clinicians, it is essential to share clinical knowledge and experience broadly through publications and educational platforms within the oncology community and beyond.

References

Abbas, A.K., Lichtman, A.H., & Pillai, S. (2016). *Basic immunology: Functions and disorders of the immune system* (5th ed.). St. Louis, MO: Elsevier.

Aguilera, T.A., & Giaccia, A.J. (2017). Molecular pathways: Oncologic pathways and their role in T-cell exclusion and immune evasion—A new role for the AXL receptor tyrosine kinase. *Clinical Cancer Research, 23,* 2928–2933. https://doi.org/10.1158/1078-0432.CCR-17-0189

Amulic, B., Cazalet, C., Hayes, G.L., Metzler, K.D., & Zychlinsky, A. (2012). Neutrophil function: From mechanism to disease. *Annual Review of Immunology, 30,* 459–489. https://doi.org/10.1146/annurev-immunol-020711-074942

Antonia, S.J., Larkin, J., & Ascierto, P.A. (2014). Immuno-oncology combinations: A review of clinical experience and future prospects. *Clinical Cancer Research, 20,* 6258–6268. https://doi.org/10.1158/1078-0432.CCR-14-1457

Bluestone, J.A., Bour-Jordan, H., Cheng, M., & Anderson, M. (2015). T cells in the control of organ-specific autoimmunity. *Journal of Clinical Investigation, 125,* 2250–2260. https://doi.org/10.1172/JCI78089

Bollino, D., & Webb, T.J. (2017). Chimeric antigen receptor–engineered natural killer and natural killer T cells for cancer immunotherapy. *Translational Research, 187,* 32–43. https://doi.org/10.1016/j.trsl.2017.06.003

Brand, A., Singer, K., Koehl, G.E., Kolitzus, M., Schoenhammer, G., Thiel, A., ... Kreutz, M. (2016). LDHA-associated lactic acid production blunts tumor immunosurveillance by T and NK cells. *Cell Metabolism, 24,* 657–671. https://doi.org/10.1016/j.cmet.2016.08.011

Buck, M.D., O'Sullivan, D., & Pearce, E.L. (2015). T cell metabolism drives immunity. *Journal of Experimental Medicine, 212,* 1345–1360. https://doi.org/10.1084/jem.20151159

Butterfield, L.H., Kaufman, H.L., & Marincola, F.M. (Eds.). (2017). *Cancer immunotherapy principles and practice.* New York, NY: Demos Medical.

Byrne, K.T., Vonderheide, R.H., Jaffee, E.M., & Armstrong, T.D. (2015). Special conference on tumor immunology and immunotherapy: A new chapter. *Cancer Immunology Research, 3,* 590–597. https://doi.org/10.1158/2326-6066.CIR-15-0106

Chang, C.-H., & Pearce, E.L. (2016). Emerging concepts of T cell metabolism as a target of immunotherapy. *Nature Immunology, 17,* 364–368. https://doi.org/10.1038/ni.3415

Chen, D.S., & Mellman, I. (2013). Oncology meets immunology: The cancer-immunity cycle. *Immunity, 39,* 1–10. https://doi.org/10.1016/j.immuni.2013.07.012

Chen, D.S., & Mellman, I. (2017). Elements of cancer immunity and the cancer-immune set point. *Nature, 541,* 321–330. https://doi.org/10.1038/nature21349

Coates, L.C., FitzGerald, O., Helliwell, P.S., & Paul, C. (2016). Psoriasis, psoriatic arthritis, and rheumatoid arthritis: Is all inflammation the same? *Seminars in Arthritis and Rheumatism, 46,* 291–304. https://doi.org/10.1016/j.semarthrit.2016.05.012

Cooper, M.D. (2015). The early history of B cells. *Nature Reviews Immunology, 15,* 191–197. https://doi.org/10.1038/nri3801

Crepeau, R.L., & Ford, M.L. (2017). Challenges and opportunities in targeting the CD28/CTLA-4 pathway in transplantation and autoimmunity. *Expert Opinion on Biological Therapy, 17,* 1001–1012. https://doi.org/10.1080/14712598.2017.1333595

de Charette, M., Marabelle, A., & Houot, R. (2016). Turning tumour cells into antigen presenting cells: The next step to improve cancer immunotherapy? *European Journal of Cancer, 68,* 134–147. https://doi.org/10.1016/j.ejca.2016.09.010

Delves, P.J., & Roitt, I.M. (2000a). The immune system. Part I. *New England Journal of Medicine, 343,* 37–49. https://doi.org/10.1056/NEJM200007063430107

Delves, P.J., & Roitt, I.M. (2000b). The immune system. Part II. *New England Journal of Medicine, 343,* 108–117. https://doi.org/10.1056/NEJM200007133430207

Disis, M.L. (2014). Mechanism of action of immunotherapy. *Seminars in Oncology, 41*(Suppl. 5), S3–S13. https://doi.org/10.1053/j.seminoncol.2014.09.004

Dunn, G.P., & Okada, H. (2015). Principles of immunology and its nuances in the central nervous system. *Neuro-Oncology, 17*(Suppl. 7), vii3–vii8. https://doi.org/10.1093/neuonc/nov175

Dunn, G.P., Old, L.J., & Schreiber, R.D. (2004). The immunobiology of cancer immunosurveillance and immunoediting. *Immunity, 21,* 137–148. https://doi.org/10.1016/j.immuni.2004.07.017

Ercolini, A.M., & Miller, S.D. (2009). The role of infections in autoimmune diseases. *Clinical and Experimental Immunology, 155,* 1–15. https://doi.org/10.1111/j.1365-2249.2008.03834.x

Fukuda, K., Kobayashi, A., & Watabe, K. (2012). The role of tumor-associated macrophage in tumor progression. *Frontiers in Bioscience, 4,* 787–798. https://doi.org/10.2741/s299

Gajewski, T.F., Woo, S.-R., Zha, Y., Spaapen, R., Zheng, Y., Corrales, L., & Spranger, S. (2013). Cancer immunotherapy strategies based on overcoming barriers within the tumor microenvironment. *Current Opinion in Immunology, 25,* 268–276. https://doi.org/10.1016/j.coi.2013.02.009

Granzin, M., Wagner, J., Köhl, U., Cerwenka, A., Huppert, V., & Ullrich, E. (2017). Shaping of natural killer cell antitumor activity by ex vivo cultivation. *Frontiers in Immunology, 8,* 458. https://doi.org/10.3389/fimmu.2017.00458

Greenwald, R.J., Freeman, G.J., & Sharpe, A.H. (2005). The B7 family revisited. *Annual Reviews of Immunology, 23,* 515–548. https://doi.org/10.1146/annurev.immunol.23.021704.115611

Hamanishi, J., Mandai, M., Matsumura, N., Abiko, K., Baba, T., & Konishi, I. (2016). PD-1/PD-L1 blockade in cancer treatment: Perspectives and issues. *International Journal of Clinical Oncology, 21,* 462–473. https://doi.org/10.1007/s10147-016-0959-z

Harris, T.J., & Drake, C.G. (2013). Primer on tumor immunology and cancer immunotherapy. *Journal for Immunotherapy of Cancer, 1,* 1–12. https://doi.org/10.1186/2051-1426-1-12

Hong, J.T., Son, D.J., Lee, C.K., Yoon, D.-Y., Lee, D.H., & Park, M.H. (2017). Interleukin 32, inflammation and cancer. *Pharmacology and Therapeutics, 174,* 127–137. https://doi.org/10.1016/j.pharmthera.2017.02.025

Hurt, B., Schulick, R., Edil, B., El Kasmi, K.C., & Barnett, C., Jr. (2017). Cancer-promoting mechanisms of tumor-associated neutrophils. *American Journal of Surgery, 214,* 938–944. https://doi.org/10.1016/j.amjsurg.2017.08.003

Kolev, M., Towner, L., & Donev, R. (2011). Complement in cancer and cancer immunotherapy. *Archivum Immunologiae et Therapiae Experimentalis, 59,* 407–419. https://doi.org/10.1007/s00005-011-0146-x

Liszewski, M., & Atkinson, J.P. (2015). Complement regulators in human disease: Lessons from modern genetics. *Journal of Internal Medicine, 277,* 294–405. https://doi.org/10.1111/joim.12338

Liu, C., Workman, C.J., & Vignali, D.A.A. (2016). Targeting regulatory T cells in tumors. *FEBS Journal, 283,* 2731–2748. https://doi.org/10.1111/febs.13656

Markanday, A. (2015). Acute phase reactants in infections: Evidence-based review and a guide for clinicians. *Open Forum Infectious Diseases, 2,* ofv098. https://doi.org/10.1093/ofid/ofv098

Mattner, J., & Wirtz, S. (2017). Friend or foe? The ambiguous role of innate lymphoid cells in cancer development. *Trends in Immunology, 38,* 29–38. https://doi.org/10.1016/j.it.2016.10.004

Mehta, A.K., Gracias, D.T., & Croft, M. (2016). TNF activity and T cells. *Cytokine, 101,* 14–18. https://doi.org/10.1016/j.cyto.2016.08.003

Merad, M., Sathe, P., Helft, J., Miller, J., & Mortha, A. (2013). The dendritic cell lineage: Ontogeny and function of dendritic cells and their subsets in the steady state and the inflamed setting. *Annual Review of Immunology, 31,* 563–604. https://doi.org/10.1146/annurev-immunol-020711-074950

Mildner, A., & Jung, S. (2014). Development and function of dendritic cell subsets. *Immunity, 40,* 642–656. https://doi.org/10.1016/j.immuni.2014.04.016

Mittal, D., Gubin, M.M., Schreiber, R.D., & Smyth, M.J. (2014). New insights into cancer immunoediting and its three component phases—elimination, equilibrium and escape. *Current Opinion in Immunology, 27,* 16–25. https://doi.org/10.1016/j.coi.2014.01.004

Muntasell, A., Ochoa, M.C., Cordeiro, L., Berraondo, P., López-Díaz de Cerio, A., Cabo, M., … Melero, I. (2017). Targeting NK-cell checkpoints for cancer immunotherapy. *Current Opinion in Immunology, 45,* 73–81. https://doi.org/10.1016/j.coi.2017.01.003

Ott, P.A., Hodi, F.S., & Robert, C. (2013). CTLA-4 and PD-1/PD-L1 blockade: New immunotherapeutic modalities with durable clinical benefit in melanoma patients. *Clinical Cancer Research, 19,* 5300–5309. https://doi.org/10.1158/1078-0432.CCR-13-0143

Panday, A., Inda, M.E., Bagam, P., Sahoo, M.K., Osorio, D., & Batra, S. (2016). Transcription factor NF-κB: An update on intervention strategies. *Archivum Immunologiae et Therapiae Experimentalis, 64,* 463–483. https://doi.org/10.1007/s00005-016-0405-y

Patel, C.H., & Powell, J.D. (2017). Targeting T cell metabolism to regulate T cell activation, differentiation and function in disease. *Current Opinion in Immunology, 46,* 82–88. https://doi.org/10.1016/j.coi.2017.04.006

Robey, E., & Fowlkes, B.J. (1994). Selective events in T cell development. *Annual Review of Immunology, 12,* 675–705. https://doi.org/10.1146/annurev.iy.12.040194.003331

Saied, A., Pillarisetty, V.G., & Katz, S.C. (2014). Immunotherapy for solid tumors—A review for surgeons. *Journal of Surgical Research, 187,* 525–535. https://doi.org/10.1016/j.jss.2013.12.018

Shalapour, S., & Karin, M. (2015). Immunity, inflammation, and cancer: An eternal fight between good and evil. *Journal of Clinical Investigation, 125,* 3347–3355. https://doi.org/10.1172/JCI80007

Sharma, P., & Allison, J.P. (2015). Immune checkpoint targeting in cancer therapy: Toward combination strategies with curative potential. *Cell, 161,* 205–214. https://doi.org/10.1016/j.cell.2015.03.030

Stephen, B., & Hajjar, J. (2017). Overview of basic immunology for clinical investigators. In A. Naing & J. Hajjar (Eds.), *Advances in Experimental Medicine and Biology: Vol. 995. Immunotherapy* (pp. 1–31). https://doi.org/10.1007/978-3-319-53156-4_1

Takeuchi, O., & Akira, S. (2010). Pattern recognition receptors and inflammation. *Cell, 140,* 805–820. https://doi.org/10.1016/j.cell.2010.01.022

Tran, E., Robbins, P.F., & Rosenberg, S.A. (2017). 'Final common pathway' of human cancer immunotherapy: Targeting random somatic mutations. *Nature Immunology, 18,* 255–262. https://doi.org/10.1038/ni.3682

Varelas, X., & Kukuruzinska, M.A. (2014). Head and neck cancer: From research to therapy and cure. *Annals of the New York Academy of Sciences, 1333,* 1–32. https://doi.org/10.1111/nyas.12613

Velcheti, V., & Schalper, K. (2016). Basic overview of current immunotherapy approaches in cancer. *ASCO Educational Book, 35,* 298–308. https://doi.org/10.14694/EDBK_156572

Villarino, A.V., Kanno, Y., & O'Shea, J.J. (2017). Mechanisms and consequences of Jak-STAT signaling in the immune system. *Nature Immunology, 18,* 374–384. https://doi.org/10.1038/ni.3691

Vivier, E., Tomasello, E., Baratin, M., Walzer, T., & Ugolini, S. (2008). Functions of natural killer cells. *Nature Immunology, 9,* 503–510. https://doi.org/10.1038/ni1582

Ward-Kavanagh, L.K., Lin, W.W., Šedý, J.R., & Ware, C.F. (2016). The TNF receptor superfamily in co-stimulating and co-inhibitory responses. *Immunity, 44,* 1005–1019. https://doi.org/10.1016/j.immuni.2016.04.019

chapter three

Cytokines in Immunotherapy

Brianna Hoffner, MSN, RN, AOCNP®

Introduction

Cytokines play an important role in cancer pathogenesis, treatment, and symptomatology. This heterogeneous group of molecules has varying identifiable functions in the oncology setting. Three cytokines were identified as early cancer immunotherapies: interferon alfa (IFN-α), interleukin (IL)-2, and granulocyte macrophage–colony-stimulating factor (GM-CSF). Although these early cytokines are still relevant in many malignancies, including melanoma and renal cell carcinoma (RCC), a new class of immunocytokines, designed for improved efficacy and decreased adverse effects, is currently under investigation for almost all cancer types. Beyond therapeutic functions, key cytokines such as IL-6 play an important role in cancer development and potential prognosis. In addition, cytokines, whether used as therapies or just present in the tumor microenvironment, contribute to the symptoms experienced by patients with cancer. This chapter will examine the function of cytokines and their interrelated chemokines.

Cytokines

Cytokines are molecular messengers that allow the cells of the immune system to communicate with one another to coordinate a self-limited response to a target antigen (Lee & Margolin, 2011). Cellular changes resulting in cancer provoke changes in local cytokine expression, leading to immune cell infiltrates and the release of additional cytokines (Dranoff, 2004). These cytokines can either trigger a specific response from another cell in the microenvironment or release a secretory factor that affects only the secreting cell (Dranoff, 2004).

Cytokines are produced by cells of innate and adaptive immunity in response to microbes and tumor antigens (Lee & Margolin, 2011). Increased levels of circulating cytokines and their receptors have been found in various cancer types, both local and metastatic disease, as compared to healthy people or those with benign tumors (Seruga, Zhang, Bernstein, & Tannock, 2008). One cytokine acts on many different cell types to mediate diverse and, at times, opposing effects—a property known as *pleiotropism* (Lee & Margolin, 2011).

Two classes of cytokines, type 1 and type 2, orient the cytokine milieu at the tumor site toward immunity or tolerance (Smyth, Cretney, Kershaw, & Hayakawa, 2004). Type 1 cytokines, such as tumor necrosis factor-alpha (TNF-α), interferon gamma (IFN-γ), and IL-2, play a role in type 1 T helper immune responses and primarily induce cell-mediated immunity (Smyth et al., 2004). Type 2 cytokines, including IL-4, IL-5, IL-6, IL-10, and IL-13, stimulate type 2 T helper immune responses and encourage humoral immunity against tumors or immune deviation to tumor tolerance (Smyth et al., 2004). As such, cytokines can play a role in tumor pathogenesis or act as an anticancer therapy (Dranoff, 2004).

Perhaps the earliest example of the use of cytokines in cancer therapy came from Dr. William Coley, a surgeon and researcher who worked in New York City in the latter part of the 19th century. Coley noted that some patients with cancer who developed bacterial infections of the skin (erysipelas) caused by *Streptococcus pyogenes* experienced tumor regression (Dranoff, 2004). Coley started to deliberately inject live *S. pyogenes* into the skin of patients with advanced cancer, resulting in a significant increase in cytokine levels and a decrease or resolution of tumors in some patients. Today, cytokines continue to play an important role in cancer therapy. As the understanding of the tumor microenvironment and host immunity evolves, so too does the role of cytokines in immunotherapy.

Chemokines

Although chemokines represent a distinctly different cell entity, similarities exist, and some interrelationships are worth mentioning. Chemokines are small, cytokine-like molecules that regulate leukocyte transport in the body and serve as the "traffic directors" of the cell (Homey, Müller, & Zlotnik, 2002). Chemokines are induced by inflammatory cytokines, growth factors, and pathogenic stimuli (Balkwill, 2004). Chemokine signaling leads to transcription of target genes involved in cell invasion, motility, survival, and interactions with the extracellular matrix. It also coordinates cell movement during inflammation and transports hematopoietic stem cells, lymphocytes, and dendritic cells (Balkwill, 2004).

Chemokine receptors allow dendritic cells carrying antigens to migrate to draining lymph nodes (Homey et al., 2002). Dendritic cells complete their maturation process within the lymph node. These cells express high levels of costimulatory molecules, produce cytokines, and present antigenic products to T cells. Dendritic cells are the only antigen-presenting cells that can prime naïve T cells and initiate an immune response, which they do through a process of recognition using major histocompatibility complexes (MHCs) and T-cell receptors (Inaba & Inaba, 2005). Mature dendritic cells present antigenic peptides on MIIC molecules to naïve T cells, thus educating the T cells to mount an immune response against that antigen. These antigen-specific T cells then use chemokine-mediated mechanisms to travel to sites of injury, infection, or tumor growth (Homey et al., 2002). In this way, the roles of chemokines and cytokines are closely related.

Types of Cytokines

Interferon Alfa

IFN-α is a type 1 cytokine used in the treatment of RCC, melanoma, hairy cell leukemia (HCL), chronic myeloid leukemia (CML), and Kaposi sarcoma. Type 1 IFNs elicit expression of MHC class I molecules on tumor cells and regulate the maturation of some dendritic cells (Lee & Margolin, 2011). The exact mechanism of IFN-α is not fully understood, but in some situations, it may act directly on the tumor, but in other cases, it may induce host mechanisms, including immunity, to inhibit the tumor (Smyth et al., 2004).

Prior to the adjuvant approval of ipilimumab for melanoma in October 2015, IFN-α was the only U.S. Food and Drug Administration (FDA)-approved adjuvant treatment option. It remains the only option for patients with node-negative disease. Based on the presumption that micrometastatic disease is the cause of relapse, adjuvant IFN can be used to recruit host immune cells to destroy micrometastatic sites and improve outcomes (Hauschild et al., 2008). Multiple studies by the Eastern Cooperative Oncology Group have evaluated the relapse-free survival and overall survival benefits of high-dose IFN-α with somewhat conflicting results. A 2004 pooled analysis of the E1684, E1690, and E1694 trials at median follow-up intervals of 2.1–12.6 years confirmed a significant increase in relapse-free survival but not overall survival for patients treated with IFN-α versus observation (Kirkwood et al., 2004). National Comprehensive Cancer Network® (NCCN®) guidelines state that adjuvant IFN has been "shown to improve disease-free survival, but there is no impact on overall survival" (NCCN, 2018, p. 7).

Multiple dosing schedules exist for IFN-α. High-dose IFN is administered as 20 MU/m² IV five days per week for four weeks followed by 10 MU/m² subcutaneously (SC) three times per week for 48 weeks (Hauschild et al., 2008). This is the only approved dosing schedule in the United States, as lower doses have not proven to be effective. Peginterferon alfa-2b is an approved alternative therapy. It is administered at 6 mcg/kg/week SC for eight weeks followed by 3 mcg/kg/week SC for up to five years (Merck and Co., Inc., 2015). The length of treatment is often limited by adverse events. In approval trials, the median time on therapy was less than two years (Merck and Co., Inc., 2015).

Because of the prolonged length of adjuvant therapy, many patients struggle with side effects and cannot tolerate treatment for the recommended duration. The most common side effects associated with IFN include fever, myalgia, nausea and vomiting, fatigue, myelosuppression, increased aspartate aminotransferase, and neuropsychiatric symptoms such as depression (Hauschild et al., 2008). Although flu-like symptoms tend to abate during therapy, other adverse events, such as fatigue, depression, and anxiety symptoms, tend to worsen over time. Much like other immunotherapies, a risk of vitiligo and hypothyroidism exists, with rare reports of sarcoidosis, lupus, rheumatoid arthritis, polymyalgia rheumatica, and psoriasis (Lee & Margolin, 2011). The staples of symptom management for IFN include dose delays, dose reductions, and frequent monitoring (Hauschild et al., 2008).

For HCL and CML, the efficacy of IFN-α is clearer. In HCL, the dose is just 2 MU/m² SC three times per week for one year, markedly lower than any melanoma dosing schedules. This schedule has shown an 77% overall response rate and a 5% complete response rate (Lee & Margolin, 2011). For patients with an intact spleen, complete response rate may be closer to 25%–35%. IFN-α is generally well tolerated at this dose and remains an effective therapy in the setting of relapse (Lee & Margolin, 2011). Similarly, hematologic remission is seen in 60%–80% of patients treated with IFN-α for early chronic phase CML (Smyth et al., 2004). Pathologic evaluation of these patients reveals upregulation of natural killer (NK) cell activity with IFN-α therapy, as well as the presence of CML peptide-specific T cells and antibodies against CML-associated antigens (Smyth et al., 2004). Additional studies suggest that IFN-α may create an anti-leukemia immune response through differentiation of dendritic cells (Smyth et al., 2004).

Interleukin-2

The type 1 cytokine IL-2 is part of a larger group of T-cell growth factors (e.g., IL-4, IL-7, IL-9, IL-15, IL-21) that play a role in the activation and expansion of CD4+ and CD8+ T cells (Lee & Margolin, 2011). IL-2 production occurs primarily by CD4+ T helper cells in secondary lymphoid organs and promotes the activation and proliferation of T and NK cells (Lee & Margolin, 2011). IL-2 also promotes antibody production and proliferation by B cells and plays a crucial role in activation-induced cell death, which is necessary for homeostasis and the elimination of autoreactive cells (Liao, Lin, & Leonard, 2013). IL-2 affects CD8+ T cells during all stages of immune response, including primary expansion, contraction, memory generation, and secondary expansion (Boyman & Sprent, 2012).

IL-2 comprises four antiparallel α-helices, all mediated by the IL-2 receptor. The IL-2 receptor includes the α(CD25), β(CD122), and γc(CD132) chains, which are specific protein structures (Lee & Margolin, 2011). An understanding of these structures is crucial, as receptor affinity can vary depending on which chain is on the cell surface. These chains have functions and roles specific to different cell types (Lee & Margolin, 2011). Upon exposure to IL-2, NK cells proliferate and have enhanced cytolytic activity and secretion of cytokines (Lee & Margolin, 2011).

Clinicians first began using high-dose IL-2 to treat metastatic melanoma and RCC in the 1980s. In a 1998 study by Rosenberg, Yang, White, and Steinberg, 33 of 409 patients (8.1%) with metastatic melanoma or kidney cancer treated with IL-2 achieved a complete response, and 37 (9%) achieved a partial response. The study also demonstrated durability of response, with 27 of the 33 complete responders (81.8%) still disease free at the time of publication, or 39–148 months from onset of treatment. Subsequent studies produced similar response rates and durability of response. A 1995 study reported a 14% objective response rate, 5% complete response rate, and 9% partial response rate (Fyfe et al., 1995). In 1999, Atkins et al. published an analysis of 270 patients with metastatic melanoma treated between 1985 and 1993. They noted a 16% objective response rate, 6% complete response rate, and 10% partial response rate. Treatment guidelines still include high-dose IL-2 as a first-line treatment option for metastatic clear cell RCC (Choueiri & Motzer, 2017).

Unfortunately, high-dose IL-2 therapy also carries significant side effects and must be given in the inpatient hospital setting. In the Atkins et al. (1999) analysis, approximately 2% of patients died from treatment toxicity, specifically sepsis. After 1990, antibiotic prophylaxis became routine for patients receiving high-dose IL-2 therapy because of this risk. Of all adverse events, hypotension is the most common, occurring in approximately 64% of patients, with grade 4 hypotension reported in 1% (Atkins et al., 1999). This hypotension is caused by a capillary leak syndrome as the result of a cytokine infusion and is often not responsive to fluid resuscitation; therefore, it may require vasopressors and an increased level of medical care, such as transfer to an intensive care unit. With this fluid imbalance, patients frequently develop dyspnea (31%), pulmonary edema (16%), and cardiac arrhythmias (17%). The kidneys are adversely affected by low blood pressure. Oliguria and increased creatinine levels are seen in 49% and 35% of patients, respectively. Gastrointestinal toxicities, such as nausea (24%), vomiting (55%), diarrhea (54%), and stomatitis (14%), are also common (Atkins et al., 1999). Many providers will not give IL-2 to patients with brain metastases because of the fear of increased intracranial pressure from edema caused by capillary leak. However, Guirguis et al. (2002) noted that IL-2 administration may be safe in a carefully selected patient population.

More recently, IL-2 has been used in adoptive cell therapy (ACT) for the treatment of patients with metastatic melanoma. In 1987, researchers noted that lymphocytes infiltrating into metastatic melanoma tumors could be grown in a medium of IL-2 in a laboratory setting and still maintain their ability to recognize melanoma cells (Rosenberg & Dudley, 2009). These tumor-infiltrating lymphocytes (TILs) were first used to treat a melanoma patient in 1988, and since then, this treatment technique has been refined significantly, although it is yet to be FDA approved. Presently, patients undergo tumor harvest so that their T lymphocytes can be grown ex vivo. Patients then receive chemotherapy, with or without total body irradiation, to induce lymphopenia and increase the presence of homeostatic endogenous cytokines such as IL-7 and IL-15 (Dudley, 2011). TILs are then infused back into the patient in combination with high-dose IL-2 administration. Response rates with ACT range 49%–72% in sequential protocols investigating increasing intensity total body irradiation (Rosenberg & Dudley, 2009).

Limitations of ACT include similar toxicity considerations as high-dose IL-2. However, patients who do not have tumors accessible for harvest have not been eligible because of the inability to generate autologous TILs. Current research focuses on alternative techniques, such as donor-derived T cells, genetically engineered T cells, and chimeric antigen receptors, which do not have the same limitations in cell recognition via the human leukocyte antigen system as T-cell receptors, therefore providing a more universal approach (Perica, Varela, Oelke, & Schneck, 2015). ACT therapy trials include melanoma, leukemia, prostate cancer, and other malignancies, demonstrating the wide-reaching potential of this therapeutic technique.

Interleukin-6

IL-6, a proinflammatory cytokine, plays an important role in the tumor microenvironment, commonly leading to tumorigenesis and the potential for antitumor effects (Fisher, Appenheimer, & Evans, 2014). Patients with advanced cancer have higher levels of IL-6 in their blood. IL-6 elevation correlates with poor survival rates in pancreatic, gastric, breast, colorectal, and lung cancers, as well as with melanoma and myeloma (Heikkilä, Ebrahim, & Lawlor, 2008). Many of the inflammatory cells in the tumor microenvironment produce IL-6, including macrophages, myeloid-derived suppressor cells, CD4+ T cells, and fibroblasts. In addition, tumor cells themselves can produce IL-6 (Fisher et al., 2014). Increased IL-6 signaling leads to dysregulation of signal transducer and activator of transcription 3 (STAT3) and Janus kinase (JAK), causing malignant cellular transformation. Protumorigenic activities of the IL-6 pathway include increased tumor cell proliferation, survival, and metastases; release of angiogenic factors such as vascular endothelial growth factor; immune suppression through development of myeloid-derived suppressor cells, macrophages, and tolerogenic dendritic cells; and increased tumor progression through reseeding of the tumor with circulating metastatic cells (Fisher et al., 2014).

Alternatively, IL-6 can act as a mediator of humoral immunity with broad effects on leukocyte survival, proliferation, differentiation, and recruitment (Fisher et al., 2014). Activation of IL-6 trans-signaling, a process that combines a soluble form of IL-6 with the IL-6 receptor alpha subunit, directly affects lymphocytes, guiding their trafficking to lymph nodes and supporting their activation, proliferation, and transformation toward subtypes that oppose the immunosuppressive tumor microenvironment (Fisher et al., 2014). IL-6 trans-signaling is triggered in the setting of fevers of 40°C (104°F)(Rose-John & Neurath, 2004). IL-6 also acts at vascular sites, increasing adhesive properties and improving trafficking of immune cells that lethally target cancer cells (Fisher et al., 2014).

Given the duality of the role of IL-6 in the tumor microenvironment, further work to direct IL-6 interactions toward tumor control is ongoing. The complexity of interactions combined with the high levels of IL-6 in tumors makes this work particularly challenging. Presently, the proinflammatory, tumor-inducing effects of IL-6 are better understood. However, with improved comprehension of the antitumor effects of IL-6 trans-signaling, the immune-mediated tumor control properties of this cytokine may be able to be harnessed more effectively.

Granulocyte Macrophage–Colony-Stimulating Factor

GM-CSF is a hematopoietic cytokine responsible for expansion and activation of granulocytes and macrophages (Kaufman, Ruby, Hughes,

& Slingluff, 2014). It is made by activated T cells, macrophages, endo-thelial cells, and stromal fibroblasts, and it acts on bone marrow to increase the production of neutrophils and monocytes (Abbas, Licht-man, & Pillai, 2017). It is also a macrophage-activating factor that pro-motes the maturation of dendritic cells. GM-CSF is probably best known for its role in neutrophil proliferation and survival in the setting of neu-tropenia following induction chemotherapy in acute myeloid leukemia (Kaufman et al., 2014).

More recently, GM-CSF has been extensively investigated in the treat-ment of melanoma, a highly immunogenic tumor. In a seminal preclin-ical melanoma study, GM-CSF–secreting tumor vaccines demonstrated 90% protection, while vaccines expressing IL-2 and IFN-γ failed to pro-vide antitumor protection (Kaufman et al., 2014). GM-CSF–secreting tumor vaccines also show promise as combination therapy with check-point inhibitors, such as cytotoxic T-lymphocyte antigen 4 and pro-grammed cell death protein 1, in the metastatic melanoma population (Kaufman et al., 2014).

In October 2015, FDA approved the first oncolytic virus therapy, tali-mogene laherparepvec (Imlygic®), for the treatment of melanoma. This intralesional therapy is a genetically engineered herpes virus with an added gene that codes for human GM-CSF. Its approval was based on the OPTiM phase 3 trial, which showed that durable response rate and median overall survival were higher in patients who received combi-nation talimogene laherparepvec and GM-CSF versus GM-CSF alone (Andtbacka et al., 2016).

Immunocytokines

Cytokines such as IFN-α and IL-2 play an important role in cancer immunotherapy but result in significant symptomatology. Recently, research to combine cytokines with recombinant antibodies has facili-tated more direct therapeutic delivery and fewer off-target effects (Pas-che & Neri, 2012). These combined molecules have been termed *immu-nocytokines.*

Pasche and Neri (2012) divided immunocytokines into three main classes. The first class includes antibody–cytokine fusions that selec-tively localize at the site of disease with effects that are largely indepen-dent of dose. Several fusion proteins with IL-2 or TNF represent this class. The second class includes immunocytokines, of which targeting performance varies with function of the injected dose, usually exhib-iting better results at higher concentrations. Examples include fusions based on GM-CSF or IL-7. Finally, some fusion proteins exist in which the cytokine component nullifies the disease-targeting performance of the parental antibody. This strategy allows for a more targeted therapy with fewer side effects. IFN-γ, for example, has had mixed clinical trial results with significant systemic toxicities when used as a single agent; however, when combined with tumor-specific antibodies, IFN-γ is stabilized in the serum, and the cytokine is targeted to tumor cells, allowing better efficacy with fewer side effects (Balachandran & Adams, 2013). In each of these instances, the immunocytokines fulfill the desired effect of an improved therapeutic index with fewer side effects.

Currently, the most advanced immunocytokines in development use IL-2. A study of one such molecule, combination IL-2 and IL-19 in patients with metastatic RCC, achieved disease stabilization in 83% of patients after two cycles (Pasche & Neri, 2012). Median progression-free survival was eight months, and toxicities were manageable and reversible. Another trial combining the same immunocytokine with dacarbazine in patients with metastatic melanoma noted an objective response in 28% of patients (Pasche & Neri, 2012). Several studies are currently ongoing in almost all tumor types (e.g., melanoma, neuroblastoma, breast, lung) to broaden and improve this area of research.

Cytokines and Cancer Symptoms

As noted, cytokines contribute significantly to the symptomatology seen in patients with cancer. Other noncytokine cancer therapies affect cytokine production and activity and result in similar symptom profiles, including fatigue, decreased appetite, depression, and cognitive impairment. For example, radiation therapy leads to the release of cytokines in various tissues. This is associated with the development of late radiation damage, including radiation-induced fibrosis and lung damage (Seruga et al., 2008). Some chemotherapy agents may also affect the expression of cytokines. Paclitaxel and docetaxel have been reported to increase expression of IL-2, IL-6, IFN-γ, and GM-CSF, while decreasing the expression of IL-1 and TNF-α in women with advanced breast cancer (Seruga et al., 2008). Tumors themselves can induce proinflammatory cytokines, leading to adverse symptomatology. Fatigue, for example, may be partially mediated by IL-6. In a 2005 quantitative review published by Balkwill, Charles, and Mantovani, a significant correlation between fatigue and circulating levels of IL-6 and IL-1RA (IL-1 receptor antagonist) was found in patients with cancer. Aerobic physical activity may reduce cancer-related fatigue through modulation of cytokines causing anti-inflammatory effects (Seruga et al., 2008). In healthy individuals, IL-6 is released intermittently from skeletal muscle during intense physical activity and has strong anti-inflammatory effects because of the inhibition of TNF-α and induction of IL-10 and

IL-1RA. Useful interventions may result from a better understanding of cytokines' role in cancer symptoms.

Cytokine expression varies with stress level. Studies investigating the effects of chronic and acute stress showed increased circulating levels of IL-6 and TNF-α compared to controls (Seruga et al., 2008). In addition, patients with cancer who are clinically depressed have much higher levels of circulating IL-6 than nondepressed patients with cancer or healthy controls. In patients undergoing treatment with IL-2 or IFN-α, decreased levels of circulating tryptophan may lead to decreased availability of serotonin, potentially related to the proinflammatory cytokine effect (Seruga et al., 2008). The effects of cytokines on fatigue, cognitive impairment, and depression are hard to discern, as these symptoms are closely interrelated with a multitude of compounding factors. But as previously noted, tangible evidence of a connection exists, and this area of investigation requires further research.

Regulation of cytokines likely plays an important role in cancer-related pain. Peripheral neuropathy is an adverse event noted in patients treated with chemotherapies and immunotherapies and can be difficult to manage. IL-1, IL-6, and TNF-α expression are upregulated in peripheral nerves, the spinal cord, and in certain regions of the brain after peripheral nerve injury (Seruga et al., 2008). In a study of patients with painful peripheral neuropathy, levels of proinflammatory cytokines increased and anti-inflammatory cytokines decreased compared to patients with painless neuropathies or healthy controls. Ongoing studies have demonstrated that biologics that target the activity of certain proinflammatory cytokines have shown clinical benefit and are generally well tolerated (Lees, Duffy, & Moalem-Taylor, 2013). TNF-α inhibitors, such as infliximab or etanercept, have shown to significantly reduce mechanical and thermal pain hypersensitivity associated with peripheral nerve injury. They are approved to treat a wide range of diseases, including rheumatoid arthritis and psoriasis (Lees et al., 2013). Other inhibitors for the treatment of peripheral neuropathy include IL-6, IL-7, and IL-1β (Lees et al., 2013).

Nursing Implications

Cytokines are important to providing cancer therapy and understanding treatment-related adverse events. As the front line in patient education, nurses must accurately describe treatment regimens (e.g., IFN, high-dose IL-2), including their mechanism of action, rationale for use, anticipated side effects, and side effect management. The tolerability of cytokine-based regimens depends largely on early and accurate identification of symptoms with appropriate interventions. As the field of immunotherapy continues to grow, so too does the role of the oncology nurse.

Summary

The role of cytokines in immunotherapy is complex and multifaceted. Cytokines such as IFN-α and IL-2 are used as cancer therapies, as well as the new classes of immunocytokines in development. The durability of these therapies is attributable to the immune-modifying nature of the treatments, as the patient's immune system is "taught" to recognize the cancer as foreign and fight against it. Many cytokines can have a stimulatory and inhibitory function depending on the setting. The expression of these cytokines may not only influence response to immune-modulating cancer therapies but may also affect the symptom profile and tolerability of therapy.

References

Abbas, A.K., Lichtman, A.H., & Pillai, S. (2017). *Cellular and molecular immunology* (9th ed.). Philadelphia, PA: Elsevier.

Andtbacka, R.H.I., Ross, M., Puzanov, I., Milhem, M., Collichio, F., Delman, K.A., ... Kaufman, H.L. (2016). Patterns of clinical response with talimogene laherparepvec (T-VEC) in patients with melanoma treated in the OPTiM phase III clinical trial. *Annals of Surgical Oncology, 23*, 4169–4177. https://doi.org/10.1245/s10434-016-5286-0

Atkins, M.B., Lotze, M.T., Dutcher, J.P., Fisher, R.I., Weiss, G., Margolin, K., ... Rosenberg, S.A. (1999). High-dose recombinant interleukin 2 therapy for patients with metastatic melanoma: Analysis of 270 patients treated between 1985 and 1993. *Journal of Clinical Oncology, 17*, 2105–2116. https://doi.org/10.1200/JCO.1999.17.7.2105

Balachandran, S., & Adams, G.P. (2013). Interferon-γ-induced necrosis: An antitumor biotherapeutic perspective. *Journal of Interferon and Cytokine Research, 33*, 171–180. https://doi.org/10.1089/jir.2012.0087

Balkwill, F. (2004). Cancer and the chemokine network. *Nature Reviews Cancer, 4*, 540–550. https://doi.org/10.1038/nrc1388

Balkwill, F., Charles, K.A., & Mantovani, A. (2005). Smoldering and polarized inflammation in the initiation and promotion of malignant disease. *Cancer Cell, 7*, 211–217. https://doi.org/10.1016/j.ccr.2005.02.013

Boyman, O., & Sprent, J. (2012). The role of interleukin-2 during homeostasis and activation of the immune system. *Nature Reviews Immunology, 12*, 180–190. https://doi.org/10.1038/nri3156

Choueiri, T.K., & Motzer, R.J. (2017). Systemic therapy for metastatic renal-cell carcinoma. *New England Journal of Medicine, 376*, 354–366. https://doi.org/10.1056/NEJMra1601333

Dranoff, G. (2004). Cytokines in cancer pathogenesis and cancer therapy. *Nature Reviews Cancer, 4*, 11–22. https://doi.org/10.1038/nrc1252

Dudley, M.E. (2011). Adoptive cell therapy for patients with melanoma. *Journal of Cancer, 2*, 360–362. https://doi.org/10.7150/jca.2.360

Fisher, D.T., Appenheimer, M.M., & Evans, S.S. (2014). The two faces of IL-6 in the tumor microenvironment. *Seminars in Immunology, 26*, 38–47. https://doi.org/10.1016/j.smim.2014.01.008

Fyfe, G., Fisher, R.I., Rosenberg, S.A., Sznol, M., Parkinson, D.R., & Louie, A.C. (1995). Results of treatment of 255 patients with metastatic renal cell carcinoma who received high-dose recombinant interleukin-2 therapy. *Journal of Clinical Oncology, 13,* 688–696. https://doi.org/10.1200/JCO.1995.13.3.688

Guirguis, L.M., Yang, J.C., White, D.E., Steinberg, S.M., Liewehr, D.J., Rosenberg, S.A., & Schwartzentruber, D.J. (2002). Safety and efficacy of high-dose interleukin-2 therapy in patients with brain metastases. *Journal of Immunotherapy, 25,* 82–87. https://doi.org/10.1097/00002371-200201000-00009

Hauschild, A., Gogas, H., Tarhini, A., Middleton, M.R., Testori, A., Dréno, B., & Kirkwood, J.M. (2008). Practical guidelines for the management of interferon-a-2b side effects in patients receiving adjuvant treatment for melanoma. *Cancer, 112,* 982–994. https://doi.org/10.1002/cncr.23251

Heikkilä, K., Ebrahim, S., & Lawlor, D.A. (2008). Systematic review of the association between circulating interleukin-6 (IL-6) and cancer. *European Journal of Cancer, 44,* 937–945. https://doi.org/10.1016/j.ejca.2008.02.047

Homey, B., Müller, A., & Zlotnik, A. (2002). Chemokines: Agents for the immunotherapy of cancer? *Nature Reviews Immunology, 2,* 175–184. https://doi.org/10.1038/nri748

Inaba, K., & Inaba, M. (2005). Antigen recognition and presentation by dendritic cells. *International Journal of Hematology, 81,* 181–187. https://doi.org/10.1532/IJH97.04200

Kaufman, H.L., Ruby, C.E., Hughes, T., & Slingluff, C.L., Jr. (2014). Current status of granulocyte-macrophage colony-stimulating factor in the immunotherapy of melanoma. *Journal for Immunotherapy of Cancer, 2,* 11. https://doi.org/10.1186/2051-1426-2-11

Kirkwood, J.M., Manola, J., Ibrahim, J., Sondak, V., Ernstoff, M.S., & Rao, U. (2004). A pooled analysis of Eastern Cooperative Oncology Group and intergroup trials of adjuvant high-dose interferon for melanoma. *Clinical Cancer Research, 10,* 1670–1677. https://doi.org/10.1158/1078-0432.CCR-1103-3

Liao, W., Lin, J.-X., & Leonard, W.J. (2013). Interleukin-2 at the crossroads of effector responses, tolerance, and immunotherapy. *Immunity, 38,* 13–25. https://doi.org/10.1016/j.immuni.2013.01.004

Lee, S., & Margolin, K. (2011). Cytokines in cancer immunotherapy. *Cancers, 3,* 3856–3893. https://doi.org/10.3390/cancers3043856

Lees, J.G., Duffy, S.S., & Moalem-Taylor, G. (2013). Immunotherapy targeting cytokines in neuropathic pain. *Frontiers in Pharmacology, 4,* 142. https://doi.org/10.3389/fphar.2013.00142

Merck and Co., Inc. (2015). *Sylatron® (peginterferon alfa-2b)* [Package insert]. Whitehouse Station, NJ: Author.

National Comprehensive Cancer Network. (2018). *NCCN Clinical Practice Guidelines in Oncology (NCCN Guidelines®): Melanoma* [v.2.2018]. Retrieved from https://www.nccn.org/professionals/physician_gls/PDF/melanoma.pdf

Pasche, N., & Neri, D. (2012). Immunocytokines: A novel class of potent armed antibodies. *Drug Discovery Today, 17,* 583–590. https://doi.org/10.1016/j.drudis.2012.01.007

Perica, K., Varela, J.C., Oelke, M., & Schneck, J. (2015). Adoptive T cell immunotherapy for cancer. *Rambam Maimonides Medical Journal, 6,* e0004.

Rose-John, S., & Neurath, M.F. (2004). IL-6 trans-signaling: The heat is on. *Immunity, 20,* 2–4. https://doi.org/10.1016/S1074-7613(04)00003-2

Rosenberg, S.A., & Dudley, M.E. (2009). Adoptive cell therapy for the treatment of patients with metastatic melanoma. *Current Opinion in Immunology, 21,* 233–240. https://doi.org/10.1016/j.coi.2009.03.002

Rosenberg, S.A., Yang, J.C., White, D.E., & Steinberg, S.M. (1998). Durability of complete responses in patients with metastatic cancer treated with high-dose interleukin-2: Identification of the antigens mediating response. *Annals of Surgery, 228,* 307–319. https://doi.org/10.1097/00000658-199809000-00004

Seruga, B., Zhang, H., Bernstein, L.J., & Tannock, I.F. (2008). Cytokines and their relationship to the symptoms and outcome of cancer. *Nature Reviews Cancer, 8,* 887–899. https://doi.org/10.1038/nrc2507

Smyth, M.J., Cretney, E., Kershaw, M.H., & Hayakawa, Y. (2004). Cytokines in cancer immunity and immunotherapy. *Immunological Reviews, 202,* 275–293. https://doi.org/10.1111/j.0105-2896.2004.00199.x

chapter four

Immune Checkpoint Inhibitors

Victoria Sherry, DNP, CRNP, AOCNP®
Susan Stonehouse-Lee, MSN, CRNP, AOCNP®

Introduction

The immune system is poised to recognize and eradicate cancer; however, this process is curbed by inhibitory receptors, known as immune checkpoints. Immune checkpoint receptors are pivotal modulators of the immune system and include a myriad of costimulatory and inhibitory pathways. Their primary function is to maintain homeostasis by protecting normal tissues from damage and preserving self-tolerance to antigens (i.e., preventing autoimmunity) when the immune system is responding to pathogens. This is accomplished by downregulating T-cell signaling to halt the overproliferation of T cells (Bauzon & Hermiston, 2014; Pardoll, 2012). Cancer cells possess the ability to hijack these checkpoint receptors as a key immune evasion strategy, allowing them to proliferate and metastasize uninhibited (Pardoll, 2012). This discovery prompted the development of immunotherapeutic agents for cancer that modulate immune checkpoint pathways or other costimulatory receptors (Disis, 2014; Pardoll, 2012).

Checkpoint Receptors

The inhibitory receptors cytotoxic T-lymphocyte antigen 4 (CTLA-4; also known as CD152) and programmed cell death protein 1 (PD-1; also known as CD279) have been identified as key immune checkpoints in cancer cell circumvention of the immune system. PD-1's associated ligands, programmed cell death-ligand 1 (PD-L1; also known as B7-H1 and CD274) and programmed cell death-ligand 2 (PD-L2; also known as B7-DC and CD273), also share this distinction (Pardoll, 2012; Topalian, Drake, & Pardoll, 2015). The relevance of these receptors has been extensively studied, and therapeutic approaches targeting the PD-1/PD-L1 and CTLA-4 pathways have been developed and tested. A plethora of additional immune checkpoints demonstrate promising targets for therapeutic blockade; however, CTLA-4 and PD-1/PD-L1 are the only pathways with available clinical information (Pardoll, 2012).

Effective activation of T cells is modulated by two signals that work together with the immune system when the body experiences a threat from an antigen. The first signal occurs when the T-cell receptor engages the cognate peptide in the context of the major histocompatibility complex (MHC) on antigen-presenting cells (APCs). The second signal occurs when inhibitory and stimulatory coreceptors on T cells localize to the immunologic synapse and engage their own specific ligands on the surface of APCs. Although inhibitory and stimulatory signaling can occur concomitantly, the net effect, either predominantly inhibitory or stimulatory, is what determines overall T-cell response, leading to either full activation or immunologic tolerance (failure to mount an immune response) (Chen & Flies, 2013). See Figure 4-1 for a list of coinhibitory and costimulatory receptors and their ligands.

Cytotoxic T-Lymphocyte Antigen 4

CTLA-4 was discovered on the surface of T cells in 1987 (Brunet et al., 1987). Its role remained a mystery until 1996, when scientists at the University of California, Berkeley made the seminal observation that inhibiting this immune checkpoint receptor could induce tumor regression (Leach, Krummel, & Allison, 1996). CTLA-4 belongs to the receptor subfamily CD28, which is an immunoglobulin (Ig) superfamily expressed at low levels on activated T cells. These receptors transmit signals in opposition to each other. CD28 promotes T-cell survival, and CTLA-4 inhibits T-cell growth. They share the same ligands, CD80 (also known as B7-1) and CD86 (also known as B7-2), which they compete for during sustained T-cell stimulus. Because CTLA-4 possesses a 500 to 2,500 times higher affinity than CD28 for its ligands, it can outcompete CD28 in binding to CD80 and CD86 (Freeman et al., 1993; Linsley et al., 1991; Teft, Kirchhof, & Madrenas, 2006; Walker & Sansom, 2011). By countering the activity of CD28, CTLA-4 downregulates the early stages of T-cell activation, acting as an "off" switch (Linsley et al., 1996; McCoy & Le Gros, 1999; Pardoll, 2012; Rudd, Taylor, & Schneider, 2009).

FIGURE 4-1 Coinhibitory and Costimulatory Receptors and Their Cognate Ligands

Dendritic cell-derived signal II can promote T-cell activation when conveyed by costimulatory molecules, or can attenuate T-cell responses when conveyed by coinhibitory molecules.

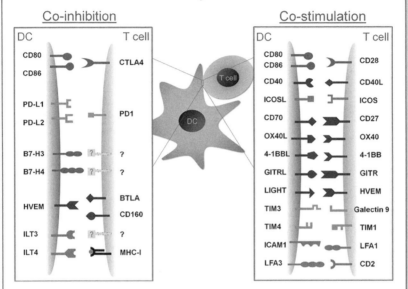

Note. From "The Nature of Activatory and Tolerogenic Dendritic Cell-Derived Signal II," by G. Bakdash, S.P. Sittig, T. van Dijk, C.G. Figdor, and I.J.M. de Vries, 2013, *Frontiers in Immunology, 4*, p. 2. Retrieved from https://www.frontiersin.org/articles/10.3389/fimmu.2013.00053/full. Copyright 2013 by Bakdash et al. Used under the CC BY license (http://creativecommons.org/licenses/by/2.0).

Programmed Cell Death Protein 1 and Its Ligands

PD-1 predated the discovery of CTLA-4 by four years; however, its function remained an enigma until the interactions between PD-1 and its ligands, PD-L1 and PD-L2, were identified as key pathways to suppress immune control (Dolan & Gupta, 2014; Ishida, Agata, Shibahara, & Honjo, 1992). The CTLA-4 and PD-l pathways operate at different stages of immune response. CTLA-4 acts earlier, and PD-1 acts later during T-cell activation. This important distinction in mechanism of action emphasizes the differences in toxicity profiles between CTLA-4 and PD-1/PD-L1 inhibitors. PD-1 inhibitor therapy usually produces less frequent and less severe immune-related adverse events (irAEs) than CTLA-4.

PD-1 is a broadly expressed immune checkpoint receptor that can be found on T cells, B cells, natural killer (NK) cells, monocytes, and tumor-infiltrating lymphocytes. It belongs to the CD28 superfamily. When PD-1 binds to its ligands, T-cell and cytokine function are down-regulated.

PD-1 binding with PD-L1 and PD-L2 in response to an antigen is critically important in maintaining homeostasis. However, this interaction in the tumor microenvironment allows an immune escape for tumor cells caused by the "turning off" of cytotoxic T cells (Kim & Eder, 2014). Blocking these checkpoint receptors makes tumor cells vulnerable to attack from cytotoxic T cells.

Each ligand has a very unique expression profile. PD-L1, referred to as the "major ligand," is more globally expressed and found on resting T cells, B cells, dendritic cells, macrophages, vascular endothelial cells, and pancreatic islet cells. Its role is to dampen T-cell function in peripheral tissues. PD-L1 is expressed on immune and tumor cells and has been detected in more than 50% of human cancers (Herbst et al., 2013).

PD-L2 is more selective and expressed mainly on the surface of dendritic cells and macrophages. Its role is less clear; however, it is responsible for T-cell activation in lymphoid organs and is expressed in certain subsets of B-cell lymphomas and gastric cancers. Approximately 20% of solid tumors harbor PD-L2 (Ansell et al., 2015; Hiraoka, 2010; Rozali, Hato, Robinson, Lake, & Lesterhuis, 2012; Taube et al., 2014; Topalian et al., 2015).

Both ligands cross-compete to bind to PD-1. Interestingly, PD-1 has a higher affinity for PD-L2 binding, but because PD-L2 has much lower levels of cell surface expression, PD-1 favors binding to PD-L1 (Rozali et al., 2012).

Checkpoint Inhibitors

Checkpoint inhibitors, also known as immunomodulators, are monoclonal antibodies (mAbs) that block the inhibitor signaling pathway, allowing for sustained T-cell activation. When T-cell activity is restored, it unleashes an immune system attack on cancer cells. A better understanding of the complex costimulatory and inhibitory pathways has prompted the development of innovative agents that modulate immune checkpoints with anti–CTLA-4, anti–PD-1, and anti–PD-L1 mAbs.

Researchers are continually looking for biomarkers on tumors that can predict clinical responses to therapy. To date, no pretreatment biomarker has been identified for anti–CTLA-4 therapy; however, post-treatment immune responses that correlate with clinical outcomes have been identified (i.e., CD8+ T cells) (Hiniker, Maecker, & Knox, 2015; Pardoll, 2012).

Similarly, no validated biomarkers for anti–PD-1 and anti–PD-L1 therapies exist; however, tumors that harbor PD-L1 have demonstrated higher response rates to these therapies. PD-L1 expression in tumors has shown to be prognostic in a variety of tumor types, including melanoma, renal cell carcinoma, and non-small cell lung cancer (NSCLC). PD-L1 expression is most frequently measured by immunohistochemistry. Several assays are approved by the U.S. Food and Drug Administration (FDA) to test tumors for PD-L1 expression. PD-L1 testing offers prognostic information that can improve a healthcare provider's ability to counsel patients. Tumors with a PD-L1 tumor proportion score (TPS) of 5% or greater respond better to PD-1/PD-L1 inhibitors than those with a TPS less than 5%; however, objective responses have been seen in patients who are PD-L1 negative (Hansen & Siu, 2016; Liu, Wang, & Bindeman, 2017).

Anti–CTLA-4 Agents

The anti–CTLA-4 mAb ipilimumab (Yervoy®) was the first-in-class checkpoint inhibitor to enter clinical testing as a T-cell potentiator (Bristol-Myers Squibb Co., 2018). In 2011, it was FDA approved for the treatment of unresectable metastatic melanoma (Hodi et al., 2010). This approval was based on the results of two separate randomized phase 3 trials that demonstrated an overall survival advantage for patients receiving ipilimumab compared to those receiving either a peptide vaccine or dacarbazine (Hodi et al., 2010; Robert et al., 2011). Ipilimumab has two dosing stratifications. In patients with unresectable or metastatic melanoma, the dose is 3 mg/kg IV administered over 90 minutes every three weeks for a maximum of four doses. This dose can be safely infused in as little as 30 minutes (Momtaz et al., 2015). In the adjuvant setting for melanoma, the dose is 10 mg/kg IV over 90 minutes every three weeks for four doses. This is followed by the same dose every 12 weeks for up to three years, or until documented progression or unacceptable toxicity occurs (Bristol-Myers Squibb Co., 2017a).

Anti–PD-1 Agents

Nivolumab (Opdivo®), a fully human immunoglobulin G4 (IgG4) mAb, blocks the PD-1 signaling pathway. It was initially approved in 2014 for the treatment of metastatic melanoma. Based on CheckMate clinical trials, it has since gained approvals for metastatic NSCLC, advanced renal cell carcinoma, classical Hodgkin lymphoma (cHL), advanced head and neck squamous cell carcinoma (HNSCC), microsatellite instability-high (MSI-H) colorectal cancer, and hepatocellular carcinoma. These studies showed improved overall response rates with durable responses (Ferris et al., 2016; Kazandjian et al., 2016; Motzer et al., 2015; Weber et al., 2015; Younes et al., 2016).

When initially approved, nivolumab was given at a recommended dose of 3 mg/kg IV over 60 minutes every two weeks. When used in combination therapy, dosing is typically adjusted to 1 mg/kg every three weeks in concert with ipilimumab for four doses. Nivolumab is then continued as a monotherapy at a dose of 3 mg/kg every two weeks. However, for most indications, the package insert has been modified to recommend a flat dose of 240 mg every two weeks or 480 mg every four weeks (Bristol-Myers Squibb Co., 2018).

Pembrolizumab (Keytruda®), another humanized IgG4 mAb against PD-1, was first approved in 2014 for patients with unresectable or metastatic melanoma. Based on the results of Keynote clinical trials, FDA granted accelerated approval of the drug for treatment of metastatic melanoma, metastatic NSCLC, HNSCC, NSCLC (chemotherapy plus pembrolizumab), urothelial carcinoma, MSI-H cancer, cHL, and gastric cancer. These trials showed durable objective response rates and acceptable toxicity profiles (Cohen et al., 2015; Reck et al., 2016; Robert et al., 2015).

Pembrolizumab is administered to adults at a flat dose of 200 mg IV every three weeks for nearly every indication. For pediatric patients with cHL and MSI-H cancer, the dose is 2 mg/kg (up to 200 mg) IV every three weeks (Merck and Co., Inc., 2017).

Anti–PD-L1 Agents

Atezolizumab (Tecentriq®) is a fully humanized IgG1 mAb that blocks the PD-L1 pathway. It was FDA approved in 2016 for the treatment of patients with locally advanced or metastatic urothelial carcinoma who have disease progression following platinum-containing chemotherapy or within 12 months of neoadjuvant or adjuvant treatment. Approval was based on the IMvigor clinical trials for urothelial carcinoma and metastatic NSCLC, which showed improvement in tumor response rate and duration of response (Barlesi et al., 2016; Hoffman-Censits et al., 2016).

Atezolizumab is administered initially as a 1,200 mg IV infusion over 60 minutes every three weeks. If the first infusion is tolerated, all subsequent infusions may be delivered over 30 minutes (Genentech, Inc., 2017).

Avelumab (Bavencio®), a fully human mAb, received FDA approval in 2017 for metastatic Merkel cell carcinoma and advanced or metastatic urothelial carcinoma. Both trials showed improvements in response rate (33% for Merkel cell carcinoma and 18.2% for urothelial carcinoma) (Apolo et al., 2017; EMD Serono, Inc., 2017). Avelumab is administered as 10 mg/kg IV over 60 minutes every two weeks until disease progression or unacceptable toxicity (EMD Serono, Inc., 2017).

Durvalumab (Imfinzi®), a human immunoglobulin G1 kappa (IgG1κ) mAb, blocks the interaction of PD-L1 with PD-1 and CD80. It was granted breakthrough therapy approval in May 2017 for locally advanced or metastatic urothelial cancer based on early clinical data from a phase 1 trial, which noted a 46% response rate in patients with PD-L1–positive advanced bladder cancer (AstraZeneca Pharmaceuticals LP, 2018). In February 2018, durvalumab was approved for unresectable stage III NSCLC that has not progressed following concurrent platinum-based chemotherapy and radiation therapy. The recommended dose of durvalumab is 10 mg/kg IV over 60 minutes every two weeks (AstraZeneca Pharmaceuticals LP, 2018).

Other Promising Checkpoint Inhibitors

Many tumors express more than one inhibitory ligand, creating an opportunity to enhance antitumor immunity through double or triple blockade of immune checkpoints.

Numerous other T-cell surface receptors have the potential to modulate an antitumor immune response. Lymphocyte-activation gene 3 (LAG-3; also known as CD223) is an inhibitory checkpoint receptor, a member of the Ig superfamily, and is expressed on activated T cells. LAG-3 has one ligand, MHC class II, which is upregulated on CD4+ regulatory T cells (Tregs) during an immune response. LAG-3 and PD-1 were found to be commonly coexpressed, which led to clinical testing evaluating both anti–LAG-3 and anti–PD-1 therapies (Huard, Gaulard, Faure, Hercend, & Triebel, 1994; Topalian et al., 2015). Another inhibitory checkpoint receptor, T-cell membrane protein 3 (TIM-3; also known as HAVCR2) is expressed on T cells, NK cells, and monocytes. It has very similar immune-modulating effects as LAG-3 (Anderson, 2016; Sánchez-Fueyo, 2003). Killer cell Ig-like receptors are important regulators of the killing activity of NK cells. NK-cell activation results in potent antitumor activity (Pardoll, 2012). B7-H3 (also known as CD276) and B7-H4 (also known as B7-S1, B7x, and VCTNI) are inhibitory ligands that belong to the B7 superfamily and downregulate T-cell responses (Kohrt et al., 2014; Linch, McNamara, & Redmond, 2015; Pardoll, 2012). The B- and T-lymphocyte attenuator (BTLA, also known as CD272) inhibits signals and includes cell surface receptors expressed by effector T cells. BTLA's ligand, HVEM, is expressed on certain tumor cells, especially melanoma. Blockade of this pathway has shown to enhance antitumor immunity (Pardoll, 2012). The adenosine A2a receptor (A2AR) drives T cells to become Tregs through engagement with its ligand, adenosine. Indoleamine 2,3-dioxygenase (IDO) is a key immunomodulatory enzyme of acquired immune tolerance in normal and pathologic conditions, particularly in the tumor microenvironment, that inhibits CD8+ T cells and enhances the suppressor activity of Tregs. IDO depletes the amino acid tryptophan, which is associated with immunosuppression involving T-cell arrest and anergy (Topalian et al., 2015).

Costimulatory Receptors

Unlike CTLA-4, PD-1, and PD-L1 pathways, which suppress T-cell activation, the absence of costimulatory checkpoint receptors renders tumors invisible to the immune system. Manipulation of these pathways is key for generating effective antitumor therapy. OX40 (ligand OX40L) is a member of the tumor necrosis factor (TNF) superfamily and is mainly expressed on CD4 and CD8 T cells (Jensen et al., 2010). Anti-OX40 mAbs have shown to amplify T-cell differentiation, leading to improved immunity against a variety of tumors (Linch et al., 2015). The 4-1BB ligand is a member of the TNF ligand family and is expressed on T cells and APCs. Therapies using the 4-1BB signaling pathway have shown promising antitumor effects in preclinical studies. The inducible T-cell costimulator protein is another member of the CD28/CTLA-4 superfamily. Its rapid T-cell upregulation is further enhanced on CTLA-4 blockade (Vonderheide et al., 2010). See Table 4-1 for a list of immune checkpoint modulators that are either approved or in clinical development.

Combination Therapies

Given the complexity of immune responses to tumors, researchers are looking beyond single-agent immunotherapy treatment and are studying mAbs in combination with chemotherapy, targeted therapy, radiation therapy, and other immunotherapies. Zitvogel, Apetoh, Ghiringhelli, and Kroemer (2011) discovered that chemotherapy may have immunostimulatory properties that can make cancer cells more susceptible to an immune attack. Targeted therapy in combination with anti–CTLA-4 mAbs was associated with significant antitumor activity; however, associated high rates of renal and hepatic toxicity need further evaluation (Hu-Lieskovan, Robert, Homet Moreno, & Ribas, 2014). A synergistic effect was noted between radiation therapy and the immune system. Preclinical data have indicated that radiation therapy can potentiate the systemic efficacy of immunotherapy by increasing

TABLE 4-1   Immune Checkpoint Modulators Either Approved or in Clinical Development

Target	Drug Name	Other Names	Pharmaceutical Company
CTLA-4	Ipilimumab*	Yervoy®	Bristol-Myers Squibb Co.
PD-1	Nivolumab*	Opdivo®, BMS-936558, MDX-1106, ONO-4538	Bristol-Myers Squibb Co.; Ono Pharmaceuticals Co. Ltd.
	Pembrolizumab*	Keytruda®, MK-3475, lambrolizumab	Merck and Co., Inc.
	Pidilizumab	CT-011	CureTech Ltd.
	MEDI0680	AMP-514	AstraZeneca Pharmaceuticals LP
PD-L1	Atezolizumab*	Tecentriq®, MPDL3280A, RG7446	Genentech, Inc.
	BMS-936559	MDX-1105	Bristol-Myers Squibb Co.
	Durvalumab*	Imfinzi®, MED14736	AstraZeneca Pharmaceuticals LP
	Avelumab	Bavencio®, MSB0010718C	EMD Serono, Inc.
PD-L2	AMP-224	–	GlaxoSmithKline plc
KIR	Lirilumab	BMS-986015, IPH2102	Bristol-Myers Squibb Co.
IDO	Indoximod	NLG-8189, D-1MT, 1-methyltryptophan	NewLink Genetics Corp.
LAG-3	BMS-986016	–	Bristol-Myers Squibb Co.
	IMP321	–	Prima BioMed Ltd.

* Indicates approved by the U.S. Food and Drug Administration

CTLA-4—cytotoxic T-lymphocyte antigen 4; PD-1—programmed cell death protein 1; PD-L1—programmed cell death-ligand 1

Note. Based on information from Disis, 2014; Topalian et al., 2015.

the expression of PD-L1 and CTLA-4 on tumor cells (Mansfield, Park, & Dong, 2015). The administration of combination immunotherapies ipilimumab and nivolumab has been clinically tested and FDA approved for melanoma. Combination therapy has demonstrated a significantly longer median progression-free survival than either agent alone and is being explored in other tumor types (Wolchok et al., 2013).

Nursing Administration

According to institutional policy, checkpoint inhibitors are administered intravenously, with or without a sterile, nonpyrogenic, low-protein-binding filter (pore size 0.2–0.22 mcm). Most checkpoint inhibitors can be administered without premedication; however, some exceptions do exist. For example, avelumab administration requires premedication, such as an antihistamine and acetaminophen, to prevent an infusion reaction during the first four doses. Subsequent infusions may omit premedication upon clinical judgment and/or presence or severity of prior infusion reactions (EMD Serono, Inc., 2017).

Infusion-related or hypersensitivity reactions have been reported with the administration of checkpoint inhibitors. As infusion reactions are uncommon, occurring in 0.4%–6% of patients across trials of checkpoint inhibitors, premedication is generally not required before administration. Mild to moderate infusion reactions can be managed by slowing the infusion rate and administering appropriate supportive care premedications (e.g., antihistamines, corticosteroids). Severe (grade 3 or 4) infusion-related reactions require permanent discontinuation of the drug (Bristol-Myers Squibb Co., 2017b; Genentech, Inc., 2017; Merck and Co., Inc., 2017).

In the metastatic setting, treatment with PD-L1 or PD-1 inhibitors is generally continued until disease progression or unacceptable toxicity. Treatment after disease progression may be considered if the patient is deriving a clinical benefit or has continued disease or symptom control despite radiologic findings. If the patient is clinically stable despite progression of disease on physical examination or radiology studies, immunotherapy should be continued, and the disease should be followed closely on scans (Wolchok et al., 2009).

Dose reduction is not recommended with checkpoint inhibitor therapy. This is unique in relation to general principles of chemotherapy and targeted therapy, where dose reductions are used to allow better tolerance and minimize the toxicity that patients experience from chemotherapy and targeted therapies. In contrast, management of irAEs requires close monitoring and follow-up. It also may require withholding or discontinuing therapy.

Adverse Effects

Checkpoint inhibitors present a unique toxicity profile. Like standard chemotherapy, common adverse events include fatigue, decreased appetite, nausea, and arthralgias (Davies, 2016). These are usually mild and tolerable for most patients; however, their mechanism of enhancing the immune system results in a spectrum of irAEs. These are caused by sustained T-cell activation or amplification of the immune system and can potentially lead to T cells attacking healthy tissue. Any organ system can be affected, but events tend to occur in areas with increased concentrations of T cells (Davies, 2016). These irAEs have emerged as a large concern with checkpoints inhibitors and present a challenge in the management of patients receiving these therapies.

Several irAEs were reported in varying degrees in the clinical trials that led to the approvals of these agents. PD-1 and PD-L1 inhibitors have a lower incidence of irAEs than CTLA-4 inhibitors. The most common irAEs occurring with ipilimumab are fatigue, diarrhea, pruritus, rash, and colitis. With PD-1 inhibitors, irAEs that occur in more than 20% of patients include fatigue, rash, pruritus, cough, diarrhea, decreased appetite, constipation, and arthralgia (Villadolid & Amin, 2015). Combination therapy with CTLA-4– and PD-L1–directed checkpoint inhibitors (e.g., nivolumab with ipilimumab) may have synergistic or additive antitumor effects. In addition to increased response benefits, patients receiving combination therapy have experienced a higher incidence of irAEs compared to agent monotherapy (Wolchok et al., 2013). The rates of grade 3 and 4 events were higher in concurrent regimens versus single-agent therapy. In a 2015 study, combination nivolumab and ipilimumab had more than twice as many reported grade 3 and 4 events than ipilimumab monotherapy (54% and 24%, respectively) (Postow et al., 2015). Toxicity may also increase when checkpoint inhibitors are combined with other systemic therapies, radiation therapies, targeted therapies, or immunotherapies (Davies, 2016; Lynch et al., 2012).

The onset of irAEs varies from patient to patient. The majority appear during the first 12 weeks of therapy, but some can occur weeks to months after discontinuation (Andrews & Holden, 2012). Such a timeline has been described for ipilimumab, with rash and diarrhea appearing in the first or second treatment, diarrhea occurring approximately six weeks into therapy, and liver or endocrine toxicities presenting after 8–12 weeks (Weber, Kähler, & Hauschild, 2012). PD-1 and PD-L1 inhibitors have a similar onset of symptoms (Weber et al., 2015). Median time to onset of pneumonitis was five months in a clinical trial of patients treated with pembrolizumab; a longer median onset of 11.6 months was reported for nephritis events (Villadolid & Amin, 2015). Patients with underlying autoimmune disorders were excluded from trials with checkpoint inhibitors because of a theoretical compromise in underlying autoimmune disease status related to immune response seen with this class of drugs. Therefore, the safety of

PD-1 and PD-L1 inhibitors and anti–CTLA-4 antibodies in the setting of autoimmune diseases is unknown.

Similarly, the safety of checkpoint inhibitors in transplant patients taking antirejection medications is unexplored (Bagley, Bauml, & Langer, 2015). Clinicians should proceed with caution when considering administration of checkpoint inhibitors in these instances; however, it should be noted that a retrospective study demonstrated that patients with preexisting autoimmune conditions can safely receive ipilimumab therapy with vigilant clinical monitoring (Johnson et al., 2016).

Education can lead to resolution of symptoms and allow for continuation of checkpoint inhibitor therapy. Patients and families should be educated on early recognition and the need to report symptoms in a timely manner, and healthcare providers should seek knowledge on prompt treatment of suspected or confirmed irAEs. Patient education materials are available online and include wallet cards and guidelines for management. The Nursing Immune-Mediated Therapy Adverse Reaction Symptom Checklist should be used to evaluate all patients prior to each drug dose (Bristol-Myers Squibb Co., 2017b). Hotlines are also accessible for medical information and to report adverse events. Pharmaceutical companies should contact physicians and providers when ipilimumab is prescribed to a patient to provide education and management strategies for adverse events (Bristol-Myers Squibb Co., 2011; Fecher, Agarwala, Hodi, & Weber, 2013).

Guidelines for ipilimumab have also been adopted for other checkpoint inhibitors (Fecher et al., 2013; Kreamer, 2014; Weber et al., 2012). Treatment for many irAEs includes corticosteroid administration. Some patients may require additional immunosuppressant medications. Other supportive care and organ system–specific therapies can be instituted. These strategies almost always reverse the irAE process and return signs and symptoms to baseline. A notable exception includes endocrine irAEs, which may require permanent hormone or steroid replacement therapy. Despite these unique side effects, checkpoint inhibitors present an acceptable safety profile. See Figure 4-2 for more information on the treatment of irAEs.

Dermatologic Toxicity

Dermatologic toxicities are common irAEs. Incidence rates of rash or pruritus can be as high as 50% for patients on ipilimumab (Hodi et al., 2010). Most dermatologic irAEs are grade 1 or 2 events; grade 3 and 4 events rarely manifest. Mucosal effects, such as mucositis, gingivitis, or sicca syndrome, have a high occurrence with anti–PD-1 antibodies. Vitiligo, although rare across various immunotherapy classes, is generally mild (grade 1) but may be permanent and cause psychological distress. This adverse event is associated with favorable treatment benefit primarily in patients with malignant melanoma (Teulings, 2015).

Rash associated with immunotherapy has a maculopapular appearance, such as that seen antibiotic use, but not necessarily like the acneform rash seen with targeted cancer therapies (see Figures 4-3 and 4-4). It can present with or without pruritus. It may also present in an area of nevi or areas of disease regression in SC tissues, suggesting a directed response toward melanocytes (Lacouture et al., 2014). Pruritus without rash is also a known toxicity.

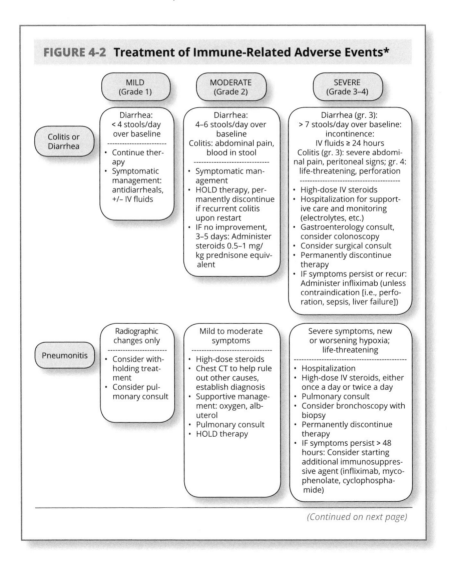

FIGURE 4-2 Treatment of Immune-Related Adverse Events*

	MILD (Grade 1)	MODERATE (Grade 2)	SEVERE (Grade 3–4)
Colitis or Diarrhea	Diarrhea: < 4 stools/day over baseline ------------------------ • Continue therapy • Symptomatic management: antidiarrheals, +/– IV fluids	Diarrhea: 4–6 stools/day over baseline Colitis: abdominal pain, blood in stool ------------------------------ • Symptomatic management • HOLD therapy, permanently discontinue if recurrent colitis upon restart • IF no improvement, 3–5 days: Administer steroids 0.5–1 mg/kg prednisone equivalent	Diarrhea (gr. 3): > 7 stools/day over baseline: incontinence: IV fluids ≥ 24 hours Colitis (gr. 3): severe abdominal pain, peritoneal signs; gr. 4: life-threatening, perforation ------------------------------------ • High-dose IV steroids • Hospitalization for supportive care and monitoring (electrolytes, etc.) • Gastroenterology consult, consider colonoscopy • Consider surgical consult • Permanently discontinue therapy • IF symptoms persist or recur: Administer infliximab (unless contraindication [i.e., perforation, sepsis, liver failure])
Pneumonitis	Radiographic changes only ------------------------ • Consider withholding treatment • Consider pulmonary consult	Mild to moderate symptoms -------------------------------- • High-dose steroids • Chest CT to help rule out other causes, establish diagnosis • Supportive management: oxygen, albuterol • Pulmonary consult • HOLD therapy	Severe symptoms, new or worsening hypoxia; life-threatening --- • Hospitalization • High-dose IV steroids, either once a day or twice a day • Pulmonary consult • Consider bronchoscopy with biopsy • Permanently discontinue therapy • IF symptoms persist > 48 hours: Consider starting additional immunosuppressive agent (infliximab, mycophenolate, cyclophosphamide)

(Continued on next page)

FIGURE 4-2 Treatment of Immune-Related Adverse Events*
(Continued)

	MILD (Grade 1)	MODERATE (Grade 2)	SEVERE (Grade 3–4)
Hepatitis	AST/ALT < 3 times ULN and/or total bilirubin < 1.5 times ULN ------------------------ • Monitor LFTs • Continue therapy	AST/ALN 3–5 times ULN; total bilirubin 1.5–3 times ULN ------------------------ • Administer steroids: 0.5–1 mg/kg prednisone equivalent • Every 3 day monitoring of LFTs • Consider hospitalization • HOLD therapy	AST/ALT > 5 times ULN; or total bilirubin > 3 times ULN ------------------------ • High-dose IV steroids, once or twice a day • Hospitalization • Hepatology/gastroenterology consult • Consider liver biopsy • Permanently discontinue therapy • IF LFT abnormalities persist: Start mycophenolate
Dermatologic Toxicity	Covering < 30% BSA, with or without symptoms (pruritus, burning, tightness) ------------------------ • Topical corticosteroids; oral antihistamines • Continue therapy	Macules/papules covering > 30% BSA with or without symptoms ------------------------ • Administer high-dose oral steroids • HOLD therapy • Consult dermatology	Stevens-Johnson syndrome, toxic epidermal necrolysis; rash complicated by full thickness dermal ulceration; or necrotic, bullous, or hemorrhagic manifestations ------------------------ • Administer high-dose IV steroids • Hospitalization • Consult dermatology; multidisciplinary team management • Consider skin biopsy • Permanently discontinue therapy

(Continued on next page)

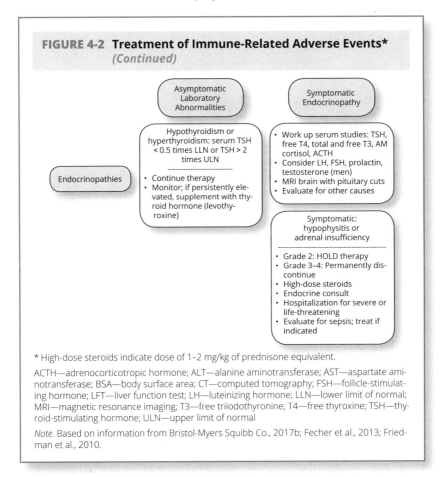

FIGURE 4-2 Treatment of Immune-Related Adverse Events* (Continued)

Asymptomatic Laboratory Abnormalities

Symptomatic Endocrinopathy

Endocrinopathies

Hypothyroidism or hyperthyroidism: serum TSH < 0.5 times LLN or TSH > 2 times ULN

• Continue therapy
• Monitor; if persistently elevated, supplement with thyroid hormone (levothyroxine)

• Work up serum studies: TSH, free T4, total and free T3, AM cortisol, ACTH
• Consider LH, FSH, prolactin, testosterone (men)
• MRI brain with pituitary cuts
• Evaluate for other causes

Symptomatic: hypophysitis or adrenal insufficiency

• Grade 2: HOLD therapy
• Grade 3–4: Permanently discontinue
• High-dose steroids
• Endocrine consult
• Hospitalization for severe or life-threatening
• Evaluate for sepsis; treat if indicated

* High-dose steroids indicate dose of 1–2 mg/kg of prednisone equivalent.

ACTH—adrenocorticotropic hormone; ALT—alanine aminotransferase; AST—aspartate aminotransferase; BSA—body surface area; CT—computed tomography; FSH—follicle-stimulating hormone; LFT—liver function test; LH—luteinizing hormone; LLN—lower limit of normal; MRI—magnetic resonance imaging; T3—free triiodothyronine; T4—free thyroxine; TSH—thyroid-stimulating hormone; ULN—upper limit of normal

Note. Based on information from Bristol-Myers Squibb Co., 2017b; Fecher et al., 2013; Friedman et al., 2010.

Dermatologic toxicities are usually managed with topical agents. Topical corticosteroids with medium to high potency are most effective. For pruritus, agents such as systemic antihistamines (e.g., diphenhydramine, hydroxyzine) are recommended, particularly if the condition is interfering with sleep. The antidepressant agent mirtazapine may help with the insomnia related to these effects (Lacouture et al., 2014). Nonpharmacologic measures to manage pruritus and rash include topical emollients, cold compresses, and oatmeal baths. For grade 1 or 2 dermatologic irAEs, therapy can typically continue without disruption; however, for more severe (grade 3 or 4) events, treatment should be delayed and high-dose corticosteroid therapy (1–2 mg/kg prednisone or equivalent) should be initiated. Grade 3 and 4 events include Stevens-Johnson syndrome and toxic epidermal necrolysis (TEN) and can develop within 48 hours of onset of symptoms/rash. Any patient with ulceration, bullae, or necrotic or hemorrhagic lesions requires urgent dermatologic evaluation,

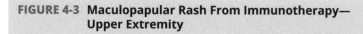

FIGURE 4-3 Maculopapular Rash From Immunotherapy— Upper Extremity

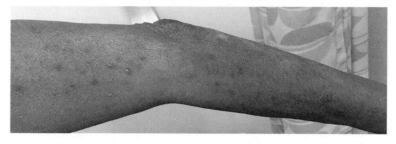

Note. Image courtesy of Victoria Sherry, DNP, CRNP, AOCNP®. Used with permission.

as well as hospital admission, with an interprofessional approach. Treatment should be permanently discontinued if Stevens-Johnson syndrome or TEN occur or if symptoms fail to improve after 12 weeks of supportive management (Friedman, Proverbs-Singh, & Postow, 2016).

Diarrhea and Colitis

Diarrhea has been noted in 44% of patients on checkpoint inhibitors, with 18% noted as grade 3 or 4 events (Robert et al., 2011). Persisting symptoms can be indicative of underlying colitis, which can lead to complications related to bowel obstruction and perforation. Other gastrointestinal effects may include bloating, cramps, gas, nausea, and abdominal pain. It is imperative that healthcare

FIGURE 4-4 Maculopapular Rash From Immunotherapy— Lower Extremity

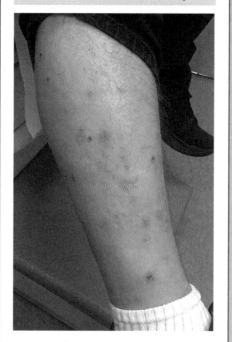

Note. Image courtesy of Victoria Sherry, DNP, CRNP, AOCNP®. Used with permission.

professionals and patients understand proper management and reporting of these gastrointestinal irAEs.

Grade 1 diarrhea (increase of two bowel movements per day more than baseline) can be managed with loperamide, oral hydration, and electrolyte replacement. Diet should be modified to exclude dairy, caffeine, spicy foods, and artificial sweeteners (sorbitol) (Davies, 2016). Other causes of diarrhea, such as infectious etiology, should simultaneously be ruled out.

If grade 2 diarrhea occurs or grade 1 diarrhea persists longer than one week, an oral steroid should be initiated (e.g., prednisone 0.5 mg/kg/day). Budesonide (9 mg/day) may reduce local inflammation; however, prophylaxis with budesonide in patients receiving ipilimumab is not recommended (Weber et al., 2009). Neither budesonide (a systemically nonabsorbed oral corticosteroid) nor systemically absorbed oral steroids affect the antitumor response in patients with metastatic disease (Downey et al., 2007).

Flexible sigmoidoscopy or colonoscopy is recommended for persistent grade 2 diarrhea and more severe (grade 3 or 4) diarrhea to evaluate for enterocolitis. Diarrhea is the most common presenting symptom of colitis. Other symptoms include abdominal pain, hematochezia, weight loss, fever, and vomiting (Haanen et al., 2017). Grade 2 (persisting more than three days), 3, or 4 colitis requires hospitalization with immediate administration of high-dose steroids (e.g., methylprednisolone 0.5–1 mg/kg/day). A gastroenterology consultation should be obtained for consideration of further workup with a computed tomography (CT) scan or colonoscopy with biopsy. Surgical consultation may also be necessary if symptoms do not begin to resolve expeditiously. Patients may develop colonic perforation with or without abscess, requiring emergent colectomy. Early surgical consultation and review are recommended for patients without resolution of symptoms, particularly those who have pain, bleeding, or distention (Haanen et al., 2017). Checkpoint inhibitors should be withheld for moderate (grade 2) or severe (grade 3) colitis and permanently discontinued for life-threatening (grade 4) colitis (Merck and Co., Inc., 2017). Infliximab may also be added for life-threatening enterocolitis or if there is an inadequate or quick response to high-dose steroids.

Pneumonitis

Pneumonitis is a serious and potentially life-threatening irAE. In clinical trials, it was seen at a rate of 1%–4%. This was increased to 6%–10% in combination therapies (Bagley et al., 2015; Naidoo et al., 2017; Rizvi et al., 2015). Pneumonitis has been observed with anti–PD-1/PD-L1 agents and more rarely with ipilimumab. Although concerning, these rates can be lower than the severe pulmonary toxicity seen with standard chemotherapy. For example, in a phase 3 study comparing nivolumab to docetaxel in previously treated patients with squamous cell lung cancer, no deaths from pneumonitis were attributable to nivolumab, but three deaths from pulmonary toxicity were attributed to docetaxel, including interstitial lung disease, pulmonary hemorrhage, and sepsis (Brahmer et al., 2015). Pneumonitis was seen at low but consistent rates in trials with nivolumab, pembrolizumab, and atezolizumab, and thus appears to be a class-related toxic effect (Gangadhar & Vonderheide, 2014). The rate of grade 3 and 4 pneumonitis is similar across tumor types; however, more treatment-related deaths due to pneumonitis have occurred in patients with NSCLC (Gettinger et al., 2016; Haanen et al., 2017; Naidoo et al., 2017).

Recognizing symptoms is crucial for prompt treatment and complete reversal or resolution of signs and symptoms. Baseline oxygen saturation and follow-up pulse oximetry at each visit have been recommended by some clinicians (Davies, 2016). Shortness of breath, cough, or pleuritic chest pain, with or without fever, must be evaluated with radiologic imaging. Grade 1 pneumonitis (with radiographic changes alone) requires closer monitoring for symptoms (i.e., every two to three days). Clinicians should consider delay of treatment as well as a sputum sample to rule out infectious etiology. If symptoms develop and grade 2 or 3 pneumonitis is suspected or confirmed, initiation of corticosteroids with subsequent corticosteroid taper is indicated. CT scan imaging features can include ground glass opacities, cryptogenic organizing, pneumonia characteristics, interstitial pattern, and hypersensitivity pneumonitis (Naidoo et al., 2017). These patients should also have a pulmonary consultation. With any grade 2 pneumonitis, therapy with a checkpoint inhibitor should be held. Therapy should be permanently discontinued with grade 3 or 4 events.

Hepatitis

Immune-related hepatitis presents asymptomatically as a rise in liver function tests. Alanine aminotransferase (ALT) and aspartate aminotransferase (AST), and to lesser extent total bilirubin, may become elevated.

Monitoring serum liver function tests at baseline and prior to each subsequent dose is required. If hepatic function is abnormal, other etiologies (e.g., alcohol consumption, liver metastasis, infectious causes, medications) should be excluded. With grade 2 hepatitis (elevation of AST or ALT greater than 2.5–5 times the upper limit of normal [ULN]; or total bilirubin greater than 1.5–3 times ULN), therapy should be withheld. The checkpoint inhibitor should be permanently discontinued if transaminases are greater than five times ULN, a concomitant rise in total bilirubin occurs, or with an elevation in total bilirubin greater than three times ULN. Consultation with hepatology and high-dose corticosteroid therapy are recommended for grade 3 or 4 events. This therapy should taper over one month after liver function tests start to normalize. If severe hepatitis persists despite high-dose corticosteroid treatment for three days, treatment with mycophenolate should be considered with a dose range of 500–1,000 mg every 12 hours (Friedman et al., 2016). The immunosuppressants tacrolimus and anti-thymocyte globulin may be beneficial in those not responsive to corticosteroids. Unlike with other gastrointestinal irAEs, infliximab is contraindicated in cases of hepatitis because of the risk of hepatotoxicity (Friedman et al., 2016). Complete resolution of immune-related hepatitis often occurs, but this may take four to eight weeks.

Endocrinopathy

Various endocrine irAEs have been observed with checkpoint inhibitors as a result of the infiltration of immune cells into the pituitary or thyroid glands. The most predominant toxicities are hypophysitis (inflammation of the pituitary gland) and hypothyroidism. Other toxicities include hyperthyroidism, hyperpituitarism, and adrenal insufficiency. Case reports of immune-related diabetes mellitus have also been observed. Hypophysitis and hypothyroidism can occur in up to 10% of patients receiving ipilimumab. Hypophysitis is an adverse event commonly related to anti–CTLA-4 therapy, whereas hypothyroidism has appeared more often in anti–PD-1 and anti–PD-L1 mAbs. Hypophysitis with combination therapy (ipilimumab and nivolumab) has been reported in 8%–10% of patients (Haanen et al., 2017; Larkin et al., 2015).

Presentation of endocrinopathies is not as straightforward as other irAEs, as symptoms are often nonspecific. Patients can present with fatigue, nausea, headache, and depression. Routine monitoring of thyroid-stimulating hormone (TSH) during therapy is recommended. If patients present with these nonspecific symptoms, further laboratory evaluation of the levels that regulate endocrine organs is warranted (Davies, 2016; Gangadhar & Vonderheide, 2014).

Hypothyroidism is usually mild, presenting with elevated levels of TSH. Patients may be asymptomatic or have symptoms associated with hypothyroidism (e.g., fatigue, hair thinning, constipation, muscle aches or weakness, cold intolerance). Replacement with thyroid hormone (levothyroxine) is generally effective and may continue after checkpoint inhibitor therapy has been discontinued.

In trials with ipilimumab for the treatment of melanoma and renal cell carcinoma, hypophysitis emerged as a distinct, though rare, adverse event related to immunotherapy. Hypophysitis is defined as inflammation of the pituitary gland that can lead to hypopituitarism, adrenal insufficiency, or potentially life-threatening adrenal crisis. Any patient with severe headaches or vision changes should undergo a dedicated pituitary cut brain magnetic resonance imaging (MRI) scan. Central nervous system metastases and immune-related hypophysitis must be ruled out. Hypophysitis may also cause visual disturbances, emotional lability, fatigue, vertigo, hypotension, confusion, memory loss, loss of libido, anorexia, temperature intolerance, hallucinations, and sensation of fevers and chills. Imaging (brain MRI) can be diagnostic for hypophysitis, showing an enlarged pituitary gland, though the pituitary gland can also appear normal on scans (Gangadhar & Vonderheide, 2014). Referral to an endocrinologist should be considered for all patients presenting with endocrine irAEs. Laboratory evaluation with TSH, free thyroxine (T4) hormone, total and free triiodothyronine (T3) hormone, cortisol, adrenocorticotropic hormone, luteinizing hormone, follicle-stimulating hormone, and testosterone (in men) can help establish a diagnosis of hypophysitis with hypopituitarism (Corsello et al., 2013).

If adrenal insufficiency manifests with sequelae of hypotension, dehydration, and electrolyte imbalances, hospitalization and stress-dose steroids should be initiated, even when ruling out other etiologies such as sepsis. Methylprednisolone 1–2 mg/kg/day or equivalent is the recommended starting dose and can be tapered once symptoms return to baseline. Some physiologic (low-dose) steroids and testosterone (in men) may be permanently required. Increased or stress-dose steroids prior to procedures may also be required. Concurrent, ongoing follow-up by an endocrinologist is optimal in long-term management of these patients.

Hyperthyroidism may also occur before patients become symptomatic and may be found with routine monitoring of thyroid function on treatment. If patients are symptomatic, this may represent acute thyroiditis secondary to immune activation. For symptomatic patients (e.g., emotional lability/anxiety, palpitations, tachycardia, tremor, increased appetite), recommended treatment is a beta-blocker and/or oral steroids (prednisolone 0.5 mg/kg and taper). Thyroiditis/Graves disease has also been observed with checkpoint inhibitor therapy and is treated with high-dose steroids (Fecher et al., 2013; Friedman et al., 2016).

Neurologic Toxicities

Neurologic symptoms associated with immunotherapy can be vague, mild, and transient (Fecher et al., 2013). If symptoms are more severe, neurologic consultation and evaluation with MRI are indicated. Neurologic toxicities occur in a range of severity, from sensory neuropathy or paresthesia, to more severe neurologic events, such as Guillain-Barré syndrome (Eggermont et al., 2015), myasthenia gravis (Johnson et al.,

2015; Loochtan, Nickolich, & Hobson-Webb, 2015), severe motor neuropathy, optic neuritis, enteric neuropathy with severe refractory constipation, inflammatory myopathy, and aseptic meningitis. These severe irAEs are very rare (less than 1% occurrence) (Bhatia, Huber, Upton, & Thompson, 2009; Tanaka et al., 2016).

Any patient presenting with severe immune-related neurotoxicities warrants immediate discontinuation of checkpoint inhibitor therapy. Treatment includes high-dose steroids, and IV Ig may be considered in concert with steroid administration. Permanent discontinuation of immune checkpoint inhibitor is warranted for all grade 3 or 4 neurologic events.

Other Toxicities

Checkpoint inhibitors may trigger a T-cell–mediated immune response in any part of the body. Less common toxicities have been observed in other body systems. Ophthalmic toxicities, particularly uveitis, may follow initiation of therapy (Weber et al., 2012). Referral to an ophthalmologist for examination and treatment with steroid eye drops is warranted for any patient with visual changes. Radiographic studies may be indicated to rule out central nervous system metastases. Checkpoint inhibitors may also result in nephritis or renal toxicity and should be held for patients with creatinine levels 1.5–6 times ULN. Treatment with high-dose steroids should continue until laboratory values return to baseline. Therapy should be permanently discontinued if creatinine level is more than 6 times ULN (Bristol-Myers Squibb Co., 2017b).

Cardiotoxicity is a rare irAE and has been reported after treatment with checkpoint inhibitor therapy. It is more common with combination ipilimumab and nivolumab compared to nivolumab alone (0.27% vs. 0.06%, respectively) (Haanen et al., 2017). Cardiotoxicity can present in a wide range of toxicities, including myocarditis, pericarditis, cardiomyopathy, arrhythmias (e.g., ventricular arrhythmia, atrial fibrillation), and hypertension. Consultation with a cardiologist is recommended if any cardiotoxicity is suspected or confirmed. For myocarditis, hospitalization and high-dose corticosteroids with 1–2 mg/kg prednisone or equivalent is recommended. Escalation to other immunosuppressive therapies is warranted if symptoms do not respond to steroids.

Other toxicities documented with checkpoint inhibitor administration include arthritis, pancreatitis, severe infection, and sepsis. In a study comparing atezolizumab to docetaxel, a higher rate of overall infections was seen in the atezolizumab arm (9.3% vs. 2.2% of grade 3 or 4 infection) (Fehrenbacher et al., 2016). Immune-related hematologic toxicities are rare but have been reported with checkpoint inhibitor therapies. Events such as neutropenia, anemia, and thrombocytopenia have been seen with checkpoint inhibitors. Other documented hematologic irAEs include thrombocytopenic purpura, hemolytic anemia, acquired hemophilia, and disseminated intravascular coagulopathy (Ahmad, Lewis, Corrie, & Iddawela, 2012; Brahmer et al., 2015). Cytopenia typically resolves with administration of high-dose steroids and discontinuation of the checkpoint inhibitor. If cytopenia persists, patients have improved with administration of IV Ig, with or without additional immune suppression (e.g., cyclosporine) (Friedman et al., 2016).

Treatment for these less common toxicities should be managed according to the package inserts for each drug, but general principles of management are similar for most irAEs. If symptoms are mild, the checkpoint inhibitor may or may not need to be held and/or administered with supportive care. If symptoms are more severe or potentially life threatening, therapy should be held, high-dose steroids should be administered, and specialty consultation or hospitalization should be considered. Immunotherapy should be held until symptoms return to baseline, but permanent discontinuation is indicated if the patient is not responsive to initial treatment or in the case of a grade 4 event.

Pregnancy and Lactation

Pregnant women should be educated on the potential fetal harms associated with immune checkpoint inhibitor therapy. Advise men and women of reproductive potential to use contraception while on immune checkpoint inhibitor therapy and for one to five months afterward (recommended duration varies by individual agent; see package insert). Infertility may result from taking these therapies. It is unknown whether PD-1/PD-L1 or CTLA-4 inhibitors cross into breast milk; women should discontinue breastfeeding while on these medications.

Summary

The landscape of cancer therapy continues to evolve and has broadened to include a new class of immunotherapy agents known as checkpoint inhibitors. Diseases that have had little to moderate gains in the recent past, such as melanoma and NSCLC, have experienced dramatically prolonged overall survival rates with checkpoint inhibitors. Clinical trials investigating combination therapies with checkpoint inhibitors (e.g., chemotherapy, targeted therapies, other immunotherapies) may provide even greater gains with various cancers in the future. Patients and families need to be aware of the signs and symptoms of toxicities related to checkpoint inhibitors and instructed to report them immediately, and clinicians need to initiate prompt evaluation and treatment to ensure the safety of these therapies.

References

Ahmad, S., Lewis, M., Corrie, P., & Iddawela, M. (2012). Ipilimumab-induced thrombocytopenia in a patient with metastatic melanoma. *Journal of Oncology Pharmacy Practice, 18,* 287–292. https://doi.org/10.1177/1078155211411001

Anderson, A.C. (2016). Tim-3: An emerging target in the cancer immunotherapy landscape. *Cancer Immunology Research, 2,* 393–399. https://doi.org/10.1158/2326-6066.CIR-14-0039

Andrews, S., & Holden, R. (2012). Characteristics and management of immune-related adverse effects associated with ipilimumab, a new immunotherapy for metastatic melanoma. *Cancer Management and Research, 4,* 299–307. https://doi.org/10.2147/CMAR.S31873

Ansell, S.M., Lesokhin, A.M., Borrello, I., Halwani, A., Scott, E.C., Gutierrez, M., … Armand, P. (2015). PD-1 blockade with nivolumab in relapsed or refractory Hodgkin's lymphoma. *New England Journal of Medicine, 372,* 311–319. https://doi.org/10.1056/NEJMoa1411087

Apolo, A.B., Infante, J.R., Balmanoukian, A., Patel, M.R., Wang, D., Kelly, K., … Gully, J.L. (2017). Avelumab, an anti-programmed death-ligand 1 antibody, in patients with refractory metastatic urothelial carcinoma: Results from a multicenter, phase Ib study. *Journal of Clinical Oncology, 35,* 2117–2124. https://doi.org/10.1200/JCO.2016.71.6795

AstraZeneca Pharmaceuticals LP. (2018). *Imfinzi® (durvalumab)* [Package insert]. Wilmington, DE: Author.

Bagley, S.J., Bauml, J.M., & Langer, C.J. (2015). PD-1/PD-L1 immune checkpoint blockade in patients with non-small cell lung cancer. *Clinical Advances in Hematology and Oncology, 13,* 676–683.

Barlesi, F., Park, K., Ciardiello, F., von Pawel, J., Gadgeel, S., Hida, T., … Rittmeyer, A. (2016). Primary analysis from OAK, a randomized phase III study comparing atezolizumab with docetaxel in 2L/3L NSCLC. *Annals of Oncology, 27*(Suppl. 6), Abstract LBA44_PR. https://doi.org/10.1093/annonc/mdw435.43

Bauzon, M., & Hermiston, T. (2014). Armed therapeutic viruses—A disruptive therapy on the horizon of cancer immunotherapy. *Frontiers in Immunology, 5,* 74. https://doi.org/10.3389/fimmu.2014.00074

Bhatia, S., Huber, B.R., Upton, M.P., & Thompson, J.A. (2009). Inflammatory enteric neuropathy with severe constipation after ipilimumab treatment for melanoma: A case report. *Journal of Immunotherapy, 32,* 203–205. https://doi.org/10.1097/CJI.0b013e318193a206

Brahmer, J., Reckamp, K.L., Bass, P., Crinò, L., Eberhardt, W.E.E., Poddubskaya, E., … Spigel, D.R. (2015). Nivolumab versus docetaxel in advanced squamous-cell non–small cell lung cancer. *New England Journal of Medicine, 373,* 123–135. https://doi.org/10.1056/NEJMoa1504627

Bristol-Myers Squibb Co. (2011). BLA 125377 YERVOY (ipilimumab) injection, for intravenous infusion: Risk evaluation and mitigation strategy. Retrieved from http://www.accessdata.fda.gov/drugsatfda_docs/label/2011/125377_REMS.pdf

Bristol-Myers Squibb Co. (2017a). *Opdivo® (nivolumab)* [Package insert]. Princeton, NJ: Author.

Bristol-Myers Squibb Co. (2017b). Opdivo® (nivolumab): Immune-mediated adverse reactions management guide. Retrieved from http://www.opdivohcp.com/servlet/servlet.FileDownload?file=00Pi000000ijs1vEAA

Bristol-Myers Squibb Co. (2018). *Yervoy® (ipilimumab)* [Package insert]. Princeton, NJ: Author.

Brunet, J.-F., Denizot, F., Luciani, M.-F., Roux-Dosseto, M., Suzan, M., Mattei, M.-G., & Golstein, P. (1987). A new member of the immunoglobulin superfamily—CTLA-4. *Nature, 328,* 267–270. https://doi.org/10.1038/328267a0

Chen, L., & Flies, D.B. (2013). Molecular mechanisms of T cell co-stimulation and co-inhibition. *Natural Reviews Immunology, 13,* 227–242. https://doi.org/10.1038/nri3405

Cohen, E.E.W., Machiels, J.-P.H., Harrington, K.J., Burtness, B., Shin, S.W., Gause, C.K., ... Tourneau, C.L. (2015). KEYNOTE-040: A phase III randomized trial of pembrolizumab (MK-3475) versus standard treatment in patients with recurrent or metastatic head and neck cancer. *Journal of Clinical Oncology, 33,* Abstract TPS6084.

Corsello, S.M., Barnabei, A., Marchetti, P., De Vecchis, L., Salvatori, R., & Torino, F. (2013). Endocrine side effects induced by immune checkpoint inhibitors. *Journal of Clinical Endocrinology and Metabolism, 98,* 1361–1375. https://doi.org/10.1210/jc.2012-4075

Davies, M. (2016). How checkpoint inhibitors are changing the treatment paradigm in solid tumors: What advanced practitioners in oncology need to know. *Journal of the Advanced Practitioner in Oncology, 7,* 500–516. https://doi.org/10.6004/jadpro.2016.7.5.3

Disis, M.L. (2014). Mechanism of action of immunotherapy. *Seminars in Oncology, 41*(Suppl. 5), S3–S13. https://doi.org/10.1053/j.seminoncol.2014.09.004

Dolan, D.E., & Gupta, S. (2014). PD-1 pathway inhibitors: Changing the landscape of cancer immunotherapy. *Cancer Control, 21,* 231–237. https://doi.org/10.1177/107327481402100308

Downey, S.G., Klapper, J.A., Smith, F.O., Yang, J.C., Sherry, R.M., Royal, R.E., ... Rosenberg, S.A. (2007). Prognostic factors related to clinical response in patients with metastatic melanoma treated by CTL-associated antigen-4 blockade. *Clinical Cancer Research, 13,* 6681–6688. https://doi.org/10.1158/1078-0432.CCR-07-0187

Eggermont, A.M.M., Chiarion-Sileni, V., Grob, J.-J., Dummer, R., Wolchok, J.D., Schmidt, H., ... Testori, A. (2015). Adjuvant ipilimumab versus placebo after complete resection of high-risk stage III melanoma (EORTC 18071): A randomised, double-blind, phase 3 trial. *Lancet Oncology, 16,* 522–530. https://doi.org/10.1016/S1470-2045(15)70122-1

EMD Serono, Inc. (2017). *Bavencio® (avelumab)* [Package insert]. Rockland, MA: Author.

Fecher, L.A., Agarwala, S.S., Hodi, F.S., & Weber, J.S. (2013). Ipilimumab and its toxicities: A multidisciplinary approach. *Oncologist, 18,* 733–743. https://doi.org/10.1634/theoncologist.2012-0483

Fehrenbacher, L., Spira, A., Ballinger, M., Kowanetz, M., Vansteenkiste, J., Mazieres, J., ... Rittmeyer, A. (2016). Atezolizumab versus docetaxel for patients with previously treated non-small-cell lung cancer (POPLAR): A multicentre, open-label, phase 2 randomised controlled trial. *Lancet, 387,* 1837–1846. https://doi.org/10.1016/S0140-6736(16)00587-0

Ferris, R.L., Blumenschein, G., Jr., Fayette, J., Guigay, J., Colevas, A.D., Licitra, L., ... Gillison, M.L. (2016). Nivolumab for recurrent squamous-cell carcinoma of the head and neck. *New England Journal of Medicine, 375,* 1856–1867. https://doi.org/10.1056/NEJMoa1602252

Freeman, G.J., Gribben, J.G., Boussiotis, V.A., Restivo, V.A., Jr., Lombard, L.A., Gray, G.S., & Nadler, L.M. (1993). Cloning of B7-2: A CTLA-4 counter-receptor that costimulates human T cell proliferation. *Science, 262,* 909–911. https://doi.org/10.1126/science.7694363

Friedman, C.F., Proverbs-Singh, T.A., & Postow, M.A. (2016). Treatment of the immune-related adverse effects of immune checkpoint inhibitors: A review. *JAMA Oncology, 2,* 1346–1353. https://doi.org/10.1001/jamaoncol.2016.1051

Gangadhar, T.C., & Vonderheide, R.H. (2014). Mitigating the toxic effects of anticancer immunotherapy. *Nature Reviews Clinical Oncology, 11,* 91–99. https://doi.org/10.1038/nrclinonc.2013.245

Genentech, Inc. (2017). *Tecentriq® (atezolizumab)* [Package insert]. South San Francisco, CA: Author.

Gettinger, S.N., Horn, L., Gandhi, L., Spigel, D.R., Antonia, S.J., Rizvi, N.A., ... Brahmer, J.R. (2016). Overall survival and long-term safety of nivolumab (anti-programmed death 1 antibody, BMS-936558, ONO-4538) in patients with previously treated advanced non-small-cell lung cancer. *Journal of Clinical Oncology, 34,* 2004–2021. https://doi.org/10.1200/JCO.2014.58.3708

Haanen, J.B.A.G., Carbonnel, F., Robert, C., Kerr, K.M., Peters, S., Larkin, J., & Jordan, K. (2017). Management of toxicities from immunotherapy: ESMO clinical practice guidelines for diagnosis, treatment and follow-up. *Annals of Oncology, 28*(Suppl. 4), iv119–iv142. https://doi.org/10.1093/annonc/mdx225

Hansen, A.R., & Siu, L.L. (2016). PD-L1 testing in cancer: Challenges in companion diagnostic development. *JAMA Oncology, 2,* 15–16. https://doi.org/10.1001/jamaoncol.2015.4685

Herbst, R.S., Gordon, M.S., Fine, G.D., Sosman, J.A., Soria, J.-C., Hamid, O., ... Hodi, F.S. (2013). A study of MPDL3280A, an engineered PD-L1 antibody in patients with locally advanced or metastatic tumors. *Journal of Clinical Oncology, 31*(Suppl. 15), 3000.

Hiniker, S.M., Maecker, H.T., & Knox, S.J. (2015). Predictors of clinical response to immunotherapy with or without radiotherapy. *Journal of Radiation Oncology, 4,* 339–345. https://doi.org/10.1007/s13566-015-0219-2

Hiraoka, N. (2010). Tumor-infiltrating lymphocytes and hepatocellular carcinoma: Molecular biology. *International Journal of Clinical Oncology, 15,* 544–551. https://doi.org/10.1007/s10147-010-0130-1

Hodi, F.S., O'Day, S.J., McDermott, D.F., Weber, R.W., Sosman, J.A., Haanen, J.B., ... Urba, W.J. (2010). Improved survival with ipilimumab in patients with metastatic melanoma. *New England Journal of Medicine, 363,* 711–723. https://doi.org/10.1056/NEJMoa1003466

Hoffman-Censits, J.H., Grivas, P., Van Der Heijden, M.S., Dreicer, R., Loriot, Y., Retz, M., ... Rosenberg, J.E. (2016). IMvigor 210, a phase II trial of atezolizumab (MPDL3280A) in platinum-treated locally advanced or metastatic urothelial carcinoma (mUC). *Journal of Clinical Oncology, 34*(Suppl. 2S), Abstract 355. https://doi.org/10.1200/jco.2016.34.2_suppl.355

Huard, B., Gaulard, P., Faure, F., Hercend, T., & Triebel, F. (1994). Cellular expression and tissue distribution of the human LAG-3-encoded protein, an MHC class II ligand. *Immunogenetics, 39,* 213–217. https://doi.org/10.1007/BF00241263

Hu-Lieskovan, S., Robert, L., Homet Moreno, B., & Ribas, A. (2014). Combining targeted therapy with immunotherapy in *BRAF*-mutant melanoma: Promise and challenges. *Journal of Clinical Oncology, 32,* 2248–2254. https://doi.org/10.1200/JCO.2013.52.1377

Ishida, Y., Agata, Y., Shibahara, K., & Honjo, T. (1992). Induced expression of PD-1, a novel member of the immunoglobulin gene superfamily, upon programmed cell death. *European Molecular Biology Organization, 11,* 3887–3895.

Jensen, S.M., Maston, L.D., Gough, M.J., Ruby, C.E., Redmond, W.L., Crittenden, M., ... Fox, B.A. (2010). Signaling through OX40 enhances antitumor immunity. *Seminars in Oncology, 37,* 524–532. https://doi.org/10.1053/j.seminoncol.2010.09.013

Johnson, D.B., Saranga-Perry, V., Lavin, P.J.M., Burnette, W.B., Clark, S.W., Uskavitch, D.R., ... Sosman, J.A. (2015). Myasthenia gravis induced by ipilimumab in patients with metastatic melanoma. *Journal of Clinical Oncology, 33,* 122–124. https://doi.org/10.1200/JCO.2013.51.1683

Johnson, D.B., Sullivan, R.J., Ott, P.A., Carlino, M.S., Khushalani, N.I., Ye, F., ... Clark, J.I. (2016). Ipilimumab therapy in patients with advanced melanoma and preexisting autoimmune disorders. *JAMA Oncology, 2,* 234–240. https://doi.org/10.1001/jamaoncol.2015.4368

Kazandjian, D., Suzman, D.L., Blumenthal, G., Mushti, S., He, K., Libeg, M., ... Pazdur, R. (2016). FDA approval summary: Nivolumab for the treatment of metastatic non-small cell lung cancer with progression on or after platinum-based chemotherapy. *Oncologist, 21,* 634–642. https://doi.org/10.1634/theoncologist.2015-0507

Kim, J.W., & Eder, J.P. (2014). Prospects for targeting PD-1 and PD-L1 in various tumor types. *Oncology, 28*(Suppl. 3), 15–28. Retrieved from http://www.cancernetwork.com/oncology-journal/prospects-targeting-pd-1-and-pd-l1-various-tumor-types/page/0/1

Kohrt, H.E., Thielens, A., Marabelle, A., Sagiv-Barfi, I., Sola, C., Chanuc, F., ... André, P. (2014). Anti-KIR antibody enhancement of anti-lymphoma activity of natural killer cells as monotherapy and in combination with anti-CD20 antibodies. *Blood, 123,* 678–686. https://doi.org/10.1182/blood-2013-08-519199

Kreamer, K.M. (2014). Immune checkpoint blockade: A new paradigm in treating advanced cancer. *Journal of the Advanced Practitioner in Oncology, 5,* 418–431.

Lacouture, M.E., Wolchok, J.D., Yosipovitch, G., Kähler, K.C., Busam, K.J., & Hauschild, A. (2014). Ipilimumab in patients with cancer and the management of dermatologic adverse events. *Journal of the American Academy of Dermatology, 71,* 161–169. https://doi .org/10.1016/j.jaad.2014.02.035

Larkin, J., Chiarion-Sileni, V., Gonzalez, R., Grob, J.J., Cowey, C.L., Lao, C.D., ... Wolchok, J.D. (2015). Combined nivolumab and ipilimumab or monotherapy in untreated melanoma. *New England Journal of Medicine, 373,* 23–34. https://doi.org/10.1056/NEJMoa1504030

Leach, D.R., Krummel, M.F., & Allison, J.P. (1996). Enhancement of antitumor immunity by CTLA-4 blockade. *Science, 271,* 1734–1736. https://doi.org/10.1126/science.271.5256 .1734

Linch, S.N., McNamara, M.J., & Redmond, W.L. (2015). OX40 agonists and combination immunotherapy: Putting the pedal to the medal. *Frontiers in Oncology, 5,* 1–14. https:// doi.org/10.3389/fonc.2015.00034

Linsley, P.S., Bradshaw, J., Greene, J.L., Peach, R., Bennett, K.L., & Mittler, R.S. (1996). Intracellular trafficking of CTLA-4 and focal localization towards sites of TCR engagement. *Immunity, 4,* 535–543. https://doi.org/10.1016/S1074-7613(00)80480-X

Linsley, P.S., Greene, J.L., Brady, W., Bajorath, J., Ledbetter, J.A., & Peach, R. (1991). Human B7-1 (CD80) and B7-2 (CD86) bind with similar avidities but distinct kinetics to CD28 and CTLA-4 receptors. *Immunity, 1,* 793–801. https://doi.org/10.1016/S1074-7613(94)80021-9

Liu, D., Wang, S., & Bindeman, W. (2017). Clinical applications of PD-L1 bioassays for cancer immunotherapy. *Journal of Hematology and Oncology, 10,* 110. https://doi.org/10 .1186/s13045-017-0479-y

Loochtan, A.I., Nickolich, M.S., & Hobson-Webb, L.D. (2015). Myasthenia gravis associated with ipilimumab and nivolumab in the treatment of small cell lung cancer. *Muscle and Nerve, 52,* 307–308. https://doi.org/10.1002/mus.24648

Lynch, T.J., Bondarenko, I., Luft, A., Serwatowski, P., Barlesi, F., Chacko, R., ... Reck, M. (2012). Ipilimumab in combination with paclitaxel and carboplatin as first-line treatment in stage IIIB/IV non–small-cell lung cancer: Results from a randomized, double-blind, multicenter phase II study. *Journal of Clinical Oncology, 30,* 2046–2054. https://doi.org /10.1200/JCO.2011.38.4032

Mansfield, A.S., Park, S.S., & Dong, H. (2015). Synergy of cancer immunotherapy and radiotherapy. *Aging, 7,* 144–145. https://doi.org/10.18632/aging.100730

McCoy, K.D., & Le Gros, G. (1999). The role of CTLA-4 in the regulation of T cell immune responses. *Immunology and Cell Biology, 77,* 1–10. https://doi.org/10.1046/j.1440-1711 .1999.00795.x

Merck and Co., Inc. (2017). *Keytruda® (pembrolizumab)* [Package insert]. Whitehouse Station, NJ: Author.

Momtaz, P., Park, V., Panageas, K.S., Postow, M.A., Callahan, M., Wolchok, J.D., & Chapman, P.B. (2015). Safety of infusing ipilimumab over 30 Minutes. *Journal of Clinical Oncology, 33,* 3454–3458. https://doi.org/10.1200/JCO.2015.61.0030

Motzer, R.J., Escudier, B., McDermott, D.F., George, S., Hammers, H.J., Srinivas, S., ... Sharma, P. (2015). Nivolumab versus everolimus in advanced renal-cell carcinoma. *New England Journal of Medicine, 373,* 1803–1813. https://doi.org/10.1056/NEJMoa1510665

Naidoo, J., Wang, X., Woo, K.M., Iyriboz, T., Halpenny, D., Cunningham, J., ... Hellmann, M.D. (2017). Pneumonitis in patients treated with anti-programmed death-1/programmed death ligand-1 therapy. *Journal of Clinical Oncology, 35,* 709–717. https://doi.org/10.1200 /JCO.2016.68.2005

Pardoll, D.M. (2012). The blockade of immune checkpoints in cancer immunotherapy. *Nature Reviews Cancer, 12,* 252–264. https://doi.org/10.1038/nrc3239

Postow, M.A., Chesney, J., Pavlick, A.C., Robert, C., Grossmann, K., McDermott, D., ... Hodi, F.S. (2015). Nivolumab and ipilimumab versus ipilimumab in untreated melanoma. *New England Journal of Medicine, 372,* 2006–2017. https:// doi.org/10.1056/NEJMoa1414428

Reck, M., Rodríguez-Abreu, D., Robinson, A.G., Hui, R., Csőszi, T., Fülöp, A., ... Brahmer, J.R. (2016). Pembrolizumab versus chemotherapy for PD-L1–positive non–small-cell lung cancer. *New England Journal of Medicine, 375,* 1823–1833. https://doi.org/10.1056 /NEJMoa1606774

Rizvi, N.A., Mazières, J., Planchard, D., Stinchcombe, T.E., Dy, G.K., Antonia, S.J., ... Rama-lingam, S.S. (2015). Activity and safety of nivolumab, an anti-PD-1 immune checkpoint inhibitor, for patients with advanced, refractory squamous non-small-cell lung cancer (CheckMate 063): A phase 2, single-arm trial. *Lancet Oncology, 16*, 257–265. https://doi .org/10.1016/S1470-2045(15)70054-9

Robert, C., Schachter, J., Long, G.V., Arance, A., Grob, J.J., Mortier, L., ... Ribas, A. (2015). Pembrolizumab versus ipilimumab in advanced melanoma. *New England Journal of Medicine, 372*, 2521–2532. https://doi.org/10.1056/NEJMoa1503093

Robert, C., Thomas, L., Bondarenko, I., O'Day, S., Weber, J., Garbe, C., ... Wolchok, J.D. (2011). Ipilimumab plus dacarbazine for previously untreated metastatic melanoma. *New England Journal of Medicine, 364*, 2517–2526. https://doi.org/10.1056/NEJMoa1104621

Rozali, E.N., Hato, S.V., Robinson, B.W., Lake, R.A., & Lesterhuis, W.J. (2012). Programmed death ligand 2 in cancer-induced immune suppression. *Clinical and Developmental Immunology, 2012*, 656340. https://doi.org/10.1155/2012/656340

Rudd, C.E., Taylor, A., & Schneider, H. (2009). CD28 and CTLA-4 coreceptor expression and signal transduction. *Immunological Reviews, 229*, 12–26. https://doi.org/10.1111 /j.1600-065X.2009.00770.x

Sánchez-Fueyo, A. (2003). Tim-3 inhibits T helper type 1-mediated auto- and alloimmune responses and promotes immunological tolerance. *Nature Immunology, 4*, 1093–1101. https://doi.org/10.1038/ni987

Tanaka, R., Maruyama, H., Tomidokoro, Y., Yanagiha, K., Hirabayashi, T., Ishii, A., ... Fujimoto, M. (2016). Nivolumab-induced chronic inflammatory demyelinating poly-radiculoneuropathy mimicking rapid-onset Guillain–Barré syndrome: A case report. *Japanese Journal of Clinical Oncology, 46*, 875–878. https://doi.org/10.1093/jjco/ hyw090

Taube, J.M., Klein, A., Brahmer, J.R., Xu, H., Pan, X., Kim, J.H., ... Anders, R.A. (2014). Association of PD-1, PD-1 ligands, and other features of the tumor immune microenviron-ment with response to anti–PD-1 therapy. *Clinical Cancer Research, 20*, 5064–5074. https:// doi.org/10.1158/1078-0432.CCR-13-3271

Teft, W.A., Kirchhof, M.G., & Madrenas, J. (2006). A molecular perspective of CTLA-4 function. *Annual Review of Immunology, 24*, 65–97. https://doi.org/10.1146/annurev .immunol.24.021605.090535

Teulings, H.-E. (2015). Vitiligo-like depigmentation in patients with stage III-IV melanoma receiving immunotherapy and its association with survival: A systematic review and meta-analysis. *Journal of Clinical Oncology, 33*, 773–781. https://doi.org/10.1200/JCO .2014.57.4756

Topalian, S.L., Drake, C.G., & Pardoll, D.M. (2015). Immune checkpoint blockade: A common denominator approach to cancer therapy. *Cancer Cell, 27*, 450–461. https:// doi.org/10.1016/j.ccell.2015.03.001

Villadolid, J., & Amin, A. (2015). Immune checkpoint inhibitors in clinical practice: Update on management of immune-related toxicities. *Translational Lung Cancer Research, 4*, 560–575. https://doi.org/10.3978/j.issn.2218-6751.2015.06.06

Vonderheide, R.H., LoRusso, P.M., Khalil, M., Gartner, E.M., Khaira, D., Soulieres, D., ... Domcheck, S.M. (2010). Tremelimumab in combination with exemestane in patients with advanced breast cancer and treatment-associated modulation of inducible costimulator expression on patient T cells. *Clinical Cancer Research, 16*, 3485–3494. https://doi.org/10 .1158/1078-0432.CCR-10-0505

Walker, L.S.K., & Sansom, D.M. (2011). The emerging role of CTLA4 as a cell-extrinsic regulator of T cell responses. *Nature Reviews Immunology, 11*, 852–863. https://doi.org /10.1038/nri3108

Weber, J.S., D'Angelo, S.P., Minor, D., Hodi, F.S., Gutzmer, R., Neyns, B., ... Larkin, J. (2015). Nivolumab versus chemotherapy in patients with advanced melanoma who progressed after anti–CTLA-4 treatment (CheckMate 037): A randomised, controlled, open-label, phase 3 trial. *Lancet Oncology, 16*, 375–384. https://doi.org/10.1016/S1470-2045(15) 70076-8

Weber, J.S., Kähler, K.C., & Hauschild, A. (2012). Management of immune-related adverse events and kinetics of response with ipilimumab. *Journal of Clinical Oncology, 30,* 2691–2697. https://doi.org/10.1200/JCO.2012.41.6750

Weber, J.S., Thompson, J.A., Hamid, O., Minor, D., Amin, A., Ron, I., ... O'Day, S. (2009). A randomized, double-blind, placebo-controlled, phase II study comparing the tolerability and efficacy of ipilimumab administered with or without prophylactic budesonide in patients with unresectable stage III or IV melanoma. *Clinical Cancer Research, 15,* 5591–5598. https://doi.org/10.1158/1078-0432.CCR-09-1024

Wolchok, J.D., Hoos, A., O'Day, S., Weber, J.S., Hamid, O., Lebbé, C., ... Hodi, F.S. (2009). Guidelines for the evaluation of immune therapy activity in solid tumors: Immune-related response criteria. *Clinical Cancer Research, 15,* 7412–7420. https://doi.org/10.1158/1078 -0432.CCR-09-1624

Wolchok, J.D., Kluger, H., Callahan, M.K., Postow, M.A., Rizvi, N.A., Lesokhin, A.M., ... Sznol, M. (2013). Nivolumab plus ipilimumab in advanced melanoma. *New England Journal of Medicine, 369,* 122–133. https://doi.org/10.1056/NEJMoa1302369

Younes, A., Santoro, A., Zinzani, P.L., Timmerman, J., Ansell, S.M., & Armand, P. (2016). CheckMate 205: Nivolumab (nivo) in classical Hodgkin lymphoma (cHL) after autologous stem cell transplant (ASCT) and brentuximab vedotin (BV)—A phase 2 study. *Journal of Clinical Oncology, 35,* Abstract 7535.

Zitvogel, L., Apetoh, L., Ghiringhelli, F., & Kroemer, G. (2011). Immunological aspects of cancer chemotherapy. *Nature Reviews Immunology, 8,* 59–73. https://doi.org/10.1038 /nri2216 *c h a p t e r f i v e*

Bacillus Calmette-Guérin

Elizabeth Prechtel Dunphy, DNP, RN, CRNP, BC, AOCN®

Introduction

Bacillus Calmette-Guérin (BCG) was the first successful immunotherapy in solid tumors and has endured in the treatment of intermediate- and high-risk non-muscle invasive bladder cancer (NMIBC) for more than 40 years. BCG's success serves as "proof of principle" that immunotherapy for urothelial cancer is effective (Morales, 2017). Although its mechanism of action in bladder cancer is not fully understood, there is a broad understanding of how BCG activates the immune system and induces an inflammatory response. The desire for further understanding of this mechanism has ignited an aggressive exploration into this exciting form of anticancer therapy. This chapter will review the history of BCG, as well as its proposed mechanism of action, antitumor effects, optimal dosing, and side effects.

History

As early as 1891, the interaction between the immune system and cancer has been recognized (Donin et al., 2017). In 1908, Albert Calmette and Camille Guérin began development of an antituberculosis vaccine at the Pasteur Institute in Paris, France (Guérin, 1980). The eventual result of this work was BCG, an attenuated *Mycobacterium bovis* strain for vaccination against *Mycobacterium tuberculosis* (Oettinger, Jørgensen, Ladefoged, Hasløv, & Andersen, 1999). Daughter strains were extracted at various times and named after their manufacturer (e.g., TICE® BCG) or site of origin (e.g., Connaught, Tokyo) (Packiam, Johnson, & Steinberg, 2017).

Other studies would further the foundation for BCG. In 1929, Pearl observed that patients with tuberculosis had fewer malignant tumors

95

during autopsy. Nearly 50 years later, Zbar and Rapp (1974) performed animal research on guinea pigs with cancer that defined the conditions necessary to obtain an antitumor effect with BCG. Such conditions include the ability to develop an immune response to mycobacteria antigens, an adequate number of living bacilli, close contact between BCG and tumor cells, and small tumor burden. In 1976, a seminal report by Morales, Eidinger, and Bruce linked BCG with superficial bladder cancer responses. These findings were replicated in prospective, randomized trials, leading to the eventual approval of intravesicular BCG in 1990 (Donin et al., 2017).

BCG has become one of the most successful immunotherapies in cancer treatment. It is the gold standard for high-risk patients with NMIBC and is superior to any single chemotherapeutic agent for reducing NMIBC recurrence and progression (Askeland, Newton, O'Donnell, & Luo, 2012; Donin et al., 2017; Sylvester, van der Meijden, Witjes, & Kurth, 2005; van der Meijden & Sylvester, 2003). A Cochrane meta-analysis of 585 patients over six randomized clinical trials noted that BCG decreased the risk of NMIBC recurrence at one year by 70% compared to transurethral resection of the bladder alone (Shelley et al., 2000).

Mechanism of Action

BCG's exact antitumor mechanism of action is not clearly defined. Rather, it is a complex cascade of immunomodulatory processes. A long-standing recognition exists that the effects of BCG are mediated by the immune system. Successful treatment depends on an intact immune system and direct contact with live BCG (Lamm et al., 1980; Packiam et al., 2017). Genetic conditions as well as BCG dose and schedule can influence antitumor effects (van der Meijden & Sylvester, 2003).

BCG works via activation of the immune system and induction of an inflammatory response (Donin et al., 2017). After BCG is instilled into the bladder, it binds to fibronectin expressed on the urothelium, allowing for attachment to the urothelium. BCG antigens are presented at the cell surfaces of urothelial and antigen-presenting cells in the context of the major histocompatibility complex class II. This presentation stimulates CD4+ T cells and induces a type 1 T helper (Th1) immune response (Zuiverloon et al., 2012). Once attached to the urothelium, the mycobacteria are internalized by urothelial and dendritic cells, which release cytokines, including interleukins (ILs), interferon gamma–inducible protein 10, tumor necrosis factor-alpha, granulocyte macrophage–colony-stimulating factor, and interferon gamma (Lou, Chen, & O'Donnell, 2003). Cell death results from direct cytotoxicity and release of apoptotic factors (Kavoussi, Brown, Ritchey, & Ratliff, 1990;

Packiam et al., 2017). This immune response results in secretion of cyto-kines. The exact role these cytokines play is not completely understood.

Evidence exists that an intact Th1 proinflammatory immune response is implicated in BCG's response to bladder cancer and immunosurveil-lance. BCG treatment failures are associated with defects in IL-2, IL-12, or interferon production (Askeland et al., 2012; Wu, Enting, Rudman, & Chowdhury, 2015).

Nursing Administration

Not every patient with superficial bladder cancer is treated with BCG. Millán-Rodríguez et al. (2000) defined risk groups by stratify-ing patients by cancer stage, tumor grade, evidence of carcinoma in situ, and number of tumors. Groups were low, intermediate, and high risk. Adjuvant treatment with BCG is recommended for patients in the intermediate- and high-risk groups.

In Morales' initial work in 1976, BCG was dosed on a weekly basis for six weeks. This schedule continues to be used (Packiam et al., 2017). Multiple trials advocate for BCG continuation beyond induction. The American Urological Association and European Association of Urol-ogy recommend maintenance therapy but give no specifics for sched-ule or duration (Packiam et al., 2017). In 2000, the Southwest Oncology Group conducted a landmark study for BCG dosing, recommend-ing three weekly instillations at three months, six months, and every six months thereafter for three years after initial induction (Lamm et al., 2000). This determination was based on improvements in response rates, recurrence-free survival, and progression-free survival (Lamm et al., 2000). The additional instillations increased the complete response rate in carcinoma in situ from the expected 68% to 84%. With mainte-nance BCG, long-term tumor recurrence in high-risk patients reduced from the expected 52% with a single six-week course to only 25%. Progression-free survival increased from 86% at four years observed with induction therapy to 92% in patients receiving maintenance BCG (Brausi et al., 2014; Lamm et al., 2000). This is reflected in the dosing for Theracys® (BCG live [intravesical]) and TICE BCG (Lamm, McGee, & Hale, 2005; Organon Teknika Corporation LLC, 2009; Sanofi-Aventis U.S., LLC, 2006).

Standard induction therapy of Theracys is 81 mg intravesical admin-istered for six consecutive weeks (Sanofi-Aventis U.S., LLC, 2006). The maintenance therapy dose is 81 mg intravesical given at 3, 6, 12, 18, and 24 months following the initial dose. Theracys is contained in an 81 mg vial of freeze-dried BCG that is reconstituted and diluted in 50 ml of sterile, preservative-free saline (Sanofi-Aventis U.S., LLC, 2006).

A TICE BCG dose is 50 mg diluted in 50 ml of sterile, preservative-free saline with a standard treatment schedule of one intravesical instillation per week for six weeks (Organon Teknika Corporation LLC, 2009). This schedule may be repeated once if tumor remission has not been achieved or if clinical circumstances warrant. Thereafter, intravesical TICE BCG administration should continue at monthly intervals for at least 6–12 months (Organon Teknika Corporation LLC, 2009).

Contraindications to treatment with intravesical BCG include known systemic hypersensitivity reaction to any component of the vaccine or after a previous administration of vaccine, immunosuppression due to congenital or acquired immune deficiencies, concurrent disease, cancer therapy or immunosuppressive therapy, symptoms or a previous history of systemic BCG reaction, concurrent febrile illness, urinary tract infection, macroscopic hematuria, and active tuberculosis (Organon Teknika Corporation LLC, 2009; Sanofi-Aventis U.S., LLC, 2006).

To avoid cross contamination, parenteral drugs cannot be prepared in areas where intravesical BCG has been prepared. All equipment, supplies, and receptacles in contact with BCG should be handled and disposed as biohazardous waste (or material). Gloves, eye protection, and precautions to avoid BCG contact with broken skin are recommended. In addition, if the preparation cannot be performed in a biocontainment hood, a mask and gown are recommended. Aseptic techniques should be used. Exposure of BCG to artificial light should be kept to a minimum (Games, 1996; Organon Teknika Corporation LLC, 2009; Sanofi-Aventis U.S., LLC, 2006).

Intravesical BCG is administered after a urethral catheter is inserted into the bladder under aseptic conditions. The bladder is drained, and a 50 ml suspension of Theracys or TICE BCG is instilled slowly by gravity. The catheter is withdrawn at the end of the instillation. It is recommended that the patient retain the suspension for as long as possible for up to two hours. During the first 15 minutes following instillation, the patient should lie prone. Thereafter, allow the patient to be in an upright position. At the end of two hours, have the patient void in a seated position (for safety reasons). Patient discharge instructions should advise an increase in fluid intake to flush the bladder in the hours following treatment (Boyd, 2003; Organon Teknika Corporation LLC, 2009; Packiam et al., 2017; Sanofi-Aventis U.S., LLC, 2006).

Any unused product, packaging, or equipment/materials for product instillation (e.g., syringes, catheters) should be disposed of in a biohazard container in accordance with local requirements applicable to biohazardous materials. For six hours after treatment, voided urine should be disinfected by adding an equal volume of household bleach (5%

hypochlorite solution) into the toilet bowl and allowing the bleach and urine to stand for 15 minutes prior to flushing (Organon Teknika Corporation LLC, 2009; Sanofi-Aventis U.S., LLC, 2006).

Side Effects

BCG induces an antitumor response in bladder cancer by drawing lymphocytes and macrophages to the bladder and stimulating a cellular immune response. Cytokines associated with this response result in bladder inflammation and flu-like symptoms. The primary side effects of BCG are local because of the route of administration. The most common adverse reactions observed with intravesical BCG treatment include transient dysuria, urinary frequency and urgency, malaise, hematuria, fever, chills, cystitis, and mild nausea. Symptoms of bladder irritability were reported in approximately 50% of patients receiving intravesical BCG. This typically occurs 4–6 hours after instillation and lasts 24–72 hours (Askeland et al., 2012; Organon Teknika Corporation LLC, 2009; Packiam et al., 2017; Sanofi-Aventis U.S., LLC, 2006). Treatment of side effects is generally based on symptoms and includes management with painkillers and antispasmodics (Packiam et al., 2017).

BCG can also have systemic side effects, including arthralgia/arthritis, rash, fatigue, fever, and systemic BCG infection. Systemic BCG infection presents with pneumonitis, hepatitis, epididymitis, prostatitis, renal abscess, or sepsis (Askeland et al., 2012; Lamm et al., 2005; Packiam et al., 2017). If a patient develops persistent fever or experiences an acute febrile illness consistent with BCG infection, permanent discontinuation of BCG instillations is recommended. Treatment for BCG infection is recommended with two or more antimycobacterial agents while a diagnostic evaluation is performed. This evaluation should include cultures (Organon Teknika Corporation LLC, 2009; Sanofi-Aventis U.S., LLC, 2006).

A systemic BCG reaction is more likely to occur if intravesical BCG is administered within two weeks of biopsy, transurethral resection, or traumatic bladder catheterization, which is associated with hematuria. If a bacterial urinary tract infection occurs, treatment should be withheld until complete resolution of the infection. Immunosuppressants can interfere with the development of an immune response to intravesical BCG and increase the risk of disseminated BCG infection. Antimicrobal therapy for other infections may interfere with the effectiveness of intravesical BCG. Intravesical treatment with BCG may induce a positive response to a tuberculin skin test (Organon Teknika Corporation LLC, 2009; Sanofi-Aventis U.S., LLC, 2006).

Summary

BCG can stimulate a robust immune response and is the standard of care for treatment after surgical resection in patients with NMIBC. Despite this, cancer can recur or patients may not tolerate side effects. Multiple immunotherapies have been investigated as adjuncts with BCG or as replacements in animal models. The widespread use of immunotherapy in bladder cancer has sparked the need for additional clinical research and scientific exploration of tumor biology and human immunology (Askeland et al., 2012). It is increasingly evident that the immune system plays an important role in tumor development, as seen by the explosion of immune-directed therapies across cancer types. Comprehensive understanding of the factors underlying antitumor immune responses will further refine the clinical benefit of immunotherapy and assist in the management of side effects related to treatment. In addition, discovery and validation of biomarkers will support the revolutionary nature of immunotherapy (Tsiatas & Grivas, 2016), not only in genitourinary malignancies, but across all cancer diagnoses.

References

Askeland, E.J., Newton, M.R., O'Donnell, M.A., & Luo, Y. (2012). Bladder cancer immunotherapy: BCG and beyond. *Advances in Urology, 2012,* 181987. https://doi.org/10.1155/2012/181987

Boyd, L.A. (2003). Intravesical bacillus Calmette-Guérin for treating bladder cancer. *Urologic Nursing, 23,* 189–199.

Brausi, M., Oddens, J., Sylvester, R., Bono, A., van de Beek, C., van Andel, G., ... Oosterlinck, W. (2014). Side effects of bacillus Calmette-Guérin (BCG) in the treatment of intermediate- and high-risk Ta, T1 papillary carcinoma of the bladder: Results of the EORTC Genito-Urinary Cancer Group randomised phase 3 study comparing one-third dose with full dose and 1 year with 3 years of maintenance BCG. *European Urology, 65,* 69–76. https://doi.org/10.1016/j.eururo.2013.07.021

Donin, N.M., Lenis, A.T., Holden, S., Drakaki, A., Pantuck, A., Belldegrun, A., & Chamie, K. (2017). Immunotherapy for the treatment of urothelial carcinoma. *Journal of Urology, 197,* 14–22. https://doi.org/10.1016/j.juro.2016.02.3005

Games, J. (1996). Nursing implications in the management of superficial bladder cancer. *Seminars in Urologic Oncology, 14*(Suppl. 1), 36–40.

Guérin, C. (1980). The history of BCG. In S.R. Rosenthal (Ed.), *B.C.G. vaccine: Tuberculosis cancer* (pp. 35–43). Littleton, MA: PSG Publishing Company.

Kavoussi, L.R., Brown, E.J., Ritchey, J.K., & Ratliff, T.L. (1990). Fibronectin-mediated Calmette-Guérin bacillus attachment to murine bladder mucosa. Requirement for expression of an antitumor response. *Journal of Clinical Investigation, 85,* 62–67. https://doi.org/10.1172/JCI114434

Lamm, D.L., Blumenstein, B.A., Crissman, J.D., Montie, J.E., Gottesman, J.E., Lowe, B.A., ... Crawford, E.D. (2000). Maintenance bacillus Calmette-Guérin immunotherapy for recurrent TA, T1 and carcinoma in situ transitional cell carcinoma of the bladder: A randomized Southwest Oncology Group Study. *Journal of Urology, 163,* 1124–1129. https://doi.org/10.1016/S0022-5347(05)67707-5

Lamm, D.L., McGee, W.R., & Hale, K. (2005). Bladder cancer: Current optimal intravesical treatment. *Urologic Nursing, 25,* 323–332.

Lamm, D.L., Thor, D.E., Harris, S.C., Reyna, J.A., Stogdill, V.D., & Radwin, H.M. (1980). Bacillus Calmette-guerin immunotherapy of superficial bladder cancer. *Journal of Urology, 124,* 38–40. https://doi.org/10.1016/S0022-5347(17)55282-9

Lou, Y., Chen, X., & O'Donnell, M.A. (2003). Role of Th1 and Th2 cytokines in BCG-induced IFN-γ production: Cytokine promotion and simulation of BCG effect. *Cytokine, 21,* 17–26. https://doi.org/10.1016/S1043-4666(02)00490-8

Millán-Rodríguez, F., Chéchile-Toniolo, G., Salvador-Bayarri, J., Palou, J., Algaba, F., & Vincente-Rodríguez, J. (2000). Primary superficial bladder cancer risk groups according to progression, mortality and recurrence. *Journal of Urology, 164,* 680–684. https://doi.org/10.1016/S0022-5347(05)67280-1

Morales, A. (2017). BCG: A throwback from the stone age of vaccines opened the path for bladder cancer immunotherapy. *Canadian Journal of Urology, 24,* 8788–8793.

Morales, A., Eidinger, D., & Bruce, A.W. (1976). Intracavitary bacillus Calmette-Guérin in the treatment of superficial bladder tumors. *Journal of Urology, 116,* 180–182. https://doi.org/10.1016/S0022-5347(17)58737-6

Oettinger, T., Jørgenson, M., Ladefoged, A., Hasløv, K., & Andersen, P. (1999). Development of the *Mycobacterium bovis* BCG vaccine: Review of the historical and biochemical evidence for a genealogical tree. *Tubercle Lung Disease, 79,* 243–250. https://doi.org/10.1054/tuld.1999.0206

Organon Teknika Corporation LLC. (2009). *TICE® BCG (BCG live [for intravesical use])* [Package insert]. Durham, NC: Author.

Packiam, V.T., Johnson, S.C., & Steinberg, G.D. (2017). Non–muscle-invasive bladder cancer: Intravesical treatments beyond bacille Calmette-Guérin. *Cancer, 123,* 390–400. https://doi.org/10.1002/cncr.30392

Pearl, R. (1929). Cancer and tuberculosis. *American Journal of Epidemiology, 9,* 97–159. https://doi.org/10.1093/oxfordjournals.aje.a121646

Sanofi-Aventis U.S., LLC. (2006). *Theracys® (BCG live [intravesical])* [Package insert]. Swiftwater, PA: Author.

Shelley, M., Court, J.B., Kynaston, H., Wilt, T.J., Fish, R., & Mason, M. (2000). Intravesical bacillus Calmette-Guérin in TA and T1 bladder cancer. *Cochrane Database of Systematic Reviews, 2000*(4). https://doi.org/10.1002/14651858.CD001986

Sylvester, R.J., van der Meijden, A.P.M., Witjes, J.A., & Kurth, K.H. (2005). Bacillus Calmette-Guérin versus chemotherapy for the intravesical treatment of patients with carcinoma in situ of the bladder: A meta-analysis of the published results of randomized clinical trials. *Journal of Urology, 174,* 86–91. https://doi.org/10.1097/01.ju.0000162059.64886.1c

Tsiatas, M., & Grivas, P. (2016). Immunobiology and immunotherapy in genitourinary malignancies. *Annals of Translational Medicine, 4,* 270. https://doi.org/10.21037/atm.2016.06.29

van der Meijden, A.P.M., & Sylvester, R.J. (2003). BCG immunotherapy for superficial bladder cancer: An overview of the past, the present and the future. *European Association of Urology Update Series, 1,* 80–86. https://doi.org/10.1016/S1570-9124(03)00016-3

Wu, Y., Enting, D., Rudman, S., & Chowdhury, S. (2015). Immunotherapy for urothelial cancer: From BCG to checkpoint inhibitors and beyond. *Expert Review of Anticancer Therapy, 15,* 509–523. https://doi.org/10.1586/14737140.2015.1015419

Zbar, B., & Rapp, H.J. (1974). Immunotherapy of guinea pig cancer with BCG. *Cancer, 34*(Suppl. 8), 1532–1540. https://doi.org/10.1002/1097-0142(197410)34:8+<1532::AID-CNCR2820340827>3.0.CO;2-H

Zuiverloon, T.C., Nieuweboer, A.J., Vékony, H., Kirkels, W.J., Bangma, C.H., & Zwarthoff, E.C. (2012). Markers predicting response to bacillus Calmette-Guérin immunotherapy in high-risk bladder cancer patients: A systematic review. *European Urology, 61,* 128–145. https://doi.org/10.1016/j.eururo.2011.09.026

chapter six

Oral Immunomodulatory Agents

Kevin Brigle, PhD, NP

Introduction

Immunomodulatory agents are a class of drugs that exert a wide range of both stimulatory and inhibitory effects on the immune system. These agents were created by the unlikely repurposing of thalidomide, a drug pulled from the world market in the 1960s because of its extraordinary fetal toxicity. Although access to prescription and distribution is rigorously controlled, the immunomodulatory properties of these agents have given them a prominent role in the successful treatment of several hematologic malignancies.

History

The resounding success of immunomodulatory drugs (IMiDs) for the treatment of cancer could not have been predicted based on the history of thalidomide, the original agent in this class of drugs. Thalidomide is a glutamic acid derivative that was initially synthesized in 1953 by the Swiss pharmaceutical company Ciba Inc. When Ciba Inc. found no pharmacologic use for the agent, the West German pharmaceutical company Chemie Grünenthal GmbH developed and marketed thalidomide as an anticonvulsant for the treatment of epilepsy (Randall, 1990). Although it was generally ineffective for this use, thalidomide had a rapid-onset sedative effect with little morning hangover. Even large doses of the drug were not lethal. Because of this, it quickly became a popular over-the-counter sleeping aid. At the height of its popularity, thalidomide was marketed as a safe, multipotent drug for a host of conditions, including irritability, stage fright, premature ejaculation, hyperthyroidism, influenza, tuberculosis, and pregnancy-related morning sickness (Lenz, 1988). By 1960, it was marketed by 14 pharmaceutical companies under 37 names in 46 countries (Matthews & McCoy, 2003). However, U.S. Food and Drug Administration (FDA) approval of thalidomide was stalled in 1961 by Dr. Frances Oldham Kelsey, who was concerned about reports of irreversible peripheral neuropathy in adults who used the drug (Fullerton & Kremer, 1961). This bothersome side effect was overshadowed by two separate reports describing serious limb and bowel defects in children born to mothers exposed to thalidomide during pregnancy (Lenz, Pfeiffer, Kosenow, & Hayman, 1962; McBride, 1961). Shortly after these publications, additional cases of fetal deformity came to light, and by 1962, the drug was pulled from the world market, remaining available only for strictly defined research purposes. Worldwide, it is estimated that 8,000–12,000 children were affected by thalidomide use, with an unknown number of associated miscarriages. These statistics vindicated Dr. Kelsey's insistence for additional data and further testing prior to FDA approval and led to the passage of rigorous new drug approval regulations in 1962. For her achievements, Dr. Kelsey was awarded the President's Award for Distinguished Federal Civilian Service that same year (Rouhi, 2005).

The story of thalidomide could have ended here; however, in 1964, a therapeutic effect from thalidomide was noted in a patient suffering from erythema nodosum leprosum (ENL), an inflammatory complication of leprosy manifested by fevers, night sweats, and painful nodular skin lesions. Thalidomide was given as a sedative, and surprisingly, the patient experienced rapid subjective and objective improvements in ENL symptoms. Over the next 12 months, similar responses were seen in five additional patients (Sheskin, 1965). These case reports led to two randomized clinical trials that confirmed the efficacy of thalidomide for treating ENL in this patient population (Iyer et al., 1971; Sheskin & Convit, 1969). Despite the success of these studies, thalidomide was not FDA approved for this indication until 1998. As part of the approval process, U.S. manufacturer Celgene Corp. developed a comprehensive and restrictive prescribing, dispensing, and monitoring program called S.T.E.P.S. (System for Thalidomide Education and Prescribing Safety) to safeguard against fetal exposure to the drug. This mandatory program controlled access to the drug, monitored compliance, and provided education to patients, prescribers, and pharmacists (Zeldis, Williams, Thomas, & Elsayed, 1999). It was later renamed the REMS (Risk Evaluation and Mitigation Strategy) program. All subsequent analogs derived from thalidomide have nearly identical programs to which patients, prescribers, and pharmacists must register.

Mechanism of Action

Although unknown in the 1960s, acute outbreaks of ENL were later found to be characterized by very high serum levels of the proinflammatory cytokine tumor necrosis factor-alpha (TNF-α). The efficacy of thalidomide in treating ENL was shown to be associated with down-regulation of TNF-α production by peripheral blood monocytes (Sampaio, Sarno, Galilly, Cohn, & Kaplan, 1991). This observation spurred interest in using thalidomide for conditions with related inflammatory symptoms, including aphthous stomatitis, Behçet disease, prurigo nodularis, rheumatoid arthritis, and graft-versus-host disease (Calabrese & Fleischer, 2000). Although thalidomide did not show the same level of efficacy with these conditions, research on the drug continued.

In the early 1990s, D'Amato, Loughnan, Flynn, and Folkman (1994) reported thalidomide as a potent inhibitor of angiogenesis, a property thought to cause the drug's teratogenic effects. This led to testing for the treatment of malignancies in which the formation of new blood vessels was a known part of the malignant phenotype.

In 1999, a landmark study by Singhal et al. reported on the efficacy and safety of single-agent thalidomide in 84 patients with highly chemotherapy-refractory myeloma. The drug showed an impressive 32% response rate, including many complete responses, but interestingly, it had no effect on the microvascular density of the patients' bone marrow. The authors suggested that thalidomide's activity might be explained by other properties of the drug that altered the activity of the immune system. Indeed, in the year prior to their publication, thalidomide was found to costimulate the proliferation and tumor-killing activity of CD8+ cytotoxic T cells and enhance the secretion of interleukin-2 and interferon lambda (Haslett, Corral, Albert, & Kaplan, 1998). Over the next decade, additional studies demonstrated that thalidomide also enhanced the activity of natural killer (NK) cells, disrupted the interaction between plasma cells and their bone marrow microenvironment, and exhibited direct antitumor effects such as cell cycle arrest (Quach et al., 2010; Sedlarikova, Kubiczkova, Sevcikova, & Hajek, 2012).

It was not until 2010 that the intracellular target of thalidomide was identified, thus providing an understanding of how the drug mediated its pleiotropic effects on the immune system. Thalidomide was found to bind cereblon, a protein that negatively regulates the growth and proliferation of B cells by tagging specific downstream regulatory proteins for destruction (Ito et al., 2010). In the presence of thalidomide, the affinity of cereblon to bind these regulatory proteins increases, resulting in enhanced inhibition of B-cell growth and proliferation. Lenalidomide and pomalidomide, more potent derivatives of thalidomide (see Figure 6-1), were synthesized in the early 2000s and have undergone extensive clinical testing. In comparison to thalidomide, these drugs exhibit increased cytokine control and antineoplastic activity with fewer side effects. Both have gained FDA approval. The differential therapeutic efficacy of these new IMiDs is based on their unique sites of cereblon protein binding (Lopez-Girona et al., 2012).

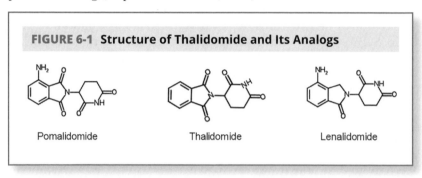

FIGURE 6-1 Structure of Thalidomide and Its Analogs

Pomalidomide   Thalidomide   Lenalidomide

Following the initial success of thalidomide in the treatment of multiple myeloma, the drug and its analogs were tested in hundreds of clinical trials for many cancer types. Although responses were seen in many B-cell malignancies, clinical trials for most other hematologic malignancies and nearly all solid tumor cancers were not successful. Based on thalidomide's mechanism of action in regulating B-cell proliferation, these results were not surprising. Thus, nearly 50 years after its original synthesis and subsequent health catastrophe, thalidomide and its analogs became classified as IMiDs because of their originally unidentified and certainly unanticipated regulation of the immune system. These properties have positioned IMiDs at the forefront of treatment in a variety of hematologic malignancies, including multiple myeloma. To date, multiple myeloma has been incurable, and patients with the disease have a relatively short survival time; however, in the decade following the introduction of IMiDs, newly diagnosed patients have seen a 50% improvement in overall survival (Kumar et al., 2008). With new drug combinations, the goal of treatment is shifting to a possible cure in a subset of patients. For those who cannot be cured, the focus is to manage this malignancy as a chronic disease with goals of long-term survival and high quality of life.

Risk Evaluation and Mitigation Strategy

Although the original REMS program was developed to protect against fetal exposure and birth defects, it later incorporated wording to alert patients, providers, and pharmacists to the increased risk of associated thromboembolic events. These serious and life-threatening events are common to IMiDs and listed as "black box" warnings in the package inserts for each drug. Warnings and requirements related to prevention of fetal harm are identical for each IMiD; however, they may differ depending on patient risk category. Because IMiDs can pass into semen, male patients are required to use at least two forms of contraception when having sex with women who are or could become pregnant. Likewise, women of child-bearing potential are instructed to use two forms of birth control and take monthly pregnancy tests. Both risk groups must take mandatory monthly surveys to attest adherence to these requirements. For women without child-bearing potential, no special requirements exist; however, they must complete a survey every six months to refresh their knowledge of drug-associated risks.

Thromboembolic events associated with IMiDs include deep vein thrombosis and pulmonary embolism. Although the mechanisms behind these events are unclear, they appear to be IMiD class effects. Thrombotic risk is increased when IMiDs are combined with other antimyeloma drugs, such as high-dose dexamethasone and carfilzomib.

As such, all patients taking an IMiD require thromboprophylaxis, the extent of which is based on thrombotic risk assessment and established guidelines. For patients with no risk factors, 325 mg daily aspirin is effective prophylaxis. However, patients with two or more risk factors require full anticoagulation with warfarin, low-molecular-weight heparin, or oral anticoagulants (Palumbo et al., 2008; Rome, Doss, Miller, & Westphal, 2008).

Clinical Applications

This section includes only FDA-approved indications for IMiDs. These agents in combination with other agents and novel therapies have been explored in numerous clinical trials and have led to additional approvals. As lenalidomide is synergistic with several agents, indications for its use can be found in the approved prescribing information of these other agents. Non–FDA-approved combinations are listed only as recommended by the National Comprehensive Cancer Network® (NCCN®, 2018a, 2018b). Based on promising clinical trials combining IMiDs with other agents, new FDA-approved indications for additional B-cell malignancies are on the horizon.

Thalidomide

Formulation

Thalidomide is available in 50, 100, 150, and 200 mg capsules. No IV formulations are used. Thalidomide undergoes biotransformation by nonenzymatic hydrolysis and enzyme-mediated hydroxylation to form more than a dozen metabolites, all of which are rapidly eliminated in the urine. Renal dysfunction does not affect drug exposure, as less than 4% of the drug is excreted in the urine as the parent compound (Melchert & List, 2007). For most thalidomide-containing regimens, the drug is taken daily with a full glass of water. Because of its sedating effects, it should be taken in the evening (Celgene Corp., 2017c).

Indication: Multiple Myeloma

For patients with newly diagnosed multiple myeloma, thalidomide is approved in combination with dexamethasone as a first-line therapy (Celgene Corp., 2017c). The starting dose is 200 mg daily but can be decreased to a minimum of 50 mg daily to manage side effects. Because of its efficacy in comparison to traditional chemotherapy, this combination became the frontline standard of care in the early 2000s, long before its FDA approval in 2005 (Cavo et al., 2005). However, since the approval of its analog lenalidomide, thalidomide has rarely been used as initial therapy in the United States because of its significant side effects and lower efficacy (Rajkumar et al., 2005). Although no longer recommended as a first-line therapy, thalidomide still has a role as a salvage therapy in relapsed multiple myeloma in combination with more traditional chemotherapy drugs (NCCN, 2018b). Because of its low level of myelosuppression in comparison to newer IMiDs, thalidomide can be an effective option in heavily pretreated patients with poor bone marrow reserve.

Indication: Erythema Nodosum Leprosum

Although few nurses will work with patients with leprosy, it is important to remember thalidomide's original indication for the treatment and maintenance of acute, moderate to severe ENL. For this indication, thalidomide is dosed at 100–300 mg daily and tapered to a minimum of 50 mg daily as symptoms subside (Celgene Corp., 2017c).

Side Effects

Thalidomide is the least myelosuppressive IMiD, but it carries the greatest risks of neuropathy and thrombosis (see Table 6-1). Peripheral neuropathy is a dose-limiting toxicity. Both onset and severity of neuropathy are related to dose and duration of drug exposure. Without proper intervention, thalidomide-induced neuropathy can become a permanent issue, even on discontinuation. Sedation, fatigue, rash, and constipation are the most common nonhematologic toxicities (Celgene Corp., 2017c).

Lenalidomide

Formulation

Lenalidomide is available in 2.5, 5, 10, 15, 20, and 25 mg capsules. No IV formulations are used. Lenalidomide undergoes limited metabolism, and its elimination is primarily renal, with 82% of the drug excreted as parent compound within 24 hours. As such, the drug must be dosed based on renal function. Recommendations are given in the prescribing information. With appropriate dosing and scheduling, it is safe to use in patients on hemodialysis; however, it should only be given following a dialysis session (Celgene Corp., 2017b). Although absorption of the drug is decreased in the presence of a high-fat meal, safety and efficacy were established without regard to food. As such, it may be taken at any time of day, with or without food, and with a full glass of water. It should, however, be taken at the same time each day. With normal renal function, the starting dose of most lenalidomide-containing regimens is 25 mg daily, with adjustments down to 2.5 mg based primarily on toxicities related to myelosuppression (neutropenia and thrombocytopenia). Because of the risk of myelosuppression, most regimens are written as 28-day cycles, with lenalidomide given on the first 21 days. This is followed by a seven-day drug-free break to give the bone marrow a short recovery time (Celgene Corp., 2017b).

TABLE 6-1 Common Adverse Events for Immunomodulatory Drugs

Adverse Event	Thalidomide	Lenalidomide	Pomalidomide
Thrombotic events	+++	++	+
Neuropathy	+++*	N/A	+
Myelosuppression	+	+++*	+++*
Infection	+	+++	+++
Rash	++	++	+
Gastrointestinal complications	+++	++	+
Sedation	+++	N/A	N/A
Fatigue	+++	+	+
Secondary malignancies	N/A	+	N/A

Side effects are scored from + to +++ relative to each other.

* Represents the dose-limiting toxicity for each drug. See prescribing information for details.

Note. Based on information from Celgene Corp., 2017a, 2017b, 2017c.

Indication: Multiple Myeloma

Of the three IMiDs, lenalidomide has the highest number of FDA-approved indications and is the only one with indications in multiple cancer types. Its most common use is in patients with multiple myeloma for which, in combination with dexamethasone, it has broad indications from initial therapy through all stages of relapse (Celgene Corp., 2017b). Although this doublet is very effective, new drug classes with potent antimyeloma activity are also receiving FDA approval. This has led to clinical trials testing combinations of these new agents with this doublet. Two such drugs, carfilzomib and ixazomib, are from the class of proteasome inhibitors (PIs). Although these PIs have excellent antimyeloma activity, their efficacy is significantly improved when combined with lenalidomide and dexamethasone (Moreau et al., 2016; Stewart et al., 2015). As such, PI-lenalidomide-dexamethasone triplet combinations have received FDA approval for the treatment of relapsed myeloma (Amgen Inc., 2017; Takeda Oncology, 2016).

Monoclonal antibodies have two agents approved for use in combination with the lenalidomide-dexamethasone doublet. One of these agents, daratumumab, gained FDA approval in 2015 based on its success as a monotherapy for heavily pretreated patients with relapsed myeloma. This antibody binds to the CD38 protein on the surface of myeloma cells, recruiting NK and T cells to attack and destroy antibody-tagged cells. As lenalidomide is known to enhance the proliferation and activity of both NK and T cells, it is not surprising that combining it with daratumumab increases efficacy (Dimopoulos et al., 2016). One year after its initial approval as a monotherapy, daratumumab received updated approval for use in combination with lenalidomide (Janssen Biotech, Inc., 2017).

The lenalidomide-dexamethasone doublet is also approved in combination with elotuzumab, an antibody directed against the CD319 protein found on the surface of myeloma cells. Unlike daratumumab, this antibody destroys myeloma cells exclusively through an NK cell–mediated pathway that requires the presence of lenalidomide to upregulate activity. As such, elotuzumab has essentially no activity as a monotherapy and is only approved in combination with lenalidomide (Bristol-Myers Squibb Co., 2017).

Despite lacking FDA approval, the regimen most widely used for the treatment of myeloma is the lenalidomide-dexamethasone doublet in combination with the PI bortezomib. This regimen has been studied in phase 2 and 3 clinical trials in patients with newly diagnosed myeloma and those in the relapsed setting (Durie et al., 2017; Kumar et al., 2012; Richardson et al., 2010; Richardson, Xie, et al., 2014). This triplet showed very high response rates, and as such, it has been adopted as the standard frontline therapy for newly diagnosed patients. It is listed by NCCN (2018b) as a preferred first-line regimen.

Because multiple myeloma is incurable, most patients will relapse multiple times and eventually die. To deepen response and improve survival, nearly all eligible patients will undergo an autologous stem cell transplantation (ASCT) following initial therapy. In the post-transplant setting, continuous treatment with a less intensive antimyeloma therapy (i.e., maintenance therapy) can delay relapse and potentially prolong overall survival. Although both thalidomide and lenalidomide have been shown as effective maintenance therapy, lenalidomide is preferred, as it has the most extensive data and is not plagued by the neuropathy seen with long-term thalidomide use (Maiolino et al., 2012; Mian et al., 2016; Ye, Huang, Pan, & Li, 2013). Patients who undergo ASCT also appear to benefit from maintenance therapy with an IMiD once induction therapy is completed (Kagoya, Nannya, & Kurokawa, 2012; Morgan et al., 2012). In the maintenance setting, lenalidomide is an FDA-approved monotherapy dosed for the standard 21 days of a 28-day cycle or as continuous, uninterrupted therapy. The maintenance dose is usually lower than that used in initial therapy, as the patient's bone marrow generally has less reserve following more aggressive induction regimens (NCCN, 2018a).

Indication: Mantle Cell Lymphoma

Mantle cell lymphoma (MCL) is a relatively rare subtype of B-cell non-Hodgkin lymphoma (NHL), typically presenting as advanced-stage disease in an older population with significant comorbidities. It is difficult to cure without a dose-intensive treatment regimen (including ASCT), which can be challenging to this patient population. Even at first relapse, the disease is often chemotherapy resistant, and subsequent chemotherapy is generally ineffective and palliative in nature. Because of their mechanism of downregulating B-cell proliferation, clinical trials were initiated using IMiDs for the treatment of relapsed/refractory B-cell NHL. Notable activity and durable responses seen in the MCL subtype (Habermann et al., 2009; Witzig et al., 2011), as well as subsequent trials in this patient population, confirmed and extended these original observations (Goy et al., 2013). Based on these data, lenalidomide received FDA approval in June 2013 as monotherapy for the treatment of multipe-relapsed MCL (Celgene Corp., 2017b). More recent studies have shown both an improved response and duration of response when lenalidomide was combined with the CD20-directed antibody rituximab (Ahmadi et al., 2014; Ruan et al., 2015). This regimen, termed R^2 (R squared), is not FDA approved but is recommended by NCCN for both first- and second-line treatment of older, less-fit patients with MCL (NCCN, 2018a).

Indication: Myelodysplastic Syndrome

The only non–B-cell malignancy for which lenalidomide is approved is in a specific subset of patients having a low- or intermediate-1-risk myelodysplastic syndrome (MDS) that carries a deletion of the long arm of chromosome 5 (5q) (Celgene Corp., 2017b). These patients are red blood cell transfusion–dependent and have an increased propensity for their malignancy to transform to acute myeloid leukemia. Treatment with lenalidomide upregulates expression of the p53 tumor suppressor gene, resulting in enhanced programed cell death of the 5q clone but not of cytogenetically normal cells (Schneider et al., 2014). In the original studies with lenalidomide, this patient population experienced increased hemoglobin levels and a durable decreased requirement for red blood cell transfusions (List et al., 2005, 2006). Raza et al. (2008) later showed that lenalidomide had clinical activity in patients with MDS without deletion of 5q, although the response was not nearly as durable or robust. In the MDS patient population, lenalidomide is initiated at 10 mg daily and adjusted downward based on hematologic parameters. In contrast to lenalidomide, neither thalidomide nor pomalidomide is particularly active in myelodysplastic cells. This is likely because of structural differences that alter their affinity for the target protein (Petzold, Fischer, & Thomä, 2016).

Side Effects

Lenalidomide has gained widespread use because of its therapeutic efficacy and low side effect profile (see Table 6-1). However, it is much more myelosuppressive than thalidomide. Cytopenia is its dose-limiting toxicity. In comparison to thalidomide, it has far less thrombotic potential and causes less fatigue. Rash, diarrhea, and constipation are its most common nonhematologic toxicities (Celgene Corp., 2017b).

A potentially more serious side effect is the increased risk of secondary primary malignancies (SPMs). These were noted in the drug's original studies, when it was used as maintenance therapy following ASCT (Attal et al., 2012; McCarthy et al., 2012). An increased number of solid tumors were reported in the lenalidomide-treated arms, but these were not significant and included many noninvasive, nonmelanoma skin cancers. However, the rate of hematologic SPMs was nearly twice as high in the lenalidomide-treated arms and included evolution to MDS and acute myeloid leukemia. This risk appeared specific to patients receiving ASCT with exposure to high-dose melphalan. A meta-analysis of a larger patient population receiving lenalidomide maintenance showed an even higher correlation to hematologic SPMs in older adult patients receiving oral melphalan as first-line treatment in lieu of ASCT (Palumbo et al., 2014). In each of these studies, mortality related to progression of myeloma was far higher than that related to SPMs. Although the benefit of increased overall survival conferred by maintenance therapy likely outweighs the risk of death secondary to SPMs, patients should be aware of this risk prior to starting maintenance therapy. Patients who choose maintenance therapy should have cancer screenings at recommended intervals and more frequent dermatologic examinations (Jones et al., 2016).

Pomalidomide

Formulation

Pomalidomide is available in 1, 2, 3, or 4 mg capsules. No IV formulations are used. It is primarily metabolized in the liver by the CYP1A2 and CYP3A4 pathways. Drug elimination is through the urine (73%) and feces (15%), with only 10% eliminated as parent compound. The recommended 28-day dosing regimen is identical to that of lenalidomide. The recommended starting dose is 4 mg, although patients with mild or moderate hepatic impairment or those with severe renal impairment requiring dialysis should start at a 3 mg dose. Pomalidomide is safe to use in patients on hemodialysis, though it should only be given following a dialysis session. Adjustments in dose are made in 1 mg decrements based primarily on toxicity related to fatigue and myelosuppression (neutropenia and thrombocytopenia). Pomalidomide may be taken at any time of the day (at the same time every day), with or without food, and with a full glass of water (Celgene Corp., 2017a).

Indication: Multiple Myeloma

In the setting of multiple myeloma, pomalidomide has more broad and robust activity than thalidomide and is also effective in patients refractory to lenalidomide (Richardson, Siegel, et al., 2014). In a pivotal phase 3 registration trial, all study patients had advanced disease and were required to have failed both bortezomib and lenalidomide. Despite this, overall response rate was 31%, and overall survival modestly improved (San Miguel et al., 2013). Based on these results, pomalidomide was approved in 2013 in combination with dexamethasone for patients with at least two prior therapies, including lenalidomide and any PI. NCCN guidelines also recommend pomalidomide's use in the second-line setting (in combination with dexamethasone) or as part of a triplet regimen (in combination with dexamethasone and a PI) (NCCN, 2018b). As with the other IMiDs, pomalidomide is currently being studied in combination with other antimyeloma agents, although no regimens have yet been approved.

Side Effects

Pomalidomide is very well tolerated. Its most common toxicities are fatigue and myelosuppression (see Table 6-1). Pomalidomide's major dose-limiting toxicity is neutropenia. The risk of infections, including sepsis and pneumonia, was as high as 34% in early studies.

Pomalidomide-induced peripheral neuropathy is relatively uncommon and mild, an important property for an agent used late in the disease course. Compared with other IMiDs, pomalidomide has the least thrombotic potential, although patients still require thromboprophylaxis. Rash, diarrhea, and anorexia are additional nonhematologic toxicities (Celgene Corp., 2017a).

Nursing Implications

With the development of IMiD-containing regimens, patients with multiple myeloma and other hematologic malignancies are surviving longer. Increased survival means increased exposure to antimyeloma drugs and their side effects (see Table 6-1). Although many of these agents are well tolerated in comparison to traditional antineoplastic therapy, treatment-related toxicity is an ever-present concern throughout the disease course. Nurses at all educational levels have a vital role in educating patients about drug-specific toxicities and encouraging prompt reporting of treatment-related symptoms. Patient- and treatment-specific comorbidities should be assessed at every opportunity, with prompt intervention when necessary.

Summary

Although the unique immunomodulatory activity of thalidomide was first recognized in the 1960s, its history of fetal toxicity led to slow incorporation into clinical trials. However, with the success of thalidomide in the first oncology clinical trials in the late 1990s, new immunomodulatory agents (lenalidomide and pomalidomide) have been synthesized. As a group, these drugs have shown significant anticancer activity in a wide variety of hematologic malignancies. Although fetal toxicity is still a concern, safeguards have been put in place to protect against this devastating side effect, and IMiDs have been used safely in thousands of patients with cancer. Research continues to find new uses for IMiDs, especially in combination with other anticancer agents. Thalidomide, a once-forgotten drug, has become the backbone of a new class of potent anticancer agents with a very bright future.

References

Ahmadi, T., Chong, E.A., Gordon, A., Aqui, N.A., Nasta, S.D., Svoboda, J., ... Schuster, S.J. (2014). Combined lenalidomide, low-dose dexamethasone, and rituximab achieves durable responses in rituximab-resistant indolent and mantle cell lymphomas. *Cancer,* *120,* 222–228. https://doi.org/10.1002/cncr.28405

Amgen Inc. (2017). *Kyprolis® (carfilzomib)* [Package insert]. Thousand Oaks, CA: Author.

Attal, M., Lauwers-Cances, V., Marit, G., Caillot, D., Moreau, P., Facon, T., ... Harousseau, J.-L. (2012). Lenalidomide maintenance after stem-cell transplantation for multiple myeloma. *New England Journal of Medicine, 366,* 1782–1791. https://doi.org/10.1056 /NEJMoa1114138

Bristol-Myers Squibb Co. (2017). *Empliciti™ (elotuzumab)* [Package insert]. Princeton, NJ: Author.

Calabrese, L., & Fleischer, A.B., Jr. (2000). Thalidomide: Current and potential clinical applications. *American Journal of Medicine, 108,* 487–495. https://doi.org/10.1016/S0002 -9343(99)00408-8

Cavo, M., Zamagni, E., Tosi, P., Tacchetti, P., Cellini, C., Cangini, D., ... Baccarani, M. (2005). Superiority of thalidomide and dexamethasone over vincristine-doxorubicin-dexamethasone (VAD) as primary therapy in preparation for autologous transplantation for multiple myeloma. *Blood, 106,* 35–39. https://doi.org/10.1182/blood-2005-02-0522

Celgene Corp. (2017a). *Pomalyst® (pomalidomide)* [Package insert]. Summit, NJ: Author.

Celgene Corp. (2017b). *Revlimid® (lenalidomide)* [Package insert]. Summit, NJ: Author.

Celgene Corp. (2017c). *Thalomid® (thalidomide)* [Package insert]. Summit, NJ: Author.

D'Amato, R.J., Loughnan, M.S., Flynn, E., & Folkman, J. (1994). Thalidomide is an inhibitor of angiogenesis. *Proceedings of the National Academy of Sciences of the United States of America, 91,* 4082–4085. https://doi.org/10.1073/pnas.91.9.4082

Dimopoulos, M.A., Oriol, A., Nahi, H., San-Miguel, J., Bahlis, N.J., Usmani, S.Z., ... Moreau, P. (2016). Daratumumab, lenalidomide, and dexamethasone for multiple myeloma. *New England Journal of Medicine, 375,* 1319–1331. https://doi.org/10.1056/NEJMoa1607751

Durie, B.G.M., Hoering, A., Abidi, M.H., Rajkumar, S.V., Epstein, J., Kahanic, S.P., ... Dispenzieri, A. (2017). Bortezomib with lenalidomide and dexamethasone versus lenalidomide and dexamethasone alone in patients with newly diagnosed myeloma without intent for immediate autologous stem-cell transplant (SWOG S0777): A randomised, open-label, phase 3 trial. *Lancet, 389,* 519–527. https://doi.org/10.1016/S0140-6736(16)31594-X

Fullerton, P.M., & Kremer, M. (1961). Neuropathy after intake of thalidomide (distaval). *BMJ, 2,* 855–858. https://doi.org/10.1136/bmj.2.5256.855

Goy, A., Sinha, R., Williams, M.E., Kalayoglu Besisik, S., Drach, J., Ramchandren, R., ... Witzig, T.E. (2013). Single-agent lenalidomide in patients with mantle-cell lymphoma who relapsed or progressed after or were refractory to bortezomib: Phase II MCL-001 (EMERGE) study. *Journal of Clinical Oncology, 31,* 3688–3695. https://doi.org/10.1200 /JCO.2013.49.2835

Habermann, T.M., Lossos, I.S., Justice, G., Vose, J.M., Wiernik, P.H., McBride, K., ... Tuscano, J.M. (2009). Lenalidomide oral monotherapy produces a high response rate in patients with relapsed or refractory mantle cell lymphoma. *British Journal of Haematology, 145,* 344–349. https://doi.org/10.1111/j.1365-2141.2009.07626.x

Haslett, P.A.J., Corral, L.G., Albert, M., & Kaplan, G. (1998). Thalidomide costimulates primary human T lymphocytes, preferentially inducing proliferation, cytokine production, and cytotoxic responses in the CD8+ subset. *Journal of Experimental Medicine, 187,* 1885–1892. https://doi.org/10.1084/jem.187.11.1885

Ito, T., Ando, H., Suzuki, T., Ogura, T., Hotta, K., Imamura, Y., ... Handa, H. (2010). Identification of a primary target of thalidomide teratogenicity. *Science, 327,* 1345–1350. https://doi.org/10.1126/science.1177319

Iyer, C.G., Languillon, J., Ramanujam, K., Tarabini-Castellani, G., De las Aguas, J.T., Bechelli, L.M., ... Sundaresan, T. (1971). WHO co-ordinated short-term double-blind trial with thalidomide in the treatment of acute lepra reactions in male lepromatous patients. *Bulletin of the World Health Organization, 45,* 719–732.

Janssen Biotech, Inc. (2017). *Darzalex® (daratumumab)* [Package insert]. Horsham, PA: Author.

Jones, J.R., Cairns, D.A., Gregory, W.M., Collett, C., Pawlyn, C., Sigsworth, R., ... Morgan, G.J. (2016). Second malignancies in the context of lenalidomide treatment: An analysis of 2732 myeloma patients enrolled to the myeloma XI trial. *Blood Cancer Journal, 6,* e506. https://doi.org/10.1038/bcj.2016.114

Kagoya, Y., Nannya, Y., & Kurokawa, M. (2012). Thalidomide maintenance therapy for patients with multiple myeloma: Meta-analysis. *Leukemia Research, 36,* 1016–1021. https://doi.org/10.1016/j.leukres.2012.04.001

Kumar, S.K., Flinn, I., Richardson, P.G., Hari, P., Callander, N., Noga, S.J., ... Rajkumar, S.V. (2012). Randomized, multicenter, phase 2 study (EVOLUTION) of combinations of bortezomib, dexamethasone, cyclophosphamide, and lenalidomide in previously untreated multiple myeloma. *Blood, 119,* 4375–4382. https://doi.org/10.1182/blood-2011-11-395749

Kumar, S.K., Rajkumar, S.V., Dispenzieri, A., Lacy, M.Q., Hayman, S.R., Buadi, F.K., ... Gertz, M.A. (2008). Improved survival in multiple myeloma and the impact of novel therapies. *Blood, 111,* 2516–2520. https://doi.org/10.1182/blood-2007-10-116129

Lenz, W. (1988). A short history of thalidomide embryopathy. *Teratology, 38,* 203–215. https://doi.org/10.1002/tera.1420380303

Lenz, W., Pfeiffer, R.A., Kosenow, W., & Hayman, D.J. (1962). Thalidomide and congenital abnormalities. *Lancet, 279,* 45–46. https://doi.org/10.1016/S0140-6736(62)92665-X

List, A., Dewald, G., Bennett, J., Giagounidis, A., Raza, A., Feldman, E., ... Knight, R. (2006). Lenalidomide in the myelodysplastic syndrome with chromosome 5q deletion. *New England Journal of Medicine, 355,* 1456–1465. https://doi.org/10.1056/NEJMoa061292

List, A., Kurtin, S., Roe, D.J., Buresh, A., Mahadevan, D., Fuchs, D., ... Zeldis, J.B. (2005). Efficacy of lenalidomide in myelodysplastic syndromes. *New England Journal of Medicine, 352,* 549–557. https://doi.org/10.1056/NEJMoa041668

Lopez-Girona, A., Mendy, D., Ito, T., Miller, K., Gandhi, A.K., Kang, J., ... Chopra, R. (2012). Cereblon is a direct protein target for immunomodulatory and antiproliferative activities of lenalidomide and pomalidomide. *Leukemia, 26,* 2326–2335. https://doi.org/10.1038/leu.2012.119

Maiolino, A., Hungria, V.T.M., Garnica, M., Oliveira-Duarte, G., Oliveira, L.C.O., Mercante, D.R., ... de Souza, C.A. (2012). Thalidomide plus dexamethasone as a maintenance therapy after autologous hematopoietic stem cell transplantation improves progression-free survival in multiple myeloma. *American Journal of Hematology, 87,* 948–952. https://doi.org/10.1002/ajh.23274

Matthews, S.J., & McCoy, C. (2003). Thalidomide: A review of approved and investigational uses. *Clinical Therapeutics, 25,* 342–395. https://doi.org/10.1016/S0149-2918(03)80085-1

McBride, W.G. (1961). Thalidomide and congenital abnormalities [Letter]. *Lancet, 278,* 1358. https://doi.org/10.1016/S0140-6736(61)90927-8

McCarthy, P.L., Owzar, K., Hofmeister, C.C., Hurd, D.D., Hassoun, H., Richardson, P.G., ... Linker, C. (2012). Lenalidomide after stem-cell transplantation for multiple myeloma. *New England Journal of Medicine, 366,* 1770–1781. https://doi.org/10.1056/NEJMoa1114083

Melchert, M., & List, A. (2007). The thalidomide saga. *International Journal of Biochemistry and Cell Biology, 39,* 1489–1499. https://doi.org/10.1016/j.biocel.2007.01.022

Mian, I., Milton, D.R., Shah, N., Nieto, Y., Popat, U.R., Kebriaei, P., ... Bashir, Q. (2016). Prolonged survival with a longer duration of maintenance lenalidomide after autologous hematopoietic stem cell transplantation for multiple myeloma. *Cancer, 122,* 3831–3837. https://doi.org/10.1002/cncr.30366

Moreau, P., Masszi, T., Grzasko, N., Bahlis, N.J., Hansson, M., Pour, L., ... Richardson, P.G. (2016). Oral ixazomib, lenalidomide, and dexamethasone for multiple myeloma. *New England Journal of Medicine, 374,* 1621–1634. https://doi.org/10.1056/NEJMoa1516282

Morgan, G.J., Gregory, W.M., Davies, F.E., Bell, S.E., Szubert, A.J., Brown, J.M., ... Child, A.J. (2012). The role of maintenance thalidomide therapy in multiple myeloma: MRC myeloma IX results and meta-analysis. *Blood, 119,* 7–15. https://doi.org/10.1182/blood-2011-06-357038

National Comprehensive Cancer Network. (2018a). *NCCN Clinical Practice Guidelines in Oncology (NCCN Guidelines®): B-cell lymphomas* [v.4.2018]. Retrieved from https://www.nccn.org/professionals/physician_gls/pdf/b-cell.pdf

National Comprehensive Cancer Network. (2018b). *NCCN Clinical Practice Guidelines in Oncology (NCCN Guidelines®): Multiple myeloma* [v.4.2018]. Retrieved from https://www.nccn.org/professionals/physician_gls/pdf/myeloma.pdf

Palumbo, A., Bringhen, S., Kumar, S.K., Lupparelli, G., Usmani, S., Waage, A., … McCarthy, P.L. (2014). Second primary malignancies with lenalidomide therapy for newly diagnosed myeloma: A meta-analysis of individual patient data. *Lancet Oncology, 15,* 333–342. https://doi.org/10.1016/S1470-2045(13)70609-0

Palumbo, A., Rajkumar, S.V., Dimopoulos, M.A., Richardson, P.G., San Miguel, J., Barlogie, B., … Hussein, M.A. (2008). Prevention of thalidomide- and lenalidomide-associated thrombosis in myeloma. *Leukemia, 22,* 414–423. https://doi.org/10.1038/sj.leu.2405062

Petzold, G., Fischer, E.S., & Thomä, N.H. (2016). Structural basis of lenalidomide-induced CK1α degradation by the CRL4(CRBN) ubiquitin ligase. *Nature, 532,* 127–130. https://doi.org/10.1038/nature16979

Quach, H., Ritchie, D., Stewart, A.K., Neeson, P., Harrison, S., Smyth, M.J., & Prince, H.M. (2010). Mechanism of action of immunomodulatory drugs (IMiDS) in multiple myeloma. *Leukemia, 24,* 22–32. https://doi.org/10.1038/leu.2009.236

Rajkumar, S.V., Hayman, S.R., Lacy, M.Q., Dispenzieri, A., Geyer, S.M., Kabat, B., … Gertz, M.A. (2005). Combination therapy with lenalidomide plus dexamethasone (rev/dex) for newly diagnosed myeloma. *Blood, 106,* 4050–4053. https://doi.org/10.1182/blood-2005-07-2817

Randall, T. (1990). Thalidomide has 37-year history. *JAMA, 263,* 1474. https://doi.org/10.1001/jama.1990.03440110028006

Raza, A., Reeves, J.A., Feldman, E.J., Dewald, G.W., Bennett, J.M., Deeg, H.J., … List, A.F. (2008). Phase 2 study of lenalidomide in transfusion-dependent, low-risk, and intermediate-1-risk myelodysplastic syndromes with karyotypes other than deletion 5q. *Blood, 111,* 86–93. https://doi.org/10.1182/blood-2007-01-068833

Richardson, P.G., Siegel, D.S., Vij, R., Hofmeister, C.C., Baz, R., Jagannath, S., … Anderson, K.C. (2014). Pomalidomide alone or in combination with low-dose dexamethasone in relapsed and refractory multiple myeloma: A randomized phase 2 study. *Blood, 123,* 1826–1832. https://doi.org/10.1182/blood-2013-11-538835

Richardson, P.G., Weller, E., Lonial, S., Jakubowiak, A.J., Jagannath, S., Raje, N.S., … Anderson, K.C. (2010). Lenalidomide, bortezomib, and dexamethasone combination therapy in patients with newly diagnosed multiple myeloma. *Blood, 116,* 679–686. https://doi.org/10.1182/blood-2010-02-268862

Richardson, P.G., Xie, W., Jagannath, S., Jakubowiak, A., Lonial, S., Raje, N.S., … Anderson, K.C. (2014). A phase 2 trial of lenalidomide, bortezomib, and dexamethasone in patients with relapsed and relapsed/refractory myeloma. *Blood, 123,* 1461–1469. https://doi.org/10.1182/blood-2013-07-517276

Rome, S., Doss, D., Miller, K., & Westphal, J. (2008). Thromboembolic events associated with novel therapies in patients with multiple myeloma: Consensus statement of the IMF nurse leadership board. *Clinical Journal of Oncology Nursing, 12*(Suppl. 3), 21–28. https://doi.org/10.1188/08.CJON.S1.21-27

Rouhi, M. (2005). Thalidomide. *Chemical and Engineering News, 83,* 122–123. https://doi.org/10.1021/cen-v083n025.p122

Ruan, J., Martin, P., Shah, B., Schuster, S.J., Smith, S.M., Furman, R.R., … Leonard, J.P. (2015). Lenalidomide plus rituximab as initial treatment for mantle-cell lymphoma. *New England Journal of Medicine, 373,* 1835–1844. https://doi.org/10.1056/NEJMoa1505237

Sampaio, E.P., Sarno, E.N., Galilly, R., Cohn, Z.A., & Kaplan, G. (1991). Thalidomide selectively inhibits tumor necrosis factor alpha production by stimulated human monocytes. *Journal of Experimental Medicine, 173,* 699–703. https://doi.org/10.1084/jem.173.3.699

San Miguel, J., Weisel, K., Moreau, P., Lacy, M., Song, K., Delforge, M., … Dimopoulos, M. (2013). Pomalidomide plus low-dose dexamethasone versus high-dose dexamethasone alone for patients with relapsed and refractory multiple myeloma (MM-003): A randomised, open-label, phase 3 trial. *Lancet Oncology, 14,* 1055–1066. https://doi.org/10.1016/S1470-2045(13)70380-2

Schneider, R.K., Ademà, V., Heckl, D., Järås, M., Mallo, M., Lord, A.M., ... Ebert, B.L. (2014). Role of casein kinase 1A1 in the biology and targeted therapy of del(5q) MDS. *Cancer Cell, 26,* 509–520. https://doi.org/10.1016/j.ccr.2014.08.001

Sedlarikova, L., Kubiczkova, L., Sevcikova, S., & Hajek, R. (2012). Mechanism of immuno-modulatory drugs in multiple myeloma. *Leukemia Research, 36,* 1218–1224. https://doi.org/10.1016/j.leukres.2012.05.010

Sheskin, J. (1965). Thalidomide in the treatment of lepra reactions. *Clinical Pharmacology and Therapeutics, 6,* 303–306. https://doi.org/10.1002/cpt196563303

Sheskin, J., & Convit, J. (1969). Results of a double blind study of the influence of thalidomide on the lepra reaction. *International Journal of Leprosy, 37,* 135–146.

Singhal, S., Mehta, J., Desikan, R., Ayers, D., Roberson, P., Eddlemon, P., ... Barlogie, B. (1999). Antitumor activity of thalidomide in refractory multiple myeloma. *New England Journal of Medicine, 341,* 1565–1571. https://doi.org/10.1056/NEJM199911183412102

Stewart, A.K., Rajkumar, S.V., Dimopoulos, M.A., Masszi, T., Špička, I., Oriol, A., ... Palumbo, A. (2015). Carfilzomib, lenalidomide, and dexamethasone for relapsed multiple myeloma. *New England Journal of Medicine, 372,* 142–152. https://doi.org/10.1056/NEJMoa1411321

Takeda Oncology. (2016). *Ninlaro® (ixazomib)* [Package insert]. Cambridge, MA: Author.

Witzig, T.E., Vose, J.M., Zinzani, P.L., Reeder, C.B., Buckstein, R., Polikoff, J.A., ... Czuczman, M.S. (2011). An international phase II trial of single-agent lenalidomide for relapsed or refractory aggressive B-cell non-Hodgkin's lymphoma. *Annals of Oncology, 22,* 1622–1627. https://doi.org/10.1093/annonc/mdq626

Ye, X., Huang, J., Pan, Q., & Li, W. (2013). Maintenance therapy with immunomodulatory drugs after autologous stem cell transplantation in patients with multiple myeloma: A meta-analysis of randomized controlled trials. *PLOS ONE, 8,* e72635. https://doi.org/10.1371/journal.pone.0072635

Zeldis, J.B., Williams, B.A., Thomas, S.D., & Elsayed, M.E. (1999). STEPS™: A comprehensive program for controlling and monitoring access to thalidomide. *Clinical Therapeutics, 21,* 319–330. https://doi.org/10.1016/S0149-2918(00)88289-2

chapter seven

Active Immunity: Vaccine Therapy

Kristine Deano Abueg, RN, MSN, OCN®, CBCN®

Introduction

The Centers for Disease Control and Prevention (CDC) defines *active immunity* as "the production of antibodies against a specific disease by the immune system" (CDC, 2016, para. 3). Active immunity is usually permanent and can be acquired either by contracting the disease or through vaccination (CDC, 2016). For obvious reasons, intentional inoculation with cancer represents an impractical and undesirable approach. Additionally, prior incidental exposure to cancer does not suggest future immunity. Tumors can develop evasion mechanisms, coaxing the immune system into labeling cancer antigens as "self" or "nonthreatening." Antigens categorized as such fail to elicit "danger signals" and ultimately result in muted or silent immune responses. Growing unchecked, these tumors can develop into malignant masses (van der Burg, Arens, Ossendorp, van Hall, & Melief, 2016).

The most common form of passive immuno-oncology, therapeutic monoclonal antibodies (mAbs) provide some antitumor benefit; however, their cytotoxicity is limited to the time of exposure to the physical drug. Moreover, mAbs target a single preselected antigen, making antigen variation and differential expression mitigating to efficacy.

Active immuno-oncology, namely vaccine therapy, harnesses the memory cell function of the immune system to cultivate sustained and adaptable immunity that can be activated by future tumor growth (Guo et al., 2013; King, 2004). Vaccines have been widely successful in reducing mortality and morbidity in numerous infectious diseases (CDC, 2016). Oncology researchers are now applying these therapies to cancer treatment. This chapter will address the role of cancer vaccines in conferring active immunity against malignant tumors.

Development of Immunity From Vaccines

Passive immuno-oncology is the introduction of manufactured or donated immunologic substances for the elimination of tumor or its associated proteins (Guo et al., 2013; King, 2004). Common examples of passive immuno-oncology include the following mAbs: rituximab, which targets CD20+ lymphoma and leukemia (Biogen, Inc. & Genentech, Inc., 2016); bevacizumab, which targets vascular endothelial growth factor (Genentech, Inc., 2009); and ado-trastuzumab emtansine, which targets HER2 molecules (Genentech, Inc., n.d.). Another example of passive immuno-oncology is the infusion of T cells, such as in adoptive cellular therapy (Perica, Varela, Oelke, & Schneck, 2015). These passive scenarios involve the ex vivo expansion of immune substances, which are then transferred into the recipient.

In contrast, active immuno-oncology involves stimulation of the recipient immune system and the in vivo expansion of antigen-specific immune cells with both cytotoxic and memory functions. As such, active immuno-oncology should theoretically offer long-term protection against future tumor growth. Vaccination, an artificial form of active immuno-oncology, is the injection of preselected molecules into a patient to elicit T-cell– and B-cell–mediated immune responses. For example, in infectious diseases, an influenza vaccination with inactive viral influenza proteins results in protective antibodies that patrol against future infections (Parmiani et al., 2014).

Therapeutic cancer vaccination includes inoculation with proteins or polysaccharides that represent existing tumor molecules, as with both manufactured and allogeneic vaccines, or with molecules harvested from the patient's own in situ tumor (Drake, 2014; Guo et al., 2013). On native in situ tumors, these substances have poor immunogenicity, or the ability to trigger an immune response, which is driven by tolerance of the tumor as self and further muted by tumor-driven immune suppression (Ding, 2014; Drake, 2014; Guo et al., 2013). Therapeutic cancer vaccines are solutions of tumor-associated molecules combined with immunostimulatory factors that, upon injection, capitalize on the host's normal immune machinery to transform tolerated molecules into immune-triggering antigens. Regardless of the vaccine formulation, the goal is to generate antitumor immune effector and memory cells that provide long-term protection against present and future tumor growth.

Vaccination begins with the injection of a solution containing processed tumor-associated antigen (TAA), the molecules displayed on the surface of individual tumor cells, and an adjuvant, an added substance that presents as a danger signal to stimulate the host's immune response. This antigen–adjuvant solution is injected into the patient's peripheral tissue or peripheral bloodstream, where it interacts with patrolling antigen-presenting cells (APCs), such as B cells, macrophages, and dendritic cells (DCs). The adjuvant produces immunostimulatory signals, triggering APC activation. The APC digests TAA, metabolizes it into shorter molecular fragments, then loads the component fragments onto the host's major histocompatibility complex (MHC). The APC displays the antigen–MHC complex on its cell surface, travels to the lymph nodes, and presents the complex to naïve CD4+ T cells, CD8+ T cells, and B cells. This triggers maturation and differentiation of naïve immune effector cells into antigen-specific CD4+ T cells, CD8+ T cells, and B cells. The antigen-specific cytotoxic T cells patrol the host for cells bearing the triggering antigen and lyse them via immune-mediated cytotoxic pathways. The memory B and T cells persist in the host's immune structures, such as the spleen and lymph nodes, where they can theoretically be reactivated in the future by antigen reexposure, thus triggering a rapid production of protective antibodies (Siegrist, 2013). In this manner, the vaccine generates a population of immune effector and memory cells capable of providing long-term immune surveillance and response against present and future tumor growth.

Vaccines can be classified as either prophylactic or therapeutic. Prophylactic vaccines are ultimately intended to prevent cancer from developing in healthy people (National Cancer Institute, 2015).

In 2006, the U.S. Food and Drug Administration (FDA) first approved the human papillomavirus (HPV) 9-valent vaccine (Gardasil® 9) for use against certain HPV strains linked to cervical cancer and HPV-associated diseases, such as genital warts and cervical intraepithelial neoplasia. Clinical trial data demonstrated a 96%–100% reduction in precancerous lesion infection rates over placebo groups (Bosch, Lorincz, Muñoz, Meijer, & Shah, 2002; Garland et al., 2007). Cervical cancer data are still emerging, but early results show a decrease in precancerous symptoms (Hariri, Markowitz, Dunne, & Unger, 2013).

Hepatitis B vaccine (Recombivax HB®) is indicated for vaccination against infection for all subtypes of hepatitis B virus (HBV), a major risk factor for hepatocellular carcinoma (HCC) (Chang, 2009). Countries that adopted universal infant vaccination against HBV have seen dramatic decreases in HBV rates and correlating decreases in HCC. For example, Taiwan has seen a reduction in chronic HBV from 10%–17% to 0.7%–1.7%, with a correlating HCC incidence decrease from 0.52–0.54 to 0.13–0.20 per 100,000 individuals (Chan, Wong, Qin, & Chan, 2016; Chang, 2009).

The remainder of this chapter will focus on the emerging therapeutic vaccines intended to "treat an existing cancer by strengthening the body's natural immune response against the cancer" (National Cancer Institute, 2015, para. 25). For additional information on HBV and

HPV vaccines, visit CDC web pages on professional resources (www.cdc
.gov/hpv/hcp/resources.html) and HBV vaccination (www.cdc.gov/
vaccines/vpd/hepb/hcp/index.html).

Considerations in Vaccine Development

Vaccines are intended to prevent future tumor growth and curtail
existing tumor through cultivation of memory cells capable of mount-
ing immune responses (National Cancer Institute, 2015). To achieve
this, vaccines must create immune components against specific TAAs
and overcome the immune-related factors that prevent naturally occurring immunity (Bilusic & Madan, 2012; Guo et al., 2013; Lollini, Cavallo,
Nanni, & Forni, 2006). Vaccine components and construction methods
are selected based on their ability to perform these goals.

Overcoming Immune Suppression

Successful cancer vaccine therapy must overcome both inherent and
tumor-induced immune suppression. The immune system involves multiple protective mechanisms to prevent attack against self (i.e., autoimmune reaction) and regulate exaggerated immune-mediated damage.
Because tumors are, in a sense, mutated self, their associated antigens
are largely self-antigens that lack robust immunogenicity. During maturation, T cells that express receptors against self-antigens are routinely edited and deleted during the clonal deletion process (Baitsch,
Fuertes-Marraco, Legat, Meyer, & Speiser, 2012; Beatty & Gladney, 2015;
Lollini et al., 2006).

Although this serves to restrict autoimmunity, clonal deletion is a
major contributing factor to tumor progression despite prior immune
activation. Moreover, self-tolerant mechanisms are often patholog-
ically enhanced in cancer (van der Burg et al., 2016). For example,
programmed cell death protein 1 (PD-1) is highly expressed on activated B cells, T cells, and natural killer (NK) cells, acting as a brake
to limit immune activity. Upon binding with its macrophage-bound
ligands, programmed cell death-ligand 1(PD-L1) and programmed cell
death-ligand 2 (PD-L2), PD-1 downregulates T-cell activation, dampen-
ing immune response. Some tumors increase their cell surface expression of PD-L1, thus downshifting T-cell activity (Gibbons-Johnson &
Dong, 2017).

Tumors can recruit immunosuppressive cells and inhibitory cytokines that further dampen a robust immune response (Beatty & Gladney, 2015; Schmidt, Nino-Castro, & Schultze, 2012). APCs, while critical to immune activation against foreign and damaged cells, also have

an inhibitory role that causes T-cell regulation (Baitsch et al., 2012). This occurs when APCs present antigen to a T cell in the absence of proinflammatory cytokines. In this situation, the T cell is taught to tolerate the antigen, thus curtailing immune response against that antigen (Schmidt et al., 2012). These observations have collectively been referred to as the *immunosuppressive microenvironment* (Beatty & Gladney, 2015; Sun, Dotti, & Savoldo, 2016). The innate regulatory mechanisms and the immunosuppressive tumor microenvironment together represent the major hurdles in vaccine development, as they hamper desired immune activation and allow for the emergence of tumors with lower immunogenicity (Beatty & Gladney, 2015). Therefore, designing therapies that shift the tumor microenvironment from an immunosuppressive to an immunostimulatory state is a main objective in cancer vaccine drug development.

Inducing Immunostimulatory Factors Tumor Sources

Vaccines have been engineered to induce or include the immunostimulatory factors necessary to stimulate the activation of APCs and the maturation of naïve T cells. The first approach to engineering a vaccine starts with the selection of a vaccine adjuvant, such as incomplete Freund adjuvant, granulocyte macrophage–colony-stimulating factor (GM-CSF), Toll-like receptor agonists, mineral salts, and polysaccharides (Banday, Jeelani, & Hruby, 2015; Slingluff, 2011; Sun et al., 2016). By themselves, these agents can recruit inflammatory cytokines and other factors that induce cell-based and humoral immune responses. Data indicate superior CD4+ T cell, CD8+ T cell, and NK cell responses when vaccines are constructed with adjuvants (Slingluff, 2011; Temizoz, Kuroda, & Ishii, 2016). Adjuvants are selected based on their ability to induce immunostimulatory factors on APCs. For example, GM-CSF induces APCs to produce key immune stimulants (e.g., cytokines, other costimulatory molecules) and stimulates APC migration to lymph nodes—both requirements for T-cell and B-cell activation (Graff & Chamberlain, 2015).

Rather than directly including an immunostimulatory factor, a second approach to vaccine engineering introduces genetic material that directs the target cell's DNA and RNA machinery to produce immunostimulatory factors. For example, in DNA-based vaccine therapy, the injected solution delivers a gene sequence that, once taken by the host's APCs, induces the production of immunostimulatory cytokines such as interleukin-2 or GM-CSF. Clinical trial data suggest that this results in increased immune activity, including increased activity of T effector cells, an influx of DCs, and recruitment of macrophages and eosinophils (Keenan & Jaffee, 2012; Wei et al., 2016). The delivery platform can also help amplify immune stimulation. In the case of virus-based vaccine therapy, the human immune system will naturally react to the presence of viral antigens by upregulation of T effector cells and B lymphocytes, thus amplifying the immunostimulatory state. Regardless of mechanism, amplification of immunostimulatory factors plays a key role in counteracting an immunosuppressive microenvironment.

Selection of Tumor-Associated Antigen in Vaccine Development

Successful active immuno-oncology induces protective immune effector cells that destroy a significant proportion of tumor volume (Buonaguro, Petrizzo, Tornessello, & Buonaguro, 2011; Siegrist, 2013). Immune cells initiate their cytotoxic effects by recognizing TAAs; therefore, the success of cancer vaccine design relies largely on the appropriate identification of representative antigens (Drake, 2014; Guo et al., 2013; Keenan & Jaffee, 2012; Li, Joshi, Singhania, Ramsey, & Murthy, 2014; Pol et al., 2015; Slingluff, 2011; Wang, Yin, Wang, & Wang, 2014).

Researchers have identified the key goals and associated challenges of antigen selection. First, the ideal TAA should be abundantly expressed on a large majority of the tumor mass. Tumor heterogeneity poses significant challenges to this goal (Buonaguro et al., 2011; Drake, 2014; Guo et al., 2013; Keenan & Jaffee, 2012; Li et al., 2014; Pol et al., 2015; Slingluff, 2011; Wang et al., 2014). *Tumor heterogeneity* is the observation that tumors express a wide variety of different morphological, genetic, and metabolic characteristics (Gay, Baker, & Graham, 2016). It exists on an intratumor level, with a single tumor displaying multiple antigens. Intertumor heterogeneity, or variation between different metastatic sites within the same patient, provides additional diversity (Gay et al., 2016). Variation is amplified when comparing tumor antigen profiles of different patients; therefore, identifying a TAA abundantly expressed in all tumor masses is a formidable challenge.

The second goal of antigen selection is avoidance of autoimmune reaction. The ideal TAA should be differentially expressed in abundance on the tumor. Conversely, it should have low expression on the host's self-cells to avoid self-directed immune attack. However, most antigens are derived from mutated self-proteins, resulting in structural similarities with host cells. This similarity is an underlying cause of poor immunogenicity, but it can also increase the risk of developing antiself immune reactions in overstimulated immune systems. Tumor heterogeneity and the self-derived nature of cancer cells are the primary challenges in antigen selection for cancer vaccines (Buonaguro et al., 2011; Drake, 2014; Guo et al., 2013). Antigen selection must carefully balance these two competing challenges.

Candidate tumor antigens for therapeutic vaccines can be classified along two dimensions. The first dimension is the antigen source, which can be either autologous, where the vaccine is based on the patient's own tumor, or allogeneic, where antigens are harvested from donor tumors. Vaccines can also be classified by the specificity of the source antigen. Cancer vaccines may either contain a single representative, defined antigen, or they may be based on a whole tumor cell and its full complement of associated antigens. Inoculation against a single defined antigen is more feasible and cost effective from a manufacturing perspective, but the antigen may be an insufficient representative of an individual patient's tumor (Helwick, 2016; Kurtz, Ravindranathan, & Zaharoff, 2014; Yamada, Sasada, Noguchi, & Itoh, 2013). Whole-cell vaccine therapy, which can be autologous or allogeneic, exposes the recipient's immune system to the full array of a tumor cell's antigens, as well as its intracellular structures. However, these vaccines may facilitate greater autoimmune side effects (Hrouda et al., 2000; Huang et al., 2014). Current clinical trials are investigating these dimensions.

Autologous Versus Allogeneic Tumor Sources

One consideration in antigen selection is the use of autologous versus allogeneic tumor sources. Autologous tumor vaccination is a highly individualized approach in which a patient's own tumor provides the antigen sources for the vaccine. An unprocessed in vivo tumor may be insufficient to stimulate an immune response, as it is inherently recognized as self by the host recipient. Therefore, the patient's own tumor is surgically harvested and rendered inactive, usually via radiation (Guo et al., 2013). The inactive tumor is then cultivated with an adjuvant, such as GM-CSF, to increase immune stimulation and is ultimately processed into an injectable vaccine. Theoretically, this approach eliminates the need to preidentify and isolate specific antigens because the patient will be exposed to the complete range of TAAs. The resulting immune response should generate antibodies against all tumor antigens (Kurtz et al., 2014; van der Burg et al., 2016; Yang, Jeang, Yang, Wu, & Hung, 2015).

An autologous approach is limited by practical issues. Autologous vaccination requires sufficient patient-specific tumor as a source for antigen development; however, available tumor tissue may be limited or not feasible in many tumor types and in situations in which tumor location prohibits biopsy. Creation of autologous vaccines requires access to highly sophisticated laboratory and pharmacy facilities, both of which come with logistical and financial burdens.

Autologous vaccines also face immunologic challenges (Guo et al., 2013; Kurtz et al., 2014; van der Burg et al., 2016; Yang et al., 2015). To counter this, these vaccines are generally prepared with an adjuvant to increase immune stimulation or are genetically engineered to increase immune response. For example, OncoVAX® is an autologous whole-cell tumor vaccine for patients with stage II or III colorectal cancer. Tumors are removed, irradiated, and processed with bacillus Calmette-Guérin, an immunomodulating adjuvant, to elicit immune response (Uyl-de Groot et al., 2005; Vermorken et al., 1999).

Allogeneic tumor vaccines, like autologous vaccines, are derived from tumor that has been harvested and processed to create an immunostimulatory agent. However, unlike their autologous counterparts, allogeneic vaccines are based on established human donor tumor cell lines. From a practical standpoint, allogeneic vaccines are much easier to create, test, and administer. They can be developed in large-scale quantities and can affect many patients, making them more amenable to clinical trial testing and subsequent commercial production. This approach also eliminates the need for prevaccination tumor from the donor/patient.

Allogeneic vaccines also come with immunologic advantages and disadvantages. Allogeneic cells can elicit a greater immune response than autogenic cells, which may be recognized as self (Hrouda et al., 2000; Sondak et al., 2002). Conversely, the donor patient's tumor may have a different antigenic profile than the recipient patient. If so, the vaccine may not generate a robust response to the key tumor drivers for the recipient patient (Sosman et al., 2002; Srivatsan et al., 2014).

Whole-Cell Vaccine Therapy

Whole-cell vaccine therapy involves the injection of harvested whole tumor cells that has been irradiated and rendered oncologically inactive. The whole-cell tumor can be from either autologous or allogeneic sources. As opposed to defined antigen vaccines, this approach eliminates the need to identify the most optimal antigen to target in a cancer type (Chiang, Coukos, & Kandalaft, 2015; Guo et al., 2013). Because tumors are widely recognized to heterogeneously express antigens, benefits include exposure to, ideally, the full complement of antigens present in the tumor (Buonaguro et al., 2011). This exposure has the theoretical likelihood to expand the T-cell arsenal against a wide variety of antigens, potentially increasing tumor kill (Keenan & Jaffee, 2012).

Tumors are widely heterogeneous. Cells within the same tumor mass can express varying levels or combinations of surface antigens; therefore, an immune response against a variety of antigens would theoretically translate to a higher proportion of tumor cell death.

Tumor composition may also change over time, as cells that bear specific target antigens are eliminated by targeted therapy or antigen-specific vaccine response. Eventually, a specific antigen may no longer be widely expressed by the tumor. Multivalency, or the ability to recognize multiple antigens, would enable the immune system to recognize alternate antigens and adapt to an evolving tumor antigen profile. This recognition implied by the whole-cell approach is frequently cited as a desirable goal in vaccine therapy (Huang et al., 2014; Kurtz et al., 2014). T cells and B cells that target a wider range of antigens may be better equipped to confront an evolving tumor mass.

The key disadvantage to whole-cell vaccine therapy is the required amount of tumor specimen for vaccine construction. If the whole cell is from autologous sources, the production of sufficient vaccine can be technically and financially challenging, which may limit its application for some patients (Huang et al., 2014; Keenan & Jaffee, 2012).

Once injected, the irradiated whole-cell tumor is phagocytosed by circulating immature APCs. The APCs, in turn, metabolize the whole-cell tumor into component antigens and process these antigens via the normal antigen presentation pathway. To further stimulate immune response, the introduced whole-cell vaccine can be genetically modified to express stimulatory cytokines such as GM-CSF, which amplifies immune stimulation by attracting effector and proinflammatory cells. GVAX is a whole-cell cancer vaccine that has been widely studied in pancreatic cancer. It includes irradiated pancreatic cancer cells from allogeneic sources modified to secrete GM-CSF (see Table 7-1) (Geary, Lemke, Lubaroff, & Salem, 2013; Ho, 2017; Sidney Kimmel Comprehensive Cancer Center, 2017).

TABLE 7-1   Comparison of Whole-Cell Versus Defined Antigen Vaccine Approaches

Vaccine Approach	Advantages	Disadvantages
Whole cell	Exposure to total antigen load Potential of increased tumor recognition Eliminates the need to identify single optimal antigen	Requires substantial tumor May increase allergic response
Defined antigen	Can be made in large quantities	Requires identification of specific antigen

Note. Based on information from Buonaguro et al., 2011; Chiang et al., 2015; Hrouda et al., 2000; Keenan & Jaffee, 2012.

Defined Antigen Vaccine Therapy

Whole-cell vaccines can contain anywhere from 10 to a few hundred proteins, but only a few are required for development of protective immunity. The remaining "unnecessary" proteins may induce an allergic response, resulting in undesired adverse events. This fact, in part, led to the development of vaccines that use isolated proteins or peptides to stimulate protective immunity (Li et al., 2014). In contrast to whole-cell vaccines, defined antigen vaccine therapies generate an immune response to one preselected TAA. This TAA should be widely expressed on the tumor but not on normal tissue. TAAs studied using vaccine therapies include epidermal growth factor receptor, HER2, and telomerase reverse transcriptase. Defined antigen vaccine therapy can be broadly subdivided into two groups, which vary depending on the antigen delivery mechanism. The first group involves peptide-based cancer vaccines, or direct injection with purified tumor proteins or peptides and an adjuvant. Circulating APCs phagocytose the foreign substance and display the tumor antigen to CD4+ and CD8+ T cells, resulting in an immune response. Clinical trial data have revealed measured regression of tumor burden and an increase in T-cell activity, but unfortunately, this has not translated into meaningful survival benefit (Pol et al., 2015; Slingluff, 2011; Yamada et al., 2013).

Instead of direct inoculation with a TAA, DNA-based vaccine therapy delivers genetic materials, such as plasmid vectors, messenger RNA, and manipulated viral vectors, that direct the host cell to produce TAA. Plasmid vectors are small, circular nucleic acid sequences common in bacteria, whereas messenger RNA synthesizes protein products. Viral vectors, such as vaccinia virus and poxvirus, are widely available and have been used in multiple clinical settings (Larocca & Schlom, 2011; Yang et al., 2015). All three genetic materials can be manufactured to incorporate specific DNA sequences. These genetic "vehicles" are injected into the patient and taken up by circulating APCs (Weide, Garbe, Rammensee, & Pascolo, 2008). Once inside the APC, the cytoplasm machinery is exploited to produce tumor antigens encoded by the introduced DNA. Ultimately, the introduced tumor antigens are presented on MHC class I molecules, stimulating the CD4+ and CD8+ T-cell pathways (Larocca & Schlom, 2011; Yang et al., 2015). Numerous clinical trials are investigating these approaches.

Combination Therapy

Combining vaccines with other cancer treatments is thought to increase the immunogenicity of tumors and potentiate the efficacy of the vaccines. For example, checkpoint inhibitors combined with therapeutic vaccines may impart a synergistic effect to induce a greater anti-tumor immune response. Previous clinical trials suggest that blockade of inhibitory checkpoints (PD-1/PD-L1 and cytotoxic T-lymphocyte antigen 4) encourages the expansion of tumor-specific T cells and stimulates the effector function (Beatty & Gladney, 2015; Curran & Allison, 2009; Gettinger, 2017; Quezada, Peggs, Curran, & Allison, 2006). Clinical trials are underway to investigate the efficacy and safety of combining vaccines with anti–PD-L1 and anti–PD-1 agents. (Curran & Allison, 2009; Ho, 2017; Kleponis, Skelton, & Zheng, 2015; Sidney Kimmel Comprehensive Cancer Center, 2017). Vaccines are also being combined with chemotherapy, radiation therapy, and targeted therapies. Data have shown that traditional cytotoxic therapies and targeted therapies can increase inflammatory factors in the local tumor environment (Antonia et al., 2006; Heery et al., 2015; Hodge, Ardiani, Farsaci, Kwilas, & Gameiro, 2012), thereby amplifying immune response. In combination therapy, each modality has a specific effect on immune function with the hope that synergy can sufficiently overcome a powerful immunosuppressive microenvironment.

Ex Vivo Dendritic Cell Therapy

DCs are important APCs that can trigger an antigen-specific T-cell response. They have critical roles in surveillance, antigen-specific differentiation and maturation, and immune activation. Immunosuppressive microenvironments can greatly impair the activity of DCs in tissue. To overcome this challenge, researchers have manipulated DCs in a laboratory setting, sheltered from both the innate immune regulation of normal tissue and the added immune suppression of tumors. This class of therapy has been termed *ex vivo dendritic cell therapy* (Nguyen, Urban, & Kalinski, 2014; Pyzer, Avigan, & Rosenblatt, 2014).

Manufactured DC vaccines exploit the natural role of DCs. Successful stimulation of T cells by DCs is a multistep process that begins in the peripheral bloodstream. Immature DCs patrol the peripheral bloodstream, capturing peptide fragments via phagocytosis and ultimately loading them with MHC class I or II molecules on the membrane surface. At this point, the maturing DCs travel to lymphoid tissue. In the presence of immunostimulatory signals, the DCs become fully mature APCs, activating the CD4+ T cells, CD8+ T cells, B cells, and NK cells circulating in the lymphoid tissue (Pyzer et al., 2014; van der Burg et al., 2016). These activated cells can then generate an antigen-specific immune response. If antigen-loaded immature DCs interact with these cells in the absence of inflammatory cytokines and other immunostimulatory signals, immune tolerance will result.

In other words, the activated cells will be taught to ignore the antigen loaded onto the DCs. Unfortunately, cancer cells can often suppress inflammatory signals and generate inhibitory signals (Pyzer et al., 2014; van der Burg et al., 2016).

Ex vivo DC therapy begins with standard leukapheresis to harvest DCs and their precursors. The DCs are isolated, incubated with commercially prepared known tumor antigen, then exposed to inflammatory cytokines designed to enhance DC maturation. In this laboratory setting, the DCs are protected from the inhibitory signals generated by in situ tumor. The mature antigen-loaded DCs are then transfused into a patient, where they circulate to lymph tissue and stimulate CD4+ and CD8+ T-cell responses specific to the loaded antigen (Anassi & Ndefo, 2011; Chiang et al., 2015). Clinical trials are ongoing for prostate, breast, lung, colorectal, and kidney cancers, as well as for leukemia, melanoma, and non-Hodgkin lymphoma.

Oncolytic Viral Therapy

Another approach, distinct from other cancer vaccines, is oncolytic viral therapy (OVT), or the injection of nontumor virus material. As a point of clarification, OVT is distinct from viral vector therapy. The intent of viral vector therapy is the expression of tumor proteins using a virus as a delivery vehicle. In contrast, OVT involves the injection of attenuated virus that preferentially targets tumor (Bartlett et al., 2013). Certain viruses, such as coxsackie, measles, or herpes simplex, preferentially target and lyse tumor cells, thereby reducing tumor burden. This tumor destruction releases tumor antigens that are phagocytosed and processed by circulating APCs, ultimately generating MHC class I and II T-cell responses (Ding, 2014; Kaufman, Kohlhapp, & Zloza, 2016; Smith, Roth, Friedman, & Gillespie, 2014). These viruses can also be genetically enhanced to promote production of immunostimulatory cytokines, which recruit APCs to the injected site and amplify immune response. As with all vaccines, the goal is sustained, cell-based immunity that can be recalled on tumor redetection.

Approved Agents

Sipuleucel-T

Sipuleucel-T (Provenge®) was the first therapeutic vaccine approved by FDA (Dendreon Corp., 2014). It is used in asymptomatic or minimally symptomatic metastatic castrate-resistant (hormone-refractory) prostate cancer. Men treated with sipuleucel-T lived an average of 4.1 months longer than men treated with placebo in randomized trials. The three-year survival rate was 38% higher than the placebo group. No difference had been observed in time to progression or prostate-specific antigen response at the time of publication (Davis et al., 2015; Dendreon Corp., 2014; Graff & Chamberlain, 2015).

A full course of sipuleucel-T comprises patient-specific mature DCs primed against a common prostate cancer antigen, prostatic acid phosphatase (PAP). This is administered as three infusions in two-week intervals. Eligible patients undergo leukapheresis at a designated apheresis center within 72 hours of each planned dose. Harvested blood is sent to an FDA-approved manufacturing facility where precursor DCs are isolated. These cells are then cultured with a complex of PAP and GM-CSF for an incubation period of 36–44 hours. GM-CSF provides additional immunostimulatory action. PAP is commonly expressed on prostate cancer cell membranes but is uncommon on normal tissue, making it an ideal target (Shore et al., 2013). The final product is a solution of mature DCs displaying PAP antigen on MHC class I and II complexes. It is suspended in 250 ml of lactated Ringer solution. The manufacturer ships this solution to the ordering physician for administration at the patient's local oncology center or physician's office. Because of the highly patient-specific action of the drug, sipuleucel-T comes in a sealed, patient-specific bag that does not require further dilution or admixture. Nurses must confirm patient identifiers listed on the bag prior to each infusion. To prevent infusion reactions, patients may be premedicated orally with acetaminophen and an antihistamine approximately 30 minutes prior to each administration. Sipuleucel-T is infused via a patent IV access (peripheral or central) without a cell filter over 60 minutes with an 18- to 22-gauge needle (Dendreon Corp., 2014). Infusions must begin and end within three hours of opening the insulated container and prior to the expiration time and date listed on the infusion bag. Patients should be observed for infusion reactions for at least 30 minutes after each dose.

Side effects are primarily the result of infusion reactions, with 71% of patients reporting chills, fever, fatigue, nausea, headache, and joint ache within 24 hours of administration (Dendreon Corp., 2014). Most side effects (95%) were described as mild to moderate and resolved within 24 hours of initiation. In the event of infusion reaction, the infusion should be interrupted and reinitiated at a slower rate once the reaction has ceased. For 1.5% of patients, symptoms were severe enough to warrant treatment discontinuation. Other adverse reactions include cerebrovascular events (3.5%) and acute myocardial infarction (0.8%) (Dendreon Corp., 2014).

Talimogene Laherparepvec

Talimogene laherparepvec (Imlygic®), or T-VEC, is the first FDA-approved OVT (Amgen Inc., 2017). It is indicated in the local treatment of unresectable cutaneous, subcutaneous, and nodal lesions in patients with melanoma recurrent after initial surgery (Mary Crowley Cancer Research, 2015). In a recent study, eligible patients were randomized 2:1 to T-VEC or GM-CSF alone. In the T-VEC arm, patients achieved higher complete or partial response for at least six months (16.3% vs. 2.15%) compared to the GM-CSF arm. No statistically significant difference in overall survival was found between the two arms (22.9 months in the T-VEC arm vs. 19 months in the GM-CSF arm) (Andtbacka et al., 2015; Kaufman & Bines, 2010). This therapy produces a weakened type 2 herpes simplex virus that is genetically modified to express GM-CSF (Andtbacka et al., 2015). GM-CSF serves to enhance immune response by recruiting phagocytic granulocytes to the injected area (Rehman, Silk, Kane, & Kaufman, 2016).

The vaccine is injected directly into cutaneous, subcutaneous, or nodal lesions that are visible, palpable, or detectable with ultrasound guidance. Dosing volume is based on lesion diameter, and injection volume is 0.1–4 ml. The manufacturer recommends using an 18- to 26-gauge needle for drug withdrawal and a 22- to 26-gauge needle for injection, which should occur in a radial fashion (see Figure 7-1) (Amgen Inc., 2017). A full treatment course includes initial intralesional injections at a concentration of 106 pfu/ml. This is followed by maintenance injections of 108 pfu/ml every two weeks for at least six months until confirmed treatment failure, unacceptable toxicity, or complete response. Injections may be reinstated if new unresectable cutaneous, subcutaneous, or nodal lesions appear after a prior complete response. Premedication, including local anesthetics, should not be injected directly into the lesion but may be applied around its periphery.

Injection sites should be covered with sterile absorbent pads and occlusive dressing for at least the first week after each treatment or longer if weeping or oozing occurs. Patients may shed live virus until the site completely heals, putting others at risk. Patients should be advised against touching the lesion, using salves or ointments, swimming, or bathing in a tub for at least two to three weeks after injection. Patients are also strongly instructed to avoid touching the injection site, any mucous membrane, or broken skin. Hand hygiene after possible exposure and before eating should be reinforced. McMahon (2016) advised using gloves to place contaminated bandages and any dried scab material in sealed plastic bags with a small amount (capful) of bleach before disposal.

The most commonly reported adverse reactions to this therapy (greater than 25%) include fatigue, chills, pyrexia, nausea, flu-like symptoms, and injection site pain. Most reactions are mild to moderate, resolving within 72 hours, and are reported most frequently during the first three months of treatment. Uncommon but serious side effects include herpetic infections (especially in immunocompromised

---

FIGURE 7-1 Injection Technique for Imlygic® (Talimogene Laherparepvec)

2.3 Administration
Follow the steps below to administer IMLYGIC to patients:

Pre-Injection
1. Clean the lesion and surrounding areas with an alcohol swab and let dry.
2. Treat the injection site with a topical or local anesthetic agent, if necessary. Do not inject anesthetic agent directly into the lesion. Inject anesthetic agent around the periphery of the lesion.

Injection
1. Inject IMLYGIC intralesionally into cutaneous, subcutaneous, and/or nodal lesions that are visible, palpable, or detectable by ultrasound guidance. Using a single insertion point, inject IMLYGIC along multiple tracks as far as the radial reach of the needle allows within the lesion to achieve even and complete dispersion. Multiple insertion points may be used if a lesion is larger than the radial reach of the needle.

  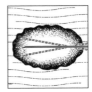

Figure 1: Injection administration for cutaneous lesions   Figure 2: Injection administration for subcutaneous lesions   Figure 3: Injection administration for nodal lesions

2. Inject IMLYGIC evenly and completely within the lesion by pulling the needle back without exiting the lesion. Redirect the needle as many times as necessary while injecting the remainder of the dose of IMLYGIC. Continue until the full dose is evenly and completely dispersed.
3. When removing the needle, withdraw it from the lesion slowly to avoid leakage of IMLYGIC at the insertion point.
4. Repeat steps 1-2 under pre-injection and steps 1-3 under injection for other lesions to be injected.
5. Use a new needle any time the needle is completely removed from a lesion and each time a different lesion is injected.

Post-Injection
1. Apply pressure to the injection site(s) with sterile gauze for at least 30 seconds.
2. Swab the injection site(s) and surrounding area with alcohol.
3. Change gloves and cover the injected lesion(s) with an absorbent pad and dry occlusive dressing.
4. Wipe the exterior of occlusive dressing with alcohol.
5. Advise patients to:
   • Keep the injection site(s) covered for at least the first week after each treatment visit or longer if the injection site is weeping or oozing.
   • Replace the dressing if it falls off.

3 DOSAGE FORMS AND STRENGTHS

   • Initial dose only: 10^6 (1 million) PFU per mL solution in 1 mL single-use vial (light green cap)
   • Subsequent doses: 10^8 (100 million) PFU per mL solution in 1 mL single-use vial (royal blue cap)

Note. From *Imlygic® (Talimogene Laherparepvec)* [Package Insert], by Amgen Inc., 2017, Thousand Oaks, CA: Author. Copyright 2017 by Amgen Inc. Reprinted with permission.

patients) and immune-mediated autoimmune disorders. Immunocompromised individuals should avoid contact with the drug, dressings, waste, or infusion equipment. Standard chemotherapy personal protective equipment should be donned when preparing or administering T-VEC (Amgen Inc., 2017; Rehman et al., 2016).

Response to treatment may be monitored by measuring injected lesion sizes. Median time to response has been reported to be four months and, as with other immunotherapies, tumor growth may precede tumor regression. Qualitative indicators of favorable response may precede objective quantitative tumor regression and include flattening, softening, eschar formation, or fading (Andtbacka et al., 2015). In the aforementioned study, objective response rates, or the proportion of patients experiencing tumor shrinkage, was 26% in the treatment group versus 11% in the control group. Overall survival for patients treated with T-VEC was reported at 23.3 months versus 18.9 months in the control group (Andtbacka et al., 2015).

Long-term immune-mediated surveillance against tumor growth is an obvious goal in cancer therapeutics. Achieving active immunity through vaccination is a growing research area. Identifying effective antigen profiles, overcoming suppressive tumor microenvironments, and optimizing immune system stimulation will lead to improved vaccine efficacy and patient survival. Ongoing clinical trials are exploring different approaches in delivering tumor antigen in the hopes of developing robust T-cell– and B-cell–mediated immune response.

Summary

Cancer vaccines are a relatively new addition to the antitumor armamentarium. Challenges to effective vaccine construction involve selecting the appropriate antigen, overcoming an inherently suppressive tumor microenvironment, and balancing the risk of autoimmune reaction. Clinically effective vaccines must translate immune activity into survival benefit. As new vaccines are developed, oncology nurses must be aware of their unique administration and monitoring needs to maximize patient safety and survival.

References

Amgen Inc. (2017). *Imlygic® (talimogene laherparepvec)* [Package insert]. Thousand Oaks, CA: Author.

Anassi, E., & Ndefo, U.A. (2011). Sipuleucel-T (Provenge) injection: The first immunotherapy agent (vaccine) For hormone-refractory prostate cancer. *Pharmacy and Therapeutics, 36,* 197–202.

Andtbacka, R.H.I., Kaufman, H.L., Collichio, F., Amatruda, T., Senzer, N., Chesney, J., … Coffin, R.S. (2015). Talimogene laherparepvec improves durable response rate in patients with advanced melanoma. *Journal of Clinical Oncology, 33,* 2780–2788. https://doi.org/10.1200/JCO.2014.58.3377

Antonia, S.J., Mirza, N., Fricke, I., Chiappori, A., Thompson, P., Williams, N., … Gabrilovic, D.I. (2006). Combination of p53 cancer vaccine with chemotherapy in patients with extensive stage small cell lung cancer. *Clinical Cancer Research, 12,* 878–887. https://doi.org/10.1158/1078-0432.CCR-05-2013

Baitsch, L., Fuertas-Marraco, S.A., Legat, A., Meyer, C., & Speiser, D.E. (2012). The three main stumbling blocks for anticancer T cells. *Trends in Immunology, 33,* 364–372. https://doi.org/10.1016/j.it.2012.02.006

Banday, A.H., Jeelani, S., & Hruby, V.J. (2015). Cancer vaccine adjuvants—Recent clinical progress and future perspectives. *Immunopharmacology and Immunotoxicology, 37,* 1–11. https://doi.org/10.3109/08923973.2014.971963

Bartlett, D.L., Liu, Z., Sathaiah, M., Ravindranathan, R., Guo, Z., He, Y., & Guo, Z.S. (2013). Oncolytic viruses as therapeutic cancer vaccines. *Molecular Cancer, 12,* 103–119. https://doi.org/10.1186/1476-4598-12-103

Beatty, G.L., & Gladney, W.L. (2015). Immune escape mechanisms as a guide for cancer immunotherapy. *Clinical Cancer Research, 21,* 687–692. https://doi.org/10.1158/1078-0432.CCR-14-1860

Bilusic, M., & Madan, R.A. (2012). Therapeutic cancer vaccines: The latest advancement in targeted therapy. *American Journal of Therapeutics, 19,* e172–e181. https://doi.org/10.1097/MJT.0b013e3182068cdb

Biogen, Inc., & Genentech, Inc. (2016). *Rituxan® (rituximab)* [Package insert]. South San Francisco, CA: Authors.

Bosch, F.X., Lorincz, A., Muñoz, N., Meijer, C.J., & Shah, K.V. (2002). The causal relation between human papillomavirus and cervical cancer. *Journal of Clinical Pathology, 55,* 244–265. https://doi.org/10.1136/jcp.55.4.244

Buonaguro, L., Petrizzo, A., Tornesello, M.L., & Buonaguro, F.M. (2011). Translating tumor antigens into cancer vaccines. *Clinical and Vaccine Immunology, 18,* 23–24. https://doi.org/10.1128/CVI.00286-10

Centers for Disease Control and Prevention. (2016). Vaccinations and immunizations: Glossary. Retrieved from https://www.cdc.gov/vaccines/terms/glossary.html

Chan, S.L., Wong, V.W.S., Qin, S., & Chan, H.L.Y. (2016). Infection and cancer: The case of hepatitis B. *Journal of Clinical Oncology, 34,* 83–90. https://doi.org/10.1200/JCO.2015.61.5724

Chang, M.-H. (2009). Cancer prevention by vaccination against hepatitis B. In H.-J. Senn, U. Kapp, & F. Otto (Eds.), *Recent Results in Cancer Research: Vol. 181. Cancer prevention II* (pp. 85–94). https://doi.org/10.1007/978-3-540-69297-3_10

Chiang, C.L.-L., Coukos, G., & Kandalaft, L.E. (2015). Whole tumor antigen vaccines: Where are we? *Vaccines, 3,* 344–372. https://doi.org/10.3390/vaccines3020344

Curran, M.A., & Allison, J.P. (2009). Tumor vaccines expressing FLT3 ligand synergize with CTLA-4 blockade to reject preimplanted tumors. *Cancer Research, 69,* 7747–7755. https://doi.org/10.1158/0008-5472.CAN-08-3289

Davis, K., Wood, S., Dill, E., Fesko, Y., Bitting, R.L., Harrison, M.R., … George, D.J. (2015). Optimizing the efficiency and quality of sipuleucel-T delivery in an academic institution. *Clinical Journal of Oncology Nursing, 19,* 297–303. https://doi.org/10.1188/15.CJON.297-303

Dendreon Corp. (2014). *Provenge® (sipuleucel-T)* [Package insert]. Seattle, WA: Author.

Ding, J. (2014). Oncolytic virus as a cancer stem cell killer: Progress and challenges. *Stem Cell Investigation, 22,* 1–7. https://doi.org/10.3978/j.issn.2306-9759.2014.12.02

Drake, C.G. (2014). The potential role of antigen spread in immunotherapy for prostate cancer. *Clinical Advances in Hematology and Oncology, 12,* 332–334.

Garland, S.M., Hernandez-Avila, M., Wheeler, C.M., Perez, G., Harper, D.M., Leodolter, S.P., … Koutsky, L.A. (2007). Quadrivalent vaccine against human papillomavirus to prevent anogenital diseases. *New England Journal of Medicine, 356,* 1928–1943. https://doi.org/10.1056/NEJMoa061760

Gay, L., Baker, A.-M., & Graham, T.A. (2016). Tumour cell heterogeneity. *F1000Research, 5*(F1000 Faculty Rev), 238. http://doi.org/10.12688/f1000research.7210.1

Geary, S.M., Lemke, C.D., Lubaroff, D.M., & Salem, A.K. (2013). Proposed mechanism of action for prostate cancer vaccines. *Nature Reviews Urology, 10,* 149–160. https://doi.org/10.1038/nrurol.2013.8

Genentech, Inc. (n.d.). *Kadcyla® (ado-trastuzumab emtansine)* [Package insert]. South San Francisco, CA: Author.

Genentech, Inc. (2009). *Avastin® (bevacizumab)* [Package insert]. South San Francisco, CA: Author.

Gettinger, S. (2017). Phase 2 study of MPDL3280A combined with CDX-1401 in NY-ESO 1 (+) IIIB, IV or recurrent non-small cell lung cancer [ClinicalTrials.gov Identifier: NCT02495636]. Retrieved from https://clinicaltrials.gov/ct2/show/NCT02495636

Gibbons-Johnson, R.M., & Dong, H. (2017). Functional expression of programmed death-ligand 1 (7-H1) by immune cells and tumor cells. *Frontiers in Immunology, 8,* 961. https://doi.org/10.3389/fimmu.2017.00961

Graff, J.N., & Chamberlain, E.D. (2015). Sipuleucel-T in the treatment of prostate cancer: An evidence-based review of its place in therapy. *Core Evidence, 10,* 1–10. https://doi.org/10.2147/CE.S54712

Guo, C., Manjili, M.H., Subjeck, J.R., Sarkar, D., Fisher, P.B., & Wang, X.-Y. (2013). Therapeutic cancer vaccines: Past, present and future. In K.D. Tew & P.B. Fisher (Eds.), *Advances in Cancer Research: Vol. 119* (pp. 421–475). https://doi.org/10.1016/B978-0-12-407190-2.00007-1

Hariri, S., Markowitz, L.E., Dunne, E.F., & Unger, E.R. (2013). Population impact of HPV vaccines: Summary of early evidence. *Journal of Adolescent Health, 53,* 679–682. https://doi.org/10.1016/j.jadohealth.2013.09.018

Heery, C.R., Ibrahim, N.K., Arlen, P.M., Mohebtash, M., Murray, J.L., Koenig, K., ... Gulley, J.L. (2015). Docetaxel alone or in combination with a therapeutic cancer vaccine (PANVAC) in patients with metastatic breast cancer: A randomized clinical trial. *JAMA Oncology, 8,* 1087–1095. https://doi.org/10.1001/jamaoncol.2015.2736

Helwick, C. (2016). Breast cancer vaccines moving forward at a fast clip. *ASCO Post.* Retrieved from http://www.ascopost.com/issues/april-10-2016/breast-cancer-vaccines-moving-forward-at-a-fast-clip

Ho, V.T. (2017). GVAX vs. placebo for MDS/AML after allo HSCT [ClinicalTrials.gov Identifier: NCT01773395]. Retrieved from https://clinicaltrials.gov/show/NCT01773395

Hodge, J.W., Ardiani, A., Farsaci, B., Kwilas, A.R., & Gameiro, S.R. (2012). The tipping point for combination therapy: Cancer vaccines with radiation, chemotherapy, or targeted small molecule inhibitors. *Seminars in Oncology, 39,* 323–339. https://doi.org/10.1053/j.seminoncol.2012.02.006

Hrouda, D., Todryk, S.M., Perry, M.J.A., Souberbielle, B.E., Kayaga, J., Kirby, R.S., & Dalgleish, A.G. (2000). Allogeneic whole-tumour cell vaccination in the rat model of prostate cancer. *British Journal of Urology International, 86,* 742–748. https://doi.org/10.1046/j.1464-410x.2000.00887.x

Huang, Z.-H., Sun, Z.-Y., Gao, Y., Chen, P.-G., Liu, Y.-F., Chen, Y.-X., & Li, Y.-M. (2014). Strategy for designing a synthetic tumor vaccine: Multi-component, multivalency and antigen modification. *Vaccines, 2,* 549–562. https://doi.org/10.3390/vaccines2030549

Kaufman, H.L., & Bines, S.D. (2010). OPTIM trial: A phase III trial of an oncolytic herpes virus encoding GM-CSF for unresectable stage III or IV melanoma. *Future Oncology, 6,* 941–949. https://doi.org/10.2217/fon.10.66

Kaufman, H.L., Kohlhapp, F.J., & Zloza, A. (2016). Oncolytic viruses: A new class of immunotherapy drugs. *Nature Reviews Drug Discovery, 14,* 642–662. https://doi.org/10.1038/nrd4663

Keenan, B.P., & Jaffee, E.M. (2012). Whole cell vaccines—Past progress and future strategies. *Seminars in Oncology, 39,* 276–286. https://doi.org/10.1053/j.seminoncol.2012.02.007

King, S.E. (2004). Therapeutic cancer vaccines: An emerging treatment option. *Clinical Journal of Oncology Nursing, 8,* 271–278. https://doi.org/10.1188/04.CJON.271-278

Kleponis, J., Skelton, R., & Zheng, L. (2015). Fueling the engine and releasing the break: Combinational therapy of cancer vaccines and immune checkpoint inhibitors. *Cancer Biology and Medicine, 12,* 201–208. http://doi.org/10.7497/j.issn.2095-3941.2015.0046

Kurtz, S.L., Ravindranathan, S., & Zaharoff, D.A. (2014). Current status of autologous breast tumor cell-based vaccines. *Expert Review of Vaccines, 13,* 1439–1445. https://doi.org/10.1586/14760584.2014.969714

Larocca, C., & Schlom, J. (2011). Viral vector-based therapeutic cancer vaccines. *Cancer Journal, 17,* 359–371. https://doi.org/10.1097/PPO.0b013e3182325e63

Li, W., Joshi, M.D., Singhania, S., Ramsey, K.H., & Murthy, A.K. (2014). Peptide vaccine: Progress and challenges. *Vaccines, 2,* 515–536. https://doi.org/10.3390/vaccines2030515

Lollini, P.-L., Cavallo, F., Nanni, P., & Forni, G. (2006). Vaccines for tumour prevention. *Nature Reviews Cancer, 6,* 204–216. https://doi.org/10.1038/nrc1815

Mary Crowley Cancer Research. (2015, October 4). FDA approves first-of-its-kind product for treatment of melanoma. Retrieved from https://www.marycrowley.org/newsroom/press-releases/fda-approves-first-its-kind-product-treatment-melanoma

McMahon, S. (2016). Minimizing hazards associated with live-virus immunotherapeutic cancer vaccines. *Clinical Journal of Oncology Nursing, 20,* 602–604. https://doi.org/10.1188/16.CJON.602-604

National Cancer Institute. (2015). Cancer vaccines. Retrieved from https://www.cancer.gov/about-cancer/causes-prevention/vaccines-fact-sheet

Nguyen, T., Urban, J., & Kalinski, P. (2014). Therapeutic cancer vaccines and combination immunotherapies involving vaccination. *Immunotargets and Therapy, 3,* 135–150. https://doi.org/10.2147/ITT.S40264

Parmiani, G., Russo, V., Maccalli, C., Parolini, D., Rizzo, N., & Maio, M. (2014). Peptide-based vaccines for cancer therapy. *Human Vaccines and Immunotherapeutics, 10,* 3175–3178. https://doi.org/10.4161/hv.29418

Perica, K., Varela, J.C., Oelke, M., & Schneck, J. (2015). Adoptive T cell immunotherapy for cancer. *Rambam Maimonides Medical Journal, 6,* e0004. https://doi.org/10.5041/RMMJ.10179

Pol, J., Bloy, N., Buqué, A., Eggermont, A., Cremer, I., Sautès-Fridman, C., ... Galluzzi, L. (2015). Trial watch: Peptide-based anticancer vaccines. *Oncoimmunology, 4,* e974411. https://doi.org/10.4161/2162402X.2014.974411

Pyzer, A.R., Avigan, D.E., & Rosenblatt, J. (2014). Clinical trials of dendritic cell-based cancer vaccines in hematologic malignancies. *Human Vaccines and Immunotherapeutics, 10,* 3125–3131. https://doi.org/10.4161/21645515.2014.982993

Quezada, S.A., Peggs, K.S., Curran, M.A., & Allison, J.P. (2006). CTLA4 blockade and GM-CSF combination immunotherapy alters the intratumor balance of effector and regulatory T cells. *Journal of Clinical Investigation, 116,* 1935–1945. https://doi.org/10.1172/JCI27745

Rehman, H., Silk, A.W., Kane, M.P., & Kaufman, H.L. (2016). Into the clinic: Talimogene laherparepvec (T-VEC), a first-in-class intratumoral oncolytic viral therapy. *Journal for Immunotherapy of Cancer, 4,* 53. https://doi.org/10.1186/s40425-016-0158-5

Schmidt, S.V., Nino-Castro, A.C., & Schultze, J.L. (2012). Regulatory dendritic cells: There is more than just immune activation. *Frontiers in Immunology, 3,* 274. https://doi.org/10.3389/fimmu.2012.00274

Shore, N.D., Mantz, C.A., Dosoretz, D.E., Fernandez, E., Myslicki, F.A., McCoy, C., ... Fishman, M.N. (2013). Building on sipuleucel-T for immunologic treatment of castration-resistant prostate cancer. *Cancer Control, 20,* 7–16. https://doi.org/10.1177/107327481302000103

Sidney Kimmel Comprehensive Cancer Center. (2017). A phase 2, multicenter study of FOLFIRINOX followed by ipilimumab with allogenic GM-CSF transfected pancreatic tumor vaccine in the treatment of metastatic pancreatic cancer [Clinicaltrials.gov Identifier: NCT01896869]. Retrieved from https://clinicaltrials.gov/show/NCT01896869NLM%20Identifie:NCT018968695

Siegrist, C.-A. (2013). Vaccine immunology. In S.A. Plotkin, W.A. Orenstein, & P.A. Offit (Eds.), *Vaccines* (6th ed., pp. 14–32). Philadelphia, PA: Elsevier Saunders.

Slingluff, C.L., Jr. (2011). The present and future of peptide vaccines for cancer: Single or multiple, long or short, alone or in combination? *Cancer Journal, 17*, 343–350. https://doi.org/10.1097/PPO.0b013e318233e5b2

Smith, T.T., Roth, J.C., Friedman, G.K., & Gillespie, G.Y. (2014). Oncolytic viral therapy: Targeting cancer stem cells. *Oncolytic Virotherapy, 3*, 21–33.

Sondak, V.K., Liu, P.-K., Tuthill, R.J., Kempf, R.A., Unger, J.M., Sosman, J.A., ... Flaherty, L.E. (2002). Adjuvant immunotherapy of resected, intermediate-thickness, node-negative melanoma with an allogeneic tumor vaccine: Overall results of a randomized trial of the Southwest Oncology Group. *Journal of Clinical Oncology, 20*, 2058–2066. https://doi.org/10.1200/JCO.2002.08.071

Sosman, J.A., Unger, J.M., Liu, P.-Y., Flaherty, L.E., Park, M.S., Kempf, R.A., ... Sondak, V.K. (2002). Adjuvant immunotherapy of resected, intermediate-thickness, node-negative melanoma with an allogeneic tumor vaccine: Impact of HLA class I antigen expression on outcome. *Journal of Clinical Oncology, 20*, 2067–2075. https://doi.org/10.1200/JCO.2002.08.072

Srivatsan, S., Patel, J.M., Bozeman, E.N., Imasuen, I.E., He, S., Daniels, D., & Selvaraj, P. (2014). Allogeneic tumor cell vaccines: The promise and limitations in clinical trials. *Human Vaccines and Immunotherapeutics, 10*, 52–63. https://doi.org/10.4161/hv.26568

Sun, C., Dotti, G., & Savoldo, B. (2016). Utilizing cell-based therapeutics to overcome immune evasion in hematologic malignancies. *Blood, 127*, 3350–3359. https://doi.org/10.1182/blood-2015-12-629089

Temizoz, B., Kuroda, E., & Ishii, K.J. (2016). Vaccine adjuvants as potential cancer immunotherapeutics. *International Immunology, 28*, 329–338. https://doi.org/10.1093/intimm/dxw015

Uyl-de Groot, C.A., Vermorken, J.B., Hanna, M.G., Jr., Verboom, P., Groot, M.J., Bonsel, B.J., ... Pinedo, M.J. (2005). Immunotherapy with autologous tumor cell-BCG vaccine in patients with colon cancer: A prospective study of medical and economic benefits. *Vaccine, 23*, 2379–2387.

van der Burg, S.H., Arens, R., Ossendorp, F., van Hall, T., & Melief, C.J.M. (2016). Vaccines for established cancer: Overcoming the challenges posed by immune evasion. *Nature Reviews Cancer, 16*, 219–233. https://doi.org/10.1038/nrc.2016.16

Vermorken, J.B., Claessen, A.M., van Tinteren, H., Gall, H.E., Ezinga, R., Meijer, S., ... Pinedo, H.M. (1999). Active specific immunotherapy for stage II and stage III human colon cancer: A randomised trial. *Lancet, 30*, 345–350. https://doi.org/10.1016/S0140-6736(98)07186-4

Wang, M., Yin, B., Wang, H.Y., & Wang, R.-F. (2014). Current advances in T-cell-based cancer immunotherapy. *Immunotherapy, 6*, 1265–1278. https://doi.org/10.2217/imt.14.86

Wei, X.X., Chan, S., Kwek, S., Lewis, J., Dao, V., Zhang, L., ... Fong, L. (2016). Systemic GM-CSF recruits effector T cells into the tumor microenvironment in localized prostate cancer. *Cancer Immunology Research, 4*, 948–958. https://doi.org/10.1158/2326-6066.CIR-16-0042

Weide, B., Garbe, C., Rammensee, H.G., & Pascolo, S. (2008). Plasmid DNA- and messenger RNA-based anti-cancer vaccination. *Immunology Letters, 115*, 33–42. https://doi.org/10.1016/j.imlet.2007.09.012

Yamada, A., Sasada, T., Noguchi, M., & Itoh, K., (2013). Next-generation peptide vaccines for advanced cancer. *Cancer Science, 104*, 15–21. https://doi.org/10.1111/cas.12050

Yang, B., Jeang, J., Yang, A., Wu, T.C., & Hung, C.-F. (2015). DNA vaccine for cancer immunotherapy. *Human Vaccines and Immunotherapies, 10*, 3153–3164. https://doi.org/10.4161/21645515.2014.980686

c h a p t e r e i g h t

Passive/Adoptive Immunotherapy

Barbara Barnes Rogers, CRNP, MN, AOCN®, ANP-BC

Introduction

Anticancer immunotherapies are generally classified as either *passive* or *active* based on their ability to activate the immune system against malignant cells. Tumor-targeting monoclonal antibodies (mAbs) and adoptively transferred T cells are considered passive forms of immunotherapy because they have intrinsic antineoplastic activity. Passive immunotherapy is advantageous because it does not rely on the immune system to initiate a response, which is beneficial for those with dysfunctional immune systems caused by tumor burden or prior therapies. A disadvantage of passive immunotherapy is that target cells can mutate, downregulate, or otherwise alter the targeted antigen, making the disease resistant to therapy (Brody, Kohrt, Marabelle, & Levy, 2011). This chapter will review the passive/adoptive immunotherapies currently in practice.

Tumor-Targeting Monoclonal Antibodies

Therapeutic mAbs are structured in a classic "Y" formation of bifunctional capacity. These structures comprise two identical fragment antigen-binding (Fab) fragments and one constant fragment crystallizable (Fc) fragment. These bind to and activate immune cells (e.g., macrophages, natural killer [NK] cells, cytotoxic T-lymphocytes) (see Figure 8-1). The mAbs are named based on human amino acid sequences (see Figure 8-2 and Table 8-1). Chimeric antibodies are engineered from the cells of nonhuman organisms, usually mice, with a portion replaced with a human sequence of amino acids. These protein sequences are modified to increase similarities to antibodies produced naturally by humans. Human antibodies contain the full human protein sequence.

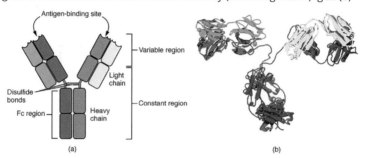

FIGURE 8-1 Structure of an Antibody

The typical four-chain structure of a generic antibody (a) and the corresponding three-dimensional structure of the antibody (immunoglobulin) IgG2 (b)

Note. From "The Adaptive Immune Response: B-Lymphocytes and Antibodies, Anatomy and Physiology," by T. Vickers, 2014. Retrieved from https://cnx.org/contentsFPtK1zmh@6.27:AY5_7yUs@4/The-Adaptive-Immune-Response-B. Used under the CC BY-SA 3.0 license (https://creativecommons.org/licenses/by-sa/3.0/deed.en).

Tumor-targeting mAbs are the most characterized form of anticancer immunotherapy. These mAbs specifically alter the signaling functions of receptors expressed on the surface of malignant cells. They also bind to and neutralize signals produced by malignant cells or stromal components of neoplastic lesions. Tumor-targeting mAbs can selectively recognize cancer cells based on tumor-associated antigen (TAA) expression by transformed cells (Galluzzi et al., 2014). Some mAb target receptors can display on both tumor and normal cells (e.g., CD20 [cluster of differentiation 20] on both normal B cells and B-cell non-Hodgkin lymphoma [NHL]).

Tumor-targeting mAbs exist in at least five functionally different variants and include the following (Galluzzi et al., 2014) (see Table 8-2):
- Naked mAbs that inhibit signaling pathways required for progression or survival of neoplastic cells (e.g., the epidermal growth factor receptor [EGFR]-specific mAb cetuximab)
- Naked mAbs that activate potentially lethal receptors on malignant cells (e.g., the tumor necrosis factor–specific mAb tigatuzumab)
- Immune conjugates coupled to toxins or radionuclides (e.g., the anti-CD33 calicheamicin conjugate gemtuzumab ozogamicin)
- Naked TAA-specific mAbs that opsonize cancer cells and activate antibody-dependent cellular cytotoxicity (ADCC), antibody-dependent cellular phagocytosis (ADCP), and complement-dependent cytotoxicity (CDC) (e.g., the CD20-specific mAb rituximab)
- Bispecific T-cell engagers (BiTEs) that are chimeric proteins of two single-chain variable fragments from distinct mAbs. One fragment tar-

FIGURE 8-2 Description of Components of Monoclonal Antibodies

Light gray indicates human component, while dark gray indicates non-human component.

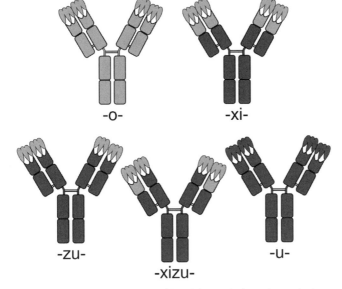

o—mouse; u—human; xi—chimeric; xizu—chimeric/humanized; zu—humanized

Note. From "Chimeric and Humanized Antibodies," by Anypodetos, 2011. Retrieved from https://commons.wikimedia.org/wiki/File:Chimeric_and_humanized_antibodies_with_CDRs.svg. Used under the CC BY-SA 3.0 license (https://creativecommons.org/licenses/by-sa/3.0/deed.en).

gets a tumor-targeting antigen, and the other is specific for a T-cell surface antigen.

These mAbs have three possible mechanisms of action: ADCC, CDC, or direct growth inhibition/apoptosis (direct cell death).

Epidermal Growth Factor Receptor–Specific Monoclonal Antibodies

EGFR is stimulated by transforming growth factor alpha (TGF-α) and epidermal growth factor (EGF). Cetuximab (Erbitux®) and panitumumab (Vectibix®), mAbs against human EGFR, act as functional antagonists of the EGF and TGF-α ligands and inhibit the EGFR-dependent signaling pathways. Blocking these pathways leads to inhibition of can-

TABLE 8-1   Nomenclature for Monoclonal Antibodies

Antibody Origin	Substem	Examples
Chimeric	-xi-	Brentuximab vedotin, cetuximab, rituximab, siltuximab
Humanized	-zu-	Ado-trastuzumab emtansine, alemtuzumab, bevacizumab, obinutuzumab, pertuzumab
Human	-u-	Denosumab, ofatumumab, panitumumab, ramucirumab

Note. Based on information from American Medical Association, n.d.

TABLE 8-2   Types of Monoclonal Antibodies

Type	Specific Target	Conjugated	Examples
Naked	Yes	No	EGFR-specific cetuximab
Naked and activates potentially lethal receptors on cancer cells	Yes	No	TNF-specific tigatuzumab
Conjugated	Yes	Yes	CD33-specific gemtuzumab ozogamicin
Naked and activates ADCC, ADCP, and CDC	Yes	No	CD20-specific rituximab
Bispecific	Two targets	No (not with currently available agents)	CD19- and CD3-specific blinatumumab

ADCC—antibody-dependent cellular cytotoxicity; ADCP—antibody-dependent cellular phagocytosis; CD—cluster of differentiation; CDC—complement-dependent cytotoxicity; EGFR—epidermal growth factor receptor; TNF—tumor necrosis factor

Note. Based on information from Galluzzi et al., 2014.

cer cell division in the G_1 phase. This is caused by a lack of transcription factors and eventually results in cell death (Holubec, Polivka, Safanda, Karas, & Liska, 2016). Both cetuximab and panitumumab induce an immune response against the cells that contain their binding receptors.

The *KRAS* mutation has been identified in lung and colon cancer. When present, signaling pathways are activated independent of EGFR, which may make the anti-EGFR mechanism ineffective (Mahipal & Grothey, 2016). Therefore, cetuximab and panitumumab are not recommended for use with *KRAS* mutations.

Although panitumumab binds to EGFR with higher activity than cetuximab, its immunoglobulin (Ig) G2 isotype has significantly lower immunogenicity and binds poorly to Fc receptor gamma. The Fc region provides the mAb the ability to interact with complement or with receptors expressed by effector immune cells. Because IgG2 mAbs bind poorly to the Fc region, they cannot induce an immune response by ADCC or other mechanisms; however, IgG1 mAbs (cetuximab) have this ability (Holubec et al., 2016).

Cetuximab

Cetuximab is a chimeric IgG1 mAb that inhibits the tyrosine kinase domain of EGFR. Because of antibody binding, the receptor internalizes, CDC occurs, and cell division is halted.

Cetuximab is approved as a single agent or combined with radiation or platinum-based therapy for the management of squamous cell carcinoma of the head and neck. It is approved as a single agent or with FOLFIRI (leucovorin, 5-fluorouracil [5-FU], and irinotecan) or irinotecan alone for the management of *KRAS* wild-type EGFR-expressing colorectal cancer (Bristol-Myers Squibb Co., 2012).

Cetuximab is administered through a low-protein-binding 0.22 mcm in-line filter at a dose of 400 mg/m² over 120 minutes for the first infusion. Subsequent infusions are administered at 250 mg/m² weekly over 60 minutes. Premedication includes a histamine-1 (H_1) blocker (e.g., diphenhydramine) IV 30–60 minutes prior to the first dose. Subsequent premedication is based on clinical judgment and the presence or severity of prior infusion reactions (Bristol-Myers Squibb Co., 2012).

In the CRYSTAL study, 1,198 patients were randomly assigned to receive infusional FOLFIRI with or without cetuximab. Overall response rate (ORR; 57% vs. 40%), progression-free survival (PFS; 9.9 months vs. 8.4 months), and overall survival (OS; 23.5 months vs. 20 months) were better in the cetuximab arm (Van Cutsem et al., 2009). This margin widened when patients with *KRAS* or *NRAS* mutations were excluded. This study led to U.S. Food and Drug Administration (FDA) approval of cetuximab for frontline therapy of metastatic colorectal cancer.

In the COIN trial, 1,630 patients were randomized to receive either FOLFOX (5-FU, leucovorin, and oxaliplatin) or XELOX (capecitabine and oxaliplatin) with or without cetuximab. Although ORR was slightly higher in the cetuximab arm (64% vs. 57%), no significant differences in PFS or OS were reported; however, patients treated with FOLFOX with cetuximab showed improvements in PFS (Maughan et al., 2011). After excluding patients with *KRAS* and *BRAF* mutations, cetuximab did not confer any survival benefit (20.1 months vs. 19.9 months). National Comprehensive Cancer Network® (NCCN®) guidelines recommend against combining capecitabine-based therapies with EGFR mAbs (NCCN, 2017).

Panitumumab

Panitumumab is a fully humanized IgG2 mAb that blocks activation of EGFR, prevents tumor formation, and eradicates established tumors (Yang et al., 1999). Mirroring cetuximab, panitumumab's proposed mechanism of antitumor effect includes induction of cell cycle arrest, promotion of apoptosis, and EGFR downregulation.

Panitumumab is indicated for the treatment of *KRAS* (exon 2 in codons 12 or 13) wild-type metastatic colorectal cancer. It can be used as a first-line monotherapy or in combination with FOLFOX following disease progression after prior treatment with fluoropyrimidine-, oxaliplatin-, and irinotecan-containing chemotherapy. Panitumumab is administered at 6 mg/kg every 14 days via IV infusion over 60 (1,000 mg or less) or 90 minutes (greater than 1,000 mg) (Amgen Inc., 2017b).

In the PRIME trial, 1,183 patients were randomized to FOLFOX4 plus panitumumab or FOLFOX4 alone for the treatment of *KRAS* (exon 2) wild-type metastatic colorectal cancer (Douillard et al., 2010). Initially, the study was designed to test treatment effect in all randomized patients. However, once *KRAS* was established as a predictive biomarker, the study was amended to compare outcomes based on *KRAS* status. Results indicated improved PFS for patients who received FOLFOX4 plus panitumumab (10 months vs. 8.6 months). A detrimental PFS was seen in those with exon 2 mutations enrolled in the FOLFOX4 plus panitumumab arm compared to those who did not receive panitumumab (7.4 months vs. 9.2 months) (Douillard et al., 2010). Although the reasons for this detrimental effect are unclear, comprehensive *KRAS* mutation testing is critical before EGFR mAbs are used in the treatment of colorectal cancer. This study led to FDA approval of panitumumab as a first-line treatment for metastatic colorectal cancer (Douillard et al., 2010).

Side Effects

Toxicity incidence for EGFR-specific mAbs varies between agents. Agent selection can be aided by considering potential incidence for each agent (Yazdi, Faramarzi, Nikfar, & Abdollahi, 2015) (see Table 8-3). Toxicities include ocular toxicity, stomatitis, diarrhea/colitis, altered liver function, hypomagnesemia, infusion reactions, and interstitial lung disease. Dermatologic toxicity will be discussed extensively in a separate section.

TABLE 8-3   Most Common Toxicities of Passive/Adoptive Immunotherapy Agents

Agent	Toxicities
EGFR-Targeted Antibodies	
Cetuximab (≥ 25%)	Cutaneous reactions (e.g., rash, pruritus, nail changes), headache, diarrhea, and infection
Panitumumab	
• Monotherapy (≥ 20%)	Skin rash (with variable presentation), paronychia, fatigue, nausea, and diarrhea
• In combination with FOLFOX (≥ 20%)	Diarrhea, stomatitis, mucosal inflammation, asthenia, paronychia, anorexia, hypomagnesemia, hypokalemia, rash, acneform dermatitis, pruritus, and dry skin
HER2–Targeted Antibodies	
Pertuzumab	
• Metastatic breast cancer (> 30%) in combination with trastuzumab + docetaxel	Diarrhea, alopecia, neutropenia, nausea, fatigue, rash, and peripheral neuropathy
• Neoadjuvant treatment of breast cancer	
— In combination with trastuzumab + docetaxel (> 30%) given for 3 cycles following 3 cycles of FEC	Fatigue, alopecia diarrhea, nausea, vomiting, and neutropenia
— In combination with docetaxel, carboplatin, and trastuzumab (> 30%)	Fatigue, alopecia, diarrhea, nausea, vomiting, neutropenia, thrombocytopenia, and anemia
— In combination with trastuzumab and docetaxel	Alopecia, diarrhea, nausea, and neutropenia
— In combination with trastuzumab and paclitaxel for 4 cycles following 4 cycles of ddAC (> 30%)	Fatigue, alopecia, diarrhea, nausea, constipation, and headache
— In combination with trastuzumab and docetaxel when given for 4 cycles following 4 cycles of FEC (> 30%)	Fatigue, alopecia, diarrhea, nausea, mucosal inflammation, vomiting, myalgias, and anemia
Trastuzumab	
• Adjuvant breast cancer (≥ 5%)	Headache, diarrhea, nausea, and chills
• Metastatic breast cancer (≥ 10%)	Fever, chills, headache, infection, congestive heart failure, insomnia, cough, and rash
• Metastatic gastric cancer (≥ 10%)	Neutropenia, diarrhea, fatigue, anemia, stomatitis, weight loss, upper respiratory tract infection, fever, thrombocytopenia, mucosal inflammation, nasopharyngitis, and dysgeusia

(Continued on next page)

TABLE 8-3   Most Common Toxicities of Passive/Adoptive Immunotherapy Agents *(Continued)*

Agent	Toxicities
VEGF-Targeted Antibodies	
Bevacizumab (≥ 25%)	Cutaneous adverse reactions (e.g., rash, pruritus, nail changes), headache, diarrhea, and infection
Ramucirumab	
• ≥ 10% single agent	Hypertension and diarrhea
• ≥ 30% and ≥ 2% higher than placebo + paclitaxel	Fatigue, neutropenia, diarrhea, and epistaxis
• ≥ 30% and ≥ 2% higher than placebo + docetaxel	Neutropenia, fatigue/asthenia, and stomatitis/mucosal inflammation
• ≥ 30% and ≥ 2% higher than placebo + FOLFIRI	Diarrhea, neutropenia, decreased appetite, epistaxis, and stomatitis
PDGFR-α–Targeted Antibody	
Olaratumab plus doxorubicin (≥ 20%)	Nausea, fatigue, musculoskeletal pain, mucositis, alopecia, vomiting, diarrhea, decreased appetite, abdominal pain, neuropathy, and headache Most common laboratory abnormalities: lymphopenia, neutropenia, thrombocytopenia, hyperglycemia, elevated activated PTT, hypokalemia, and hypophosphatemia
CD20-Targeted Antibodies	
Obinutuzumab	
• Previously untreated CLL (≥ 10%)	Infusion reactions, neutropenia, thrombocytopenia, and diarrhea
• Relapsed/refractory NHL (≥ 10%)	Infusion reactions, neutropenia, cough, constipation, pyrexia, upper respiratory tract infection, arthralgia, sinusitis, asthenia, and urinary tract infection
• Previously untreated NHL (≥ 10%)	Infusion reaction, neutropenia, upper respiratory tract infection, cough, constipation, diarrhea, headache, herpes virus infection, arthralgias, insomnia, pneumonia, thrombocytopenia, decreased appetite, alopecia, and pruritus

(Continued on next page)

TABLE 8-3   Most Common Toxicities of Passive/Adoptive Immunotherapy Agents *(Continued)*

Agent	Toxicities
CD20-Targeted Antibodies *(cont.)*	
Ofatumumab	
• Previously untreated CLL (≥ 10%)	Infusion reactions and neutropenia
• Relapsed CLL (≥ 10%)	Infusion reactions, neutropenia, leukopenia, and febrile neutropenia
• Extended treatment CLL (≥ 10%)	Infusion reactions, neutropenia, and upper respiratory tract infection
• Refractory CLL (> 10%)	Neutropenia, pneumonia, pyrexia, cough, diarrhea, anemia, fatigue, dyspnea, rash, nausea, bronchitis, and upper respiratory tract infection
Rituximab	NHL (≥ 25%)—infusion reaction, fever, lymphocytopenia, chills, infection, asthenia CLL (≥ 25%)—infusion reaction and neutropenia
Rituximab and hyaluronidase (> 20%)	FL (≥ 20%)—infection, neutropenia, nausea, constipation, cough, and fatigue DLBCL (≥ 20%)—infection, neutropenia, alopecia, nausea, and anemia CLL (≥ 20%)—infection, neutropenia, nausea, thrombocytopenia, pyrexia, vomiting, and injection-site erythema
SLAMF7-Targeted Antibody	
Elotuzumab (≥ 20%)	Fatigue, diarrhea, pyrexia, constipation, cough, peripheral neuropathy, nasopharyngitis, upper respiratory tract infection, decreased appetite, and pneumonia
CD38-Targeted Antibody	
Daratumumab (≥ 20%)	Infusion reaction, neutropenia, thrombocytopenia, fatigue, nausea, diarrhea, constipation, vomiting, muscle spasms, arthralgia, back pain, pyrexia, chills, dizziness, insomnia, cough, dyspnea, peripheral edema, peripheral sensory neuropathy, and upper respiratory tract infection

(Continued on next page)

TABLE 8-3   Most Common Toxicities of Passive/Adoptive Immunotherapy Agents *(Continued)*

Agent	Toxicities
IL-6–Targeted Antibody	
Siltuximab (> 10%)	Pruritus, increased weight, rash, hyperuricemia, and upper respiratory tract infection
CD52-Targeted Antibody	
Alemtuzumab (≥ 10%)	Rash, headache, pyrexia, nasopharyngitis, nausea, urinary tract infection, fatigue, insomnia, upper respiratory tract infection, herpes viral infection, urticaria, pruritus, thyroid gland disorders, fungal infection, arthralgia, pain in extremity, back pain, diarrhea, sinusitis, oropharyngeal pain, paresthesia, dizziness, abdominal pain, flushing, and vomiting
RANKL-Targeted Antibody	
Denosumab • Bone metastasis for solid tumors (≥ 25%)	Arthralgia, back pain, pain in extremity, and musculoskeletal pain
• Multiple myeloma (> 10%)	Diarrhea, nausea, anemia, back pain, thrombocytopenia, peripheral edema, hypocalcemia, upper respiratory tract infection, rash, and headache
Antibody–Drug Conjugates	
Ado-trastuzumab emtansine (≥ 25%)	Fatigue, nausea, musculoskeletal pain, hemorrhage, thrombocytopenia, headache, increased transaminases, constipation, and epistaxis
Brentuximab vedotin (≥ 20%)	Neutropenia, peripheral sensory neuropathy, nausea, fatigue, constipation, diarrhea, vomiting, and pyrexia
Radioimmunotherapy	
Ibritumomab tiuxetan (≥ 10%)	Cytopenias, fatigue, nasopharyngitis, nausea, abdominal pain, asthenia, cough, diarrhea, and pyrexia
Bispecific T-Cell Engager Antibody	
Blinatumomab (≥ 20%)	Infections (bacteria + pathogen unspecified), pyrexia, headache, infusion reactions, anemia, febrile neutropenia, thrombocytopenia, and neutropenia

(Continued on next page)

TABLE 8-3   Most Common Toxicities of Passive/Adoptive Immunotherapy Agents *(Continued)*

Agent	Toxicities
Chimeric Antigen Receptor T Cells	
Axicabtagene ciloleucel (≥ 20%)	Cytokine release syndrome, fever, hypotension, encephalopathy, tachycardia, fatigue, headache, decreased appetite, chills, diarrhea, febrile neutropenia, infections (pathogen unspecified), nausea, hypoxia, tremor, cough, vomiting, dizziness, constipation, and cardiac arrhythmias
Tisagenlecleucel (> 20%)	Cytokine release syndrome, hypogammaglobulinemia, infections (pathogen unspecified), pyrexia, decreased appetite, headache, encephalopathy, hypotension, bleeding episodes, tachycardia, nausea, diarrhea, vomiting, viral infectious disorders, hypoxia, fatigue, acute kidney injury, and delirium

CD—cluster of differentiation; CLL—chronic lymphocytic leukemia; ddAC—dose-dense doxorubicin and cyclophosphamide; DLBCL—diffuse large B-cell lymphoma; EGFR—epidermal growth factor receptor; FEC—5-fluorouracil, epirubicin, cyclophosphamide; FL—follicular lymphoma; FOLFOX—5-fluorouracil, leucovorin, oxaliplatin; HER2—human epidermal growth factor receptor 2; IL—interleukin; NHL—non-Hodgkin lymphoma; PDGFR-α—platelet-derived growth factor receptor alpha; PTT—partial thromboplastin time; RANKL—receptor activator of nuclear factor kappa-B ligand; SLAMF7—signaling lymphocytic activation molecule F7; VEGF—vascular endothelial growth factor

Note. Based on information from Amgen Inc., 2017a, 2017b, 2018; Bristol-Myers Squibb Co., 2012, 2017; Eli Lilly and Co., 2017a, 2017b; Gemzyme Corp., 2017; Genentech, Inc., 2016a, 2016b, 2017a, 2017b, 2017c, 2017d, 2017e; Janssen Biotech, Inc., 2014, 2017; Novartis Pharmaceuticals Corp., 2016, 2017; Seattle Genetics, Inc., 2017; Wyeth Pharmaceuticals Inc., 2017a, 2017b.

Ocular Toxicity

Ocular toxicity in the form of keratosis or ulcerative keratosis has been reported with panitumumab. Corneal abnormalities (e.g., keratoconjunctivitis, corneal ulceration) are direct toxic effects of EGFR agents. The incidence of all-grade ocular toxicity is 4%–18%, with less than 1% representing grade 3 symptoms (Dy & Adjei, 2013).

Patients should be monitored for all signs of ocular toxicity. Artificial tears can be applied if necessary, and antibacterial ointment should be used if infection is noted. Ophthalmologic evaluation is recommended for patients with visual changes, persistent eye pain, photosensitivity, or other drug-induced ocular changes, such as trichiasis. If patients exhibit grade 3 symptoms, treatment is withheld (Wen & Li, 2016). At first symptom occurrence, the drug is withheld for one to two weeks, but once improvement is noted, the agent can be given at the same dose. If symptoms show no improvement, the drug is discontinued. With second or subsequent occurrence, drug dose is modified based on package insert instructions (Bristol-Myers Squibb Co., 2012).

Stomatitis

Stomatitis has an incidence of 7%–32% with EGFR inhibitors (Amgen Inc., 2017b; Bristol-Myers Squibb Co., 2012). Alcohol- or peroxide-based mouthwashes should be avoided. If infection is noted, antifungal agents should be prescribed. Refer to the Oncology Nursing Society's Putting Evidence Into Practice resources on mucositis treatment for other recommendations (www.ons.org/practice-resources/pep).

Diarrhea and Colitis

Frequency of all-grade diarrhea and colitis with EGFR-specific mAbs is 20%–66%, with grade 3 or higher incidence at 2%–16%. Diarrhea presents as widespread inflammation of the mucosa, and its cause should be determined (e.g., drug related, *Clostridium difficile*, gastrointestinal virus). Patients who develop diarrhea related to mAb therapy should be treated with antimotility agents, such as loperamide and diphenoxylate/atropine (Wen & Li, 2016).

Altered Liver Function

Approximately 38%–43% of patients receiving cetuximab exhibit elevated transaminase levels (Wen & Li, 2016). Liver function tests should be evaluated at baseline and at least monthly if transaminase is elevated during treatment. No specific guidelines exist for the management of altered liver function tests; however, some authors recommend holding treatment if aspartate aminotransferase (AST) and alanine aminotransferase (ALT) are above the upper limit of normal (Wen & Li, 2016).

Hypomagnesemia

All-grade hypomagnesemia frequency is 11%–55%, with 4%–17% incidence of grade 3 or 4 (Bristol-Myers Squibb Co., 2012; Wen & Li, 2016). Based on toxicity reports from various studies, hypomagnesemia appears more frequently with cetuximab. A noted association exists between total treatment duration and defective renal magnesium reabsorption. Age and baseline serum magnesium levels are negatively associated with hypomagnesemia. Older adult patients are more likely to experience more severe magnesium wasting. Those with high baseline magnesium levels have altered magnesium regulation and are also more likely to experience hypomagnesemia (Tejpar et al., 2007). Patients should be monitored before treatment, periodically during treatment, and up to eight weeks after treatment (Enokida et al., 2016). Oral supplementation of magnesium can be used; however, the effectiveness of magnesium repletion by the oral route has been questioned. Patients with grade 2 hypomagnesemia should be given a weekly IV infusion of magnesium sulfate (Wen & Li, 2016).

When EGFR agents are administered with chemotherapy, severe diarrhea and dehydration can occur, which can affect electrolyte status. Optimal repletion of magnesium levels is based on diarrhea management (Douillard et al., 2010; Schwartzberg et al., 2014). Other electrolyte abnormalities observed with EGFR agents include hypokalemia and hypocalcemia.

Infusion Reactions

Infusion reactions occur in approximately 4% of patients receiving panitumumab and 15%–20% receiving cetuximab. Of infusion reactions associated with cetuximab, 1%–5% may be severe. Infusion reactions may be fatal and are usually manifested by fever and chills, dyspnea, bronchospasm, and hypotension. The incidence of grade 3 and 4 infusion reactions is lower in patients receiving panitumumab than cetuximab (Yazdi et al., 2015). All patients on cetuximab should receive an H_1 blocker (e.g., diphenhydramine) based on package insert instructions. No such recommendations exist for panitumumab. If the reaction is minor (grade 1 or 2), it can be restarted with a 50% reduction in the rate of the infusion.

Interstitial Lung Disease

Fatal and nonfatal cases of interstitial lung disease, including pulmonary fibrosis, have been reported in 1% of patients receiving panitumumab. Lung infiltrates and pneumonitis associated with panitumumab have also been reported (Polito, 2010). Panitumumab should be interrupted or discontinued when patients exhibit pulmonary symptoms.

Dermatologic Toxicity Management

EGFR is also present in healthy skin tissue. It is expressed in the epidermis, hair follicles, and sebaceous and eccrine glands of the skin (Pugliese, Neal, & Kwong, 2015). Dermatologic, or skin-specific, toxicity occurs in 49%–95% of patients (Dy & Adjei, 2013). Approximately 5%–18% experience toxicity of grade 3 or higher. Skin toxicities have been equated with improved responses from EGFR inhibitors.

Rash

Rash is related to impaired quality of life, especially in younger patients, because of discomfort and impact on self-image. Rash associated with EGFR-targeted therapies includes pruritic papulopustular eruption in seborrheic distribution (areas of the skin with greater density of sebaceous glands) of the scalp, face, retroarticular skin, chest, shoulders, and upper back (see Figure 8-3). It develops between the first and second weeks of treatment, gradually worsens, and peaks between weeks 4 and 6 (Kyllo & Anadkat, 2014). Papules and pustules typically resolve after the eighth week of treatment and can leave behind erythema and postinflammatory hyperpigmentation. Although rash can mimic inflammatory acne, the term *acneform* is not used as frequently because comedones do not develop with EGFR inhibitor-related eruption; therefore, management is distinct from acne vulgaris (Pugliese et al., 2015). Photosensitivity is also common in patients receiving EGFR inhibitors.

Infection

Secondary infections of lesions are common with *Staphylococcus aureus*. Methicillin-sensitive *Staphylococcus aureus* (MSSA) is the most common pathogen; however, methicillin-resistant *Staphylococcus aureus* (MRSA), tetracycline-resistant MSSA, and clindamycin-resistant MSSA can also occur (Eilers et al., 2010). Herpetic infection is another possibility. Bacterial cultures and viral studies should be performed for patients exhibiting worsening, atypical, or recalcitrant eruptions, especially if heavily crusted or active beyond eight weeks.

Skin Changes

Xerosis, or dry skin, has an incidence up to 47%. It is progressive, becoming most prominent one to three months after treatment (Valentine et al., 2015). Xerosis can exacerbate papulopustular eruption and pruritus. The epidermal barrier may become less intact, leading to painful fissuring of the skin, especially of the hands and feet. Significant fissuring of the fingertips is common with cetuximab.

Skin changes can also affect the area around the nails. These changes usually develop one to two months after initiation of EGFR inhibitor treatment; however, they can develop up to six months after the initiation of treatment, even after discontinuation. Acute paronychia is characterized by painful erythematous swelling of the nail folds. Pyogenic granuloma is manifested by vascular papules with a tendency to bleed. These lesions are usually sterile; however, suspicious eruptions should be cultured because of the high frequency of secondary infection with bacteria and yeast.

Alopecia

Prolonged, untreated inflammation can result in scarring hair loss and should be treated with topical steroids and antibiotics. Nonscar-

FIGURE 8-3 Management of Dermatologic Toxicities Associated With Epidermal Growth Factor Receptor (EGFR) Inhibitors

Papulopustular Eruption
- Avoid sun exposure.
  - Sunscreen (SPF 30 or higher): Apply frequently as outlined on product label.
  - Use physical sun blockers (e.g., hats, long sleeves).
- Avoid gel- or alcohol-containing skin products.
- Use emollients or moisturizer (fragrance free).
- Clean skin with mild cleansing gels.
- Use mild topical steroids (e.g., 1% hydrocortisone cream) 2–3 times a day for dry skin.
- Avoid hot showers.
  - Take daily 10-minute antiseptic soaks (bleach soak with ¼ cup household bleach in full bathtub or 1 teaspoon bleach in 1 gallon of water) to decrease crusting and bacterial burden of the skin.
- Take a tetracycline antibiotic (e.g., doxycycline 100 mg twice daily, or minocycline 100 mg once or twice daily) during treatment.
- Treatment of papulopustular rash
  - Apply topical antibiotic (e.g., clindamycin 1% lotion twice daily, dapsone 5% gel twice daily, mupirocin 2% ointment twice daily).
  - Use topical antifungals.
  - Use systemic antibiotics (e.g., doxycycline, minocycline, tetracycline, cephalexin, sulfamethoxazole/trimethoprim).
  - Use topical steroids for pruritus or tender skin rashes (e.g., triamcinolone 0.1%, hydrocortisone 2.5%).
  - Take oral corticosteroids for more severe rashes.
  - Make a dose adjustment or hold treatment of EGFR inhibitor for grade 3 rash.
  - Hold or discontinue EGFR inhibitor for dermatologic or soft tissue toxicity associated with severe or life-threatening inflammatory or infectious complications.
- Scalp involvement
  - Use over-the-counter antidandruff shampoo (containing 2% ketoconazole 2%, 1% pyrithione zinc, selenium sulfide, 0.5% coal tar extract, or 3% salicylic acid) to reduce crusting and pruritus.
  - Lather onto scalp.
  - Leave on for 5–10 minutes.
  - Apply topical fluocinolone oil for pruritus.

Xerosis
- Apply cyanoacrylate to fissure and pinch skin together to decrease pain and allow faster healing.

(Continued on next page)

FIGURE 8-3 Management of Dermatologic Toxicities Associated With Epidermal Growth Factor Receptor (EGFR) Inhibitors *(Continued)*

Pruritus
• Treat underlying xerosis.
 – Use moisturizers, especially hygroscopic moisturizers (e.g., urea cream, colloidal oatmeal).
 – Avoid soap.
 – Apply oily calamine or menthol in aqueous cream for itching.
 – Apply topical agents (e.g., camphor, menthol, pramoxine, doxepin).
• Use oral antihistamines (e.g., cetirizine 10 mg daily, hydroxyzine 25–75 mg in evening).
• Take gabapentin 300 mg every 8 hours.
• Take aprepitant 125 mg on day 1, 80 mg on day 3, and 80 mg on day 5 during treatment.

Hair Changes
• Scarring hair loss
 – Use topical steroids.
 – Use topical or oral antibiotics (prevention).
• Nonscarring hair loss: minoxidil
• Excess hair growth of face
 – Apply eflornithine cream.
 – Use hair removal procedures (e.g., laser hair removal, threading).
• Eyelash overgrowth
 – Trim eyelashes.
 – Apply antibiotic ointment for trichiasis that leads to corneal abrasions.

Nail Changes
• Apply topical antibiotics twice daily (e.g., mupirocin 2% ointment, gentamicin ophthalmic drops).
• Apply topical antifungals (e.g., ciclopirox 0.77% cream or 8% solution, ketoconazole 2% cream).
• Use systemic antibiotics.
• Use antiseptic soaks (e.g., vinegar or dilute bleach soaks).
• Use topical steroids (e.g., triamcinolone 0.1% ointment, fluocinonide ointment, clobetasol ointment).
• Use topical adapalene.

Note. Based on information from Aw et al., 2017; Pugliese et al., 2015; Wen & Li, 2016.

ring alopecia can be treated with minoxidil. Excess hair growth on the face can be treated with eflornithine cream or via hair removal methods, including laser hair removal and threading. Eyelash overgrowth will resolve with treatment discontinuation. While the patient is receiving treatment, eyelashes can be trimmed. An antibiotic ointment can be used if trichiasis (ingrowth of eyelashes) leads to corneal abrasions (Day, Abramson, Patel, Warren, & Menter, 2014).

Current data support the use of tetracyclines as the most effective treatment strategy for EGFR-associated dermatologic toxicity (Baas et al., 2012). Oral minocycline or doxycycline is used prophylactically during EGFR-targeted treatment.

The STEPP trial evaluated preemptive treatment, including the use of sunscreen, a moisturizer, 1% hydrocortisone cream daily, and doxycycline 100 mg orally twice daily, prior to the initiation of panitumumab treatment (Lacouture et al., 2010). This phase 2, open-label, randomized trial showed a decreased incidence of grade 2 or higher skin toxicities, from 62% to 29%.

A similar study indicated that preemptive treatment helped prevent grade 2 or higher rash but not overall occurrence (Jatoi et al., 2008). Appropriate prophylaxis duration is not clear in the absence of lesions; however, treatment should be discontinued after six weeks (Baas et al., 2012; Peuvrel & Dréno, 2014). Similar interventions have been found useful in the prevention of dermatologic toxicity associated with cetuximab. Management of rash associated with EGFR agents includes the use of topical and systemic antibiotics and steroids and avoidance of irritating agents. Antidandruff shampoo can be useful for scalp rash. EGFR inhibitors should be withheld or discontinued with the presence of dermatologic or soft tissue toxicities associated with severe or life-threatening inflammatory or infectious complications.

HER2-Targeted Monoclonal Antibodies

Human epidermal growth factor receptor 2 (HER2) belongs to the tyrosine kinase receptor family and mediates critical signaling functions in normal and malignant breast tissue. It is also important in cell proliferation and differentiation. On the surface of epithelial cells, HER2 is expressed at low levels; however, expression increases in breast cancer (15%–30%). HER2 stimulates HER2 phosphorylation and the activation of downstream signaling pathways that stimulate tumor growth. Increased HER2 levels in breast cancer inhibit apoptosis and promote cell proliferation, angiogenesis, and metastasis (Maximiano, Magalhães, Guerreiro, & Morgado, 2016). Clinically, increased HER2 levels equate to high-grade tumors, increased growth rates, early systemic metastasis, and decreased rates of disease-free survival and OS (Maximiano et al., 2016). HER2 overexpression is needed for this target to be useful in the treatment of breast cancer; therefore, international guidelines recommend screening for this biomarker (i.e., overexpression of HER2) through immunohistochemistry or in situ hybridization in all newly diagnosed cases of invasive breast cancer.

Trastuzumab

Trastuzumab (Herceptin®) is a humanized mAb directed against HER2 through high-affinity binding to its extracellular domain. The immunologic mechanism of ADCC has been considered a key factor in trastuzumab efficacy. Numerous studies have indicated trastuzumab's ability to target immune cells in tumor sites that overexpress HER2, though its exact mechanism remains obscure.

Trastuzumab can be included in either a neoadjuvant or adjuvant setting for the management of early-stage or advanced breast cancer (Petrelli & Barni, 2012). This strategy provides better outcomes than chemotherapy alone and includes higher pathologic complete response rates and lower risk of disease relapse and patient death. Trastuzumab has been shown to have limited therapeutic responses against brain metastases and resistant diseases associated with breast cancer (Gradishar, 2013).

HER2 is also amplified in gastric cancer, but it often stains heterogeneously; therefore, a threshold of 10% positive cells is considered appropriate (30% in breast cancer). Trastuzumab is approved for the management of adenocarcinoma of the stomach or gastroesophageal junction.

Trastuzumab is administered intravenously. Some studies have reviewed the safety and efficacy of subcutaneous (SC) administration; however, this method is not yet approved in the United States. Various dosing schedules are used in breast cancer treatment and depend on the other administered agents. If administered as adjuvant therapy, dosing should be started within two to six weeks after surgery, as administration more than 12 weeks after surgery has been associated with a clinically significant decrease in efficacy. For metastatic breast cancer, the initial dose is 4 mg/kg over 90 minutes followed by 2 mg/kg over 30 minutes weekly until disease progression. For metastatic gastric cancer, the initial dose is 8 mg/kg over 90 minutes followed by 6 mg/kg over 30–90 minutes every three weeks (Genentech, Inc., 2017c).

Studies by the National Surgical Adjuvant Breast and Bowel Project and the North Central Cancer Treatment Group support trastuzumab use in HER2-positive early breast cancer (Perez et al., 2011). A 2014 study update noted a 37% decrease in the risk of death and an increase in 10-year OS rate, from 75.2% to 84%, with the addition of trastuzumab to chemotherapy. In addition, there was a 40% improvement in disease-free survival and an increase in 10-year disease-free survival rate, from 62.2% to 73.7% (Perez et al., 2011, 2014).

The NOAH trial found improved therapeutic outcomes with the use of neoadjuvant chemotherapy concurrently with trastuzumab compared to neoadjuvant chemotherapy alone in patients with HER2-positive locally advanced breast cancer. The trastuzumab arm significantly improved event-free survival (71% vs. 56%) and complete response rates (Gianni et al., 2012).

Trastuzumab can be used concomitantly or sequentially with chemotherapy agents. Because of the therapeutic differences between combinations, the best approach is not clear; however, concomitant administration is trending. Anti-HER2 treatment is recommended early to all patients with HER2-positive metastatic breast cancer. Patients treated with endocrine therapy can concurrently receive anti-HER2 therapy. Several retrospective studies have attempted to clarify the optimal duration of trastuzumab therapy. In the majority, trastuzumab alone or in combination with a different chemotherapy agent was continued beyond disease progression. Enrollment in prospective trials is slow, as many physicians and patients refuse to accept randomization to discontinue trastuzumab after disease progression (Fountzilas et al., 2003; Gelmon et al., 2004; Tripathy et al., 2004).

Several studies have shown HER2 overexpression and amplification in gastric cancer; however, frequency of positivity has varied from 6% to 30%. The ToGA study evaluated trastuzumab plus chemotherapy versus chemotherapy alone in patients with HER2-positive advanced gastric/gastroesophageal cancers. Results showed that patients with higher HER2 expression (immunohistochemistry +3 or above) treated with trastuzumab had prolonged OS (16 months vs. 11.8 months). These findings led to FDA approval of trastuzumab for the treatment of HER2-positive metastatic gastric cancer (Bang et al., 2010).

Pertuzumab

Pertuzumab (Perjeta®) is a recombinant humanized mAb directed against the HER2 extracellular dimerization domain. It prevents dimerization of HER2 with other members of the HER family (e.g., HER1, HER3, HER4) and inhibits the downstream signaling of two key pathways that regulate cell survival and growth (HER dimerization inhibitor).

Evidence exists that dual-targeted HER2 therapies against HER2-amplified breast cancer have increased effectiveness over single blockade. HER2 inhibitor combinations (e.g., trastuzumab with pertuzumab) provide higher response rates and increased pathologic complete responses (Moya-Horno & Cortés, 2015). Multiple studies have confirmed improved response rates when trastuzumab and pertuzumab are combined with chemotherapy in the management of breast cancer (Gianni et al., 2012; Schneeweiss et al., 2013; Swain et al., 2013).

Pertuzumab is indicated in combination with trastuzumab and docetaxel for treatment of patients with HER2-positive metastatic breast cancer who have not received prior anti-HER2 therapy or chemotherapy for metastatic disease. This combination is also used as neoadjuvant treatment for patients with HER2-positive, locally advanced, inflammatory, or early-stage breast cancer. Pertuzumab safety as part of a doxorubicin-containing regimen has not been established, including when used for more than six cycles in early-stage breast cancer treatment (Genentech, Inc., 2017d).

Initial pertuzumab treatment includes an 840 mg IV infusion over 60 minutes. This is followed every three weeks with a 420 mg IV infusion over 30–60 minutes. Trastuzumab, when used in combination with pertuzumab, should be initially dosed at an 8 mg/kg IV infusion over 90 minutes. This is followed every three weeks by a 6 mg/kg IV infusion over 30–90 minutes (Genentech, Inc., 2017d).

Pertuzumab, trastuzumab, and docetaxel should be administered sequentially. Pertuzumab and trastuzumab can be given in any order; however, docetaxel should be administered after both. An observation period of 30–60 minutes is recommended after each pertuzumab infusion and prior to any subsequent infusion of trastuzumab or docetaxel (Genentech, Inc., 2017d).

In the CLEOPATRA trial, the addition of pertuzumab to trastuzumab and docetaxel showed improved PFS (12.4 months vs. 18.5 months) and OS (23.6% vs. 17.2%) over trastuzumab and docetaxel alone in the management of breast cancer (Baselga et al., 2012). This study led to FDA approval of pertuzumab in combination with trastuzumab and docetaxel for patients with HER2-positive metastatic breast cancer who have not received prior anti-HER2 treatment or chemotherapy for metastatic disease. Based on the results of the NeoSphere and TRYPHAENA trials, where pathologic complete response was improved, pertuzumab in combination with trastuzumab and docetaxel was FDA approved as neoadjuvant treatment for patients with HER2-positive tumors that are more than 2 cm in diameter or with positive lymph nodes (Moya-Horno & Cortés, 2015).

Side Effects

The most common adverse reactions with HER2-targeted mAbs are infusion reactions, which are reported in approximately 40% of patients receiving trastuzumab and 13% receiving pertuzumab. Most infusion reactions are mild to moderate and frequently occur with the first infusion (Barroso-Sousa, Santana, Testa, de Melo Gagliato, & Maon, 2013; Thompson et al., 2014). Thompson et al. (2014) reported that high body mass index, high disease stage, and the use of premedication were significantly associated with the incidence of infusion reactions from trastuzumab. Infusion reactions with maintenance doses of trastuzumab are rare and do not appear to be dose related (Thompson et al., 2014).

Side effects include gastrointestinal reactions (e.g., nausea and vomiting, diarrhea, constipation), hematologic reactions (usually neutropenia), infections, rash, erythema, headaches, asthenia, arthralgia, and myalgia (Garnock-Jones, Keating, & Scott, 2010; Genentech, Inc., 2017c, 2017d; Lambert & Chari, 2014). Although hepatotoxicity is rare, periodic monitoring of liver function is necessary during trastuzumab therapy (Ishizuna, Ninomiya, Ogawa, & Tsuji, 2014).

Cardiac and pulmonary toxicity are considered the most critical toxicities of HER2-targeted mAbs. Severe, occasionally fatal pulmonary toxicity has been reported with trastuzumab. Symptoms include dyspnea, interstitial pneumonitis, pulmonary infiltrates, pleural effusions, noncardiac pulmonary edema, pulmonary insufficiency and hypoxia, acute respiratory distress syndrome, and pulmonary fibrosis (Genentech, Inc., 2017c, 2017d). An important risk marker for the development of pulmonary events is the presence of shortness of breath at rest. Patients with shortness of breath at rest should not receive trastuzumab. Pulmonary toxicities reported with trastuzumab include acute respiratory distress syndrome, bronchiolitis obliterans, interstitial pneumonitis, pleural effusions, and pulmonary infiltrates/fibrosis/edema (Baldo, 2013).

Cardiotoxicity associated with HER2-targeted mAbs ranges from asymptomatic left ventricular systolic dysfunction to heart failure. This toxicity is common and related to fatal outcomes; however, cardiac dysfunction is not dose related and is often reversible. Cardiotoxic events have been noted in those receiving trastuzumab alone or in combination with taxanes after receiving an anthracycline-containing treatment. These events are also likely increased in those receiving pertuzumab after receiving anthracycline agents or radiation therapy. The incidence of cardiac dysfunction with trastuzumab ranges from 3% to 64% in single-agent or combination regimens (Chen & Ai, 2016).

Risk factors for cardiotoxicity include anthracycline use, high body mass index, hypertension, antihypertensive therapy, coronary artery disease, congestive heart failure, left ventricular ejection fraction (LVEF) lower than 55%, and older age (Ewer & Ewer, 2016; Jawa et al., 2016).

Multiple guidelines warn against the concomitant administration of trastuzumab and anthracyclines because of the overlapping toxicity affecting the heart. In a meta-analysis of the risk of cardiotoxicity with concurrent administration of anthracyclines and trastuzumab in the neoadjuvant and metastatic settings, no indication of increased risk of cardiotoxicity was found, even when agents were administered for a short time (Du et al., 2014). Other studies did not confirm these findings. Combination trastuzumab with anthracycline therapy is approved by FDA; however, combination trastuzumab with taxanes is safer and more effective than sequential treatment. For most patients, an anthracycline-based regimen followed by a taxane- and trastuzumab-based regimen is the preferred treatment (Foldi et al., 2018).

Although recommendations have been published regarding survivorship issues in the adult population with cancer, formal guidelines for prevention, surveillance, and treatment of related cardiotoxicities are not available. No specific monitoring recommendations are available.

The European Society of Cardiology heart failure guidelines recommend pre- and post-therapy LVEF evaluation, as well as discontinuation of chemotherapy and initiation of heart failure therapy, once left ventricular dysfunction (LVD) is noted (Ponikowski et al., 2016). The Canadian Trastuzumab Working Group recommends baseline and three-month interval imaging for all patients receiving trastuzumab (Hamo et al., 2016). The American Society of Echocardiography indicated the usefulness of echocardiograms before, during, and after cardiotoxic anticancer agents. No specific recommendations exist regarding follow-up frequency and duration (Plana et al., 2014).

The American Society of Clinical Oncology recommends the use of an echocardiogram in patients who have symptoms (Armenian et al., 2017); however, it also indicates that no recommendation can be made regarding the frequency and duration of surveillance in patients with increased risk of cardiotoxicity associated with cancer treatment. Additional studies, including a cardiac magnetic resonance imaging scan, multigated acquisition (MUGA) scan, or cardiac biomarkers, can be included in the workup of patients with potential cardiac dysfunction. Referral to a cardiologist is also recommended (Armenian et al., 2017).

In most cases, cardiac dysfunction improves after receiving treatment for heart failure. It is considered acceptable to reintroduce trastuzumab after patient recovery from cardiac dysfunction (Chen & Ai, 2016). Cardiac function should be monitored during treatment. For trastuzumab, patients should have LVEF evaluated by MUGA scan or echocardiogram at baseline, every three months during treatment, and at the end of treatment. An evaluation should be completed every six months for at least two years after treatment. With pertuzumab, patients should be monitored with an echocardiogram or MUGA scan every three months in the metastatic setting and every six weeks in the neoadjuvant setting (Genentech, Inc., 2017d).

Treatment with HER2-targeted mAbs needs to be interrupted or discontinued altogether in the presence of cardiotoxicity, severe infusion reactions, or pulmonary toxicity (Barroso-Sousa et al., 2013; Genentech, Inc., 2017c). Trastuzumab should be held for a 16% or greater decrease in pretreatment LVEF (Genentech, Inc., 2017c). Pertuzumab should be held for an LVEF less than 45% or if LVEF is between 45% and 49% but greater than 10% below baseline (Genentech, Inc., 2017d).

Combination pertuzumab and trastuzumab is well tolerated. Toxicities are mild to moderate and include diarrhea (64%), asthenia (33%), and nausea (27%) (Baselga et al., 2010). In the TOC3487 trial, 54% of patients experienced a reduction in LVEF after receiving trastuzumab as treatment for metastatic disease (Moya-Horno & Cortés, 2015). All patients had prior anthracycline therapy, and the majority had prior trastuzumab in the adjuvant setting. Because of cardiotoxicity concerns, the study was stopped early. In the CLEOPATRA trial, the most common toxicities among those who received pertuzumab, trastuzumab, and docetaxel versus those who received trastuzumab and docetaxel were diarrhea (66.8% vs. 46.3%), rash (33.7% vs. 24.2%), mucosal inflammation (27.8% vs. 19.9%), febrile neutropenia (13.8% vs. 7.6%), and dry skin (10.6% vs. 4.3%) (Baselga et al., 2012). A meta-analysis of six trials evaluated cardiotoxicity between anti-HER2 monotherapy and combination therapy with or without chemotherapy in breast cancer in any treatment setting (metastatic or adjuvant). Results showed that dual HER2 blockade does not significantly increase the risk of cardiac adverse events as compared with anti-HER2 monotherapy (Valachis, Nearchou, Polyzos, & Lind, 2013).

Vascular Endothelial Growth Factor Receptor Inhibitors

Solid tumors are highly vascularized and overexpress vascular endothelial growth factor type A (VEGF-A). Angiogenesis, the formation of new capillaries and blood vessels, is important in the growth of malignancies and metastases (Lee, Alwan, Sun, McLean, & Urban, 2016). VEGF is a potent proangiogenic factor expressed in most solid tumors. VEGF and VEGF receptors play an important role in physiologic and pathologic angiogenesis (Vennepureddy, Singh, Rastogi, & Terjanian, 2017). Multiple triggering pathways are prompted by the activation of VEGF and VEGF receptors, resulting in the survival, proliferation, and migration of endothelial cells. VEGF overexpression has been associated with enhanced progression of tumors and a dimmer prognosis for patients with several types of solid tumors. Studies have shown that anti-VEGF antibodies administered alone or in combination with chemotherapy can suppress angiogenesis and tumor growth (Roviello et al., 2017). Antiangiogenic inhibitors that block VEGF/VEGF-2 pathways have had varying levels of success (Tian et al., 2016).

Bevacizumab

Bevacizumab is a recombinant humanized Ig mAb directed against VEGF-A and angiogenesis. It improves varying levels of efficacy and survival in many malignancies. Minimal data exist on the predictive biomarkers that guide this therapy (Roviello et al., 2017).

Bevacizumab is FDA approved for the management of non-small cell lung cancer (NSCLC), metastatic colorectal cancer, metastatic renal cell carcinoma, advanced cervical cancer, recurrent glioblastoma, and platinum-resistant ovarian, fallopian tube, and primary peritoneal cancer (Genentech, Inc., 2017a). Previously, bevacizumab was approved for the treatment of HER2-negative breast cancer; however, this approval was revoked in November 2011 because the treatment lacked significant benefits. In the AVAGAST trial, bevacizumab was evaluated as first-line treatment for advanced gastric and gastroesophageal junction cancers. Although ORR and PFS were improved, OS, the study's primary endpoint, was not (Ohtsu et al., 2011); therefore, bevacizumab is not recommended in the management of gastric cancer at this time.

Bevacizumab dosing is based on disease and chemotherapy agent combinations (see Table 8-4). It is tolerable as a single agent and in combination with cytotoxic chemotherapy. Bevacizumab was first approved in 2004 as first-line treatment for management of metastatic colorectal cancer. In their landmark article, Hurwitz et al. (2004) conducted a randomized study of 813 patients receiving IFL (irinotecan, bolus 5-FU, leucovorin) with either bevacizumab or a placebo. PFS (10.6 months vs. 6.2 months) and survival (20.3 months vs. 15.6 months) were higher in the bevacizumab group.

Since this initial approval, bevacizumab's efficacy has been noted for other malignancies (e.g., second- and third-line treatment of epithelial ovarian cancer and primary peritoneal cancer) (Burger, Sill, Monk, Greer, & Sorosky, 2007). The AVOREN trial showed improved PFS with combination bevacizumab and interferon alfa-2a over interferon alfa-2a alone (10.2 months vs. 5.4 months) in patients with metastatic renal cell carcinoma (Melichar, Procházková-Študentová, & Vitásková, 2012).

Based on two studies, FDA approved bevacizumab in 2009 as a single agent for the management of glioblastoma multiforme with progressive disease following prior therapy. One trial randomized patients to receive bevacizumab plus irinotecan or bevacizumab alone. All patients received prior surgery, radiation therapy, and temozolomide. Partial responses were seen in 25.9% of patients, with a median response duration of 4.2 months in the single-agent group. The second study was a single-arm, single-institution study evaluating the efficacy and safety of bevacizumab in patients with recurrent high-grade gliomas. Patients were split into two cohorts, including those with glioblastoma and those with anaplastic astrocytoma. Only information from the glioblastoma cohort was submitted to FDA for this review. Partial responses were noted in 19.6% of patients, and the median duration of response was 3.9 months (Cohen, Shen, Keegan, & Pazdur, 2009).

In 2006, the Eastern Cooperative Oncology Group reported a randomized study of 878 patients with advanced or recurrent NSCLC with

TABLE 8-4   Dosing for Bevacizumab

Site of Disease	Dosing
Metastatic colorectal cancer	5 mg/kg IV every 2 weeks with bolus IFL 10 mg/kg IV every 2 weeks with FOLFOX4 5 mg/kg IV every 2 weeks or 7.5 mg/kg IV every 3 weeks with fluoropyrimidine-irinotecan– or fluoro-pyrimidine-oxaliplatin–based chemotherapy after progression on a first-line bevacizumab-containing regimen
Nonsquamous non-small cell lung cancer	15 mg/kg IV every 3 weeks with carboplatin/paclitaxel
Glioblastoma	10 mg/kg IV every 2 weeks
Metastatic renal cell carcinoma	10 mg/kg IV every 2 weeks with interferon alfa
Persistent, recurrent, or metastatic cervical cancer	15 mg/kg IV every 3 weeks with paclitaxel/cisplatin or paclitaxel/topotecan
Platinum-resistant recurrent epithelial ovarian, fallopian tube, or primary peritoneal cancer	10 mg/kg IV every 2 weeks with paclitaxel, pegylated liposomal doxorubicin, or weekly topotecan 15 mg/kg IV every 3 weeks with topotecan given every 3 weeks
Platinum-sensitive recurrent epithelial ovarian, fallopian tube, or primary peritoneal cancer	15 mg/kg IV every 3 weeks in combination with carboplatin/paclitaxel for 6–8 weeks followed by 15 mg/kg IV every 3 weeks as a single agent 15 mg/kg IV every 3 weeks in combination with carboplatin/gemcitabine for 6–10 cycles followed by 15 mg/kg IV every 3 weeks as a single agent

FOLFOX4—5-fluorouracil, leucovorin, oxaliplatin; IFL—irinotecan, 5-fluorouracil, leucovorin
Note. Based on information from Genentech, Inc., 2017a.

either stage IIIB or IV disease. Patients received combination paclitaxel and carboplatin alone or with bevacizumab. They were treated with both every 21 days. The bevacizumab arm showed improved median survival (6.2 months vs. 4.2 months) and response rates (35% vs. 15%) compared to paclitaxel and carboplatin alone (Sandler et al., 2006).

After the results of the AVAGAST trial, debate formed around the variances in response rates seen between geographic regions. A subgroup analysis indicated that patients in the North America and Latin America regions appeared to have a survival benefit with the addition of bevacizumab, but those from Asia (Japan and Korea) seemingly did not. Patients from Europe had intermediate results. These regions also had varying median OS (Asia, 12.1 months; Europe, 8.6 months; North and

Latin America, 6.8 months). This geographic indication was supported by the AVATAR study in China (Shen et al., 2015).

Ramucirumab

Ramucirumab is a fully humanized recombinant IgG1 mAb that inhibits angiogenesis in tumor cells by targeting the VEGF-2 receptor (Vennepureddy et al., 2017). It has been approved for the treatment of the following situations (Eli Lilly and Co., 2017a):

- Advanced or metastatic gastric or gastroesophageal junction adeno-carcinoma with disease progression on or after prior fluoropyrimidine or platinum-containing chemotherapy. Administer as a single agent or in combination with paclitaxel.
- Metastatic NSCLC with disease progression on or after platinum-based chemotherapy. Administer in combination with docetaxel.
- Metastatic colorectal cancer with disease progression on or after prior therapy with bevacizumab, oxaliplatin, and a fluoropyrimidine. Administer in combination with FOLFIRI.

Ramucirumab dosing is based on indication (Eli Lilly and Co., 2017a). For gastric cancer, ramucirumab is used as a single agent or in combination with weekly paclitaxel. A dose of 8 mg/kg IV is infused over 60 minutes every two weeks. When given in combination, ramucirumab should be administered prior to paclitaxel. For NSCLC, the recommended dose is a 10 mg/kg IV infusion over 60 minutes on day 1 of a 21-day cycle prior to docetaxel infusion. For colorectal cancer, the recommended dose is an 8 mg/kg IV infusion over 60 minutes every two weeks prior to FOLFIRI administration. Ramucirumab should be continued until disease progression or unacceptable toxicity in these indications.

Prior to each ramucirumab infusion, all patients must be premedicated with an IV H_1 blocker (e.g., diphenhydramine hydrochloride). Patients who have experienced a grade 1 or 2 infusion-related reaction should also be premedicated with dexamethasone (or equivalent) and acetaminophen (Eli Lilly and Co., 2017a).

Ramucirumab was approved for its indicated treatments based on the results of the several clinical trials (Vennepureddy et al., 2017). The REGARD trial was a phase 3 study that included 355 patients with gastric or gastroesophageal junction adenocarcinoma. Patients who received ramucirumab had longer median OS (5.2 months vs. 3.8 months) and six-month PFS (41.8% vs. 31.6%) compared to placebo. Response rates were low (4%); however, the overall rate of stable disease was more than twice that of placebo (45% vs. 21%) (Fuchs et al., 2014). The RAINBOW trial included 665 patients with advanced gastric or gastroesophageal junction adenocarcinomas who received paclitaxel plus either ramucirumab or placebo. Results showed prolonged OS in the ramucirumab arm (9.63 months vs. 7.26 months) and significant improvements in response rate and PFS (Wilke et al., 2014).

As with bevacizumab, geographic differences have been noted with ramucirumab. The REGARD trial showed similar survival in Asian and non-Asian patients; however, OS was not improved in Asian patients in the RAINBOW trial. Lower levels of VEGF-A have been noted in Asian cohorts in the AVAGAST trial. The difference in VEGF-A levels potentially explains the poorer results in the Asian cohorts of these trials. It remains unclear if geographic region is purely a surrogate for differences in disease biology (Davidson, Smyth, & Cunningham, 2016).

Side Effects

Some VEGF inhibitor toxicities have been linked to the inhibition of specific targets (e.g., hypertension and VEGF). This association with other side effects (e.g., stomatitis, diarrhea) is less clear. The most common side effects associated with bevacizumab include hypertension, proteinuria, hemorrhage, wound healing disruption, gastrointestinal perforations, arterial thrombosis events, and venous thrombosis events, all of which are thought to be related to VEGF targets (Wu, Shui, Shen, & Chen, 2016). The most common side effects from ramucirumab are fatigue (51%), headache (51%), peripheral edema (35%), diarrhea (35%), nausea (32%), respiratory infections (32%), abdominal pain (30%), arthralgia (27%), cough (27%), and dyspnea (27%) (Vennepureddy et al., 2017).

Hemorrhagic Events

Hemorrhagic events, such as epistaxis, gastrointestinal hemorrhage/bleeding, and pulmonary hemorrhage, have been reported in 7.1%–48.9% of patients treated with ramucirumab (Tian et al., 2016). These events are caused by antiangiogenic inhibitor impairment, which inhibits endothelial cell repair and causes defects of the plasma membrane or underlying matrix (Tian et al., 2016). Some tumor-dependent intrinsic mechanisms are related to certain adverse events. For example, Tian et al. (2016) noted that the lowest incidence of hemorrhage in their study was in patients with hepatocellular cancer, whereas the highest incidence was in patients with metastatic breast cancer.

Gastrointestinal Perforations

When bevacizumab was combined with either FOLFOX or FOLFIRI in phase 2 trials, gastrointestinal perforations were uncommon (1%–3%) but severe, leading to a black box warning label by FDA on package inserts (Genentech, Inc., 2017a; Giantonio et al., 2007; Hurwitz et al., 2004). Gastrointestinal perforations lead to higher rates of peritonitis, infection, and death caused by leakage from the gastrointestinal tract into the peritoneal cavity. The cause of gastrointestinal perforations with bevacizumab is not clear. The median time to a perforation is 3.35 months, although the majority occur within six months. Patients younger than age 65 years or with an intact primary intra-abdominal tumor are at increased risk for perforations. A meta-analysis by Hapani, Chu, and Wu (2009) noted that risk of gastrointestinal perforation varied with bevacizumab dose and tumor type, with higher risk found with colorectal cancer and renal cell carcinoma. Risk predictors for gastrointestinal perforations in patients with ovarian cancer include rectovaginal nodularity, history of bowel surgery, and bowel obstruction (Richardson et al., 2010). Limiting treatment to those without these predictors subsequently may limit perforation risk (Simpkins, Belinson, & Rose, 2007).

Venous Thromboembolism

Venous thromboembolism (VTE), an additional potential side effect of bevacizumab, has been reported in approximately 13% of cancers (10%–15% grade 3 or 4). VTE can occur with both high and low doses of bevacizumab (Nalluri, Chu, Keresztes, Zhu, & Wu, 2008). Recurrent VTE has been reported in patients receiving bevacizumab who previously experienced a VTE and were placed on anticoagulation therapy (Genentech, Inc., 2017a). Scappaticci et al. (2007) reported that bevacizumab combined with chemotherapy was associated with an increased risk for arterial thromboembolic events but not VTE. Arterial thromboembolic events were associated with prior arterial thromboembolic events or in patients aged 65 years and older.

Proteinuria

Because VEGF-A is expressed on glomerular epithelial cells and endothelial cells, it has the potential to compromise the integrity of kidney repair of glomerular vessels; therefore, bevacizumab may cause increased glomerular permeability and escape of high-molecular-weight proteins in the urine (George, Zhou, & Toto, 2007; Lee et al., 2016; Shord, Bressler, Tierney, Cuellar, & George, 2009). Overall incidence of all-grade proteinuria is 20% (Genentech, Inc., 2017a). Nephrotic syndrome occurrence is reported in less than 1% of those receiving bevacizumab. In prior clinical trials, 5.4% of patients who received bevacizumab in combination with chemotherapy experienced grade 2 or higher proteinuria, which resolved in 74.2% of patients (Genentech, Inc., 2017a). Bevacizumab was able to be reinitiated in 41.7% of these patients, though 47.8% experienced a second proteinuric episode. Monitoring includes a urine dipstick with urinalysis (Genentech, Inc., 2017a). If patients are noted to have a 2+ or greater protein level on the urine dipstick, they are recommended for 24-hour urine collection. Urine protein-to-creatinine (UPC) ratios are not recommended at this time; however, some practitioners do routinely complete them. These practices monitor proteinuria based on patient risk. Certain groups, such as patients with gastrointestinal malignancies, are considered low risk and are not routinely monitored for proteinuria while receiving bevacizumab. High-risk groups, such as patients with gynecologic malignancies, have an overall incidence of 35% and are routinely monitored (Lee et al., 2016). UPC ratio is obtained at baseline and monthly prior to each cycle of bevacizumab. It is used because of its timing with 24-hour collection of urinary protein. The accuracy of urine dipstick techniques for the detection of proteinuria is poor.

Platelet-Derived Growth Factor Alpha Inhibitors

Platelet-derived growth factor (PDGF) stimulates cell proliferation and is present in platelets, smooth muscle cells, endothelial cells, and inflammatory cells (Vincenzi et al., 2017). Platelet-derived growth factor receptor alpha (PDGFR-α) regulates angiogenesis in normal and pathologic conditions and stimulates the production of VEGF. It is expressed and active in several human malignancies such as glioblastoma, ependymoma, rhabdomyosarcoma, prostate cancer, hepatocellular carcinoma, cholangiocarcinoma, and breast cancer (Vincenzi et al., 2017). PDGFR-α has been correlated with aggressive disease and worsened patient survival in some malignancies.

Olaratumab is a fully human IgG1 mAb that binds PDGFR-α and inhibits PDFG binding to the receptor. It also reduces proliferation and growth of several cancer cell lines. Its pharmacokinetic characteristics are not affected by age, sex, race, mild to moderate renal impairment, or mild to moderate hepatic impairment.

Olaratumab is indicated in combination with doxorubicin for the treatment of adult patients with soft tissue sarcoma. The histologic subtype of the soft tissue sarcoma should be one in which an anthracycline-containing regimen is appropriate and not considered curative with radiation therapy or surgery (Eli Lilly and Co., 2017b). Its recommended dose is a 15 mg/kg IV infusion over 60 minutes on days 1 and 8 of a 21-day cycle. It is administered until disease progression or unacceptable toxicity. For the first eight cycles, olaratumab is administered with doxorubicin. Premedications include diphenhydramine 25–50 mg IV and dexamethasone 10–20 mg IV on day 1 of cycle 1.

In 2016, Tap et al. conducted a study of 133 anthracycline-naïve adult patients with locally advanced or metastatic soft tissue sarcomas. Patients were randomly assigned to receive either a maximum of eight cycles of 75 mg/m^2 doxorubicin (day 1) plus olaratumab (days 1 and 8) or doxorubicin alone. Patients receiving olaratumab were offered the option to continue olaratumab alone until disease progression after finishing the eight doxorubicin cycles. Leiomyosarcoma represented the largest group on the trial. The combination treatment showed improved median PFS (6.6 months vs. 4.1 months) and OS (26.5 months vs. 14.7 months) compared to doxorubicin alone. No difference was found in the objective response rate between the two groups (Tap et al., 2016).

Common side effects of olaratumab include fatigue, constipation, diarrhea, nausea, and pyrexia. Infusion reactions can occur but have not been related with treatment discontinuation. Drug-related adverse events are usually grade 1 or 2. The most common grade 3 side effect is deep vein thrombosis. When olaratumab is combined with doxorubicin, toxicities are reported in more than 20% of patients and include nausea, fatigue, musculoskeletal pain, mucositis, vomiting, diarrhea, decreased appetite, abdominal pain, neuropathy, and headache (Eli Lilly and Co., 2017b).

CD20-Targeted Monoclonal Antibodies

CD20 is a transmembrane protein that serves as a calcium channel to initiate intracellular signals. It is present during all stages of B-cell development, except in pro-B cells and antibody-producing plasma cells (Teo, Chew, & Phipps, 2016). CD20 is expressed in 90% of all B-cell NHLs and is also found with chronic lymphocytic leukemia (CLL). It is not internalized or downmodulated following antibody binding (Liu et al., 1987). CD20 antibodies are used to treat various autoimmune diseases—in which B cells are an important component—and hematologic malignancies, in which CD20-bearing B-cell lymphocytes are increased. Use of CD20-targeted mAbs leads to rapid cell lysis.

Rituximab

Rituximab (Rituxan®) is a chimeric anti-CD20 mAb used alone or in combination with chemotherapy for the management of follicular lymphoma, NHL, and CLL. It is also used as maintenance therapy for follicular lymphoma and may be used as a single agent for the management of low-grade lymphomas in patients who may not tolerate chemotherapy and have difficulty obtaining an approved oral agent treatment. Rituximab induces CDC and ADCC and exerts a direct antiproliferative effect (Robak, Blonski, & Robak, 2016).

The dosing schedule for rituximab was primarily developed empirically, and extensive studies to determine dosing are not available. No dose-limiting toxicity was found, and no clear dose–response relationship exists. A 375 mg/m^2 standard dose is administered via IV infusion weekly as a single agent for four consecutive weeks and is followed in two-month intervals (Cartron et al., 2014; Robak et al., 2016). Clinical response rates appear related to dose. In a study by O'Brien et al. (2001), clinical response rate was 22% for those treated with a 500–825 mg/m^2 dose, 43% for a 1,000–1,500 mg/m^2 dose, and 75% for a 2,250 mg/m^2 dose. Response rate was lower in those with CLL (i.e., 36% in CLL and 60% in other B-cell lymphoid leukemias) (O'Brien et al., 2001). Rate of administration for the first infusion is slower because of an increased risk of infusion reactions. The first infusion can take four to six hours depending on patient tolerance. If the patient does not experience an infusion reaction, subsequent infusions can be administered over 90 minutes.

With chemotherapy, rituximab is usually administered at the beginning of each cycle (Pavanello, Zucca, & Ghielmini, 2017). With CLL, a higher dose (500 mg/m^2) may be necessary because CLL cells present a lower level of surface CD20 (Pavanello et al., 2017).

Premedication with acetaminophen and an antihistamine is recommended prior to each rituximab infusion. For patients on a chemotherapy regimen, the glucocorticoid component should be administered prior to infusion (Genentech, Inc., 2016b).

For the first rituximab infusion, initiate at a rate of 50 mg/hr. In the absence of reaction, increase in 50 mg/hr increments every 30 minutes (400 mg/hr maximum). For subsequent infusions, initiate at a rate of 100 mg/hr. In the absence of reaction, increase in 100 mg/hr increments every 30 minutes (400 mg/hr maximum).

For previously untreated follicular NHL and diffuse large B-cell lymphoma, if a patient did not experience a grade 3 or 4 infusion-related adverse event during cycle 1, a 90-minute infusion can be administered in cycle 2 with a glucocorticoid-containing chemotherapy regimen. Initially, 20% of the total dose is given in the first 30 minutes, then the remaining 80% over the next 60 minutes. If 90-minute infusion is tolerated in cycle 2, the same rate can be used for the remainder of the treatment regimen. Patients who have clinically significant cardiovascular disease or a circulating lymphocyte count greater than or equal to 5,000/mm^3 before cycle 2 should not be given the 90-minute infusion (Genentech, Inc., 2016b).

SC rituximab (Rituxan Hycela™) was FDA approved in 2017 and offers a faster and easier administration method than IV infusion; however, it requires larger volumes, from 11.7 ml (NHL) to 13.4 ml (CLL), and is highly concentrated (Genentech, Inc., 2017e). To combat this, the agent contains human hyaluronidase alfa, an enzyme that temporarily degrades the extracellular matrix and allows large volume absorption. Degradation is temporary, reversing within 24 hours after injection, and causes minimal tissue distortion, edema, and tissue irritation (Carlson, Cox, Bedwell, & Ku, 2015; MacDonald, Crosbie, Christofides, Assaily, & Wiernikowski, 2017). Studies indicate that the safety profiles for IV and SC formulations are similar; however, the IV formulation has increased rates of gastrointestinal toxicities, and the SC formulation has increased local site reactions. Many patients have indicated preference for SC administration (Rummel et al., 2015, 2016).

In 1994, Maloney et al. published the first trial (phase 1) to investigate rituximab, which included 15 patients with relapsed low-grade B-cell NHL. A single-agent IV infusion was administered at escalating doses, resulting in tumor regression in half of the patients. CD20 B cells remained depleted for up to three months, and minimal short-term side effects were noted. Subsequent studies showed durable remissions in half of the patients with indolent but chemotherapy-resistant lymphoma (McLaughlin et al., 1998).

Coiffier et al. (1998) conducted a phase 2 trial of single-agent rituximab in patients with more aggressive lymphomas. In this study, 54 patients received rituximab once a week for eight consecutive weeks at either 375 mg/m^2 or 500 mg/m^2. No significant difference in OS or response rate between the two groups was found; however, a slightly higher number of infusion reactions (e.g., anaphylaxis, fevers, bronchospasm, hypotension) were seen with the higher dose (Coiffier et al., 1998). Weekly rituximab at 375 mg/m^2 was subsequently determined to be the most tolerable and effective schedule. Additional trials have determined that maintenance rituximab improves OS (Vidal et al., 2012), and rituximab combined with CHOP (cyclophosphamide, hydroxydaunorubicin, vincristine [Oncovin®], prednisone) chemotherapy improved PFS and OS over CHOP alone (Coiffier et al., 2010).

Ofatumumab

Ofatumumab (Arzerra®) is a fully human IgG1 mAb approved for the treatment of CLL. It is used in combination with fludarabine and cyclophosphamide for patients with relapsed CLL. Ofatumumab is also used in combination with chlorambucil for previously untreated patients with CLL for whom fludarabine-based therapy is considered inappropriate. Other uses include extended treatment for patients with recurrent or progressive CLL who are in complete or partial response after two lines of therapy and those with CLL refractory to fludarabine and alemtuzumab (Novartis Pharmaceuticals Corp., 2016). Ofatumumab induces CDC more effectively than rituximab and has more stable CD20 binding (Robak, 2008).

Ofatumumab is usually administered at a flat dosing of 300 mg IV on day 1 of cycle 1 and 1,000 mg IV on day 8. Thereafter, it is administered at 1,000 mg every 28 days. Extended treatment is an exception to this schedule. Although it includes a similar regimen on the first eight days, the 1,000 mg dose thereafter is moved from every 28 days to every eight weeks (except cycle 2, when it is seven weeks). With refractory CLL, ofatumumab is administered at 300 mg on day 1 of cycle 1 and 2,000 mg on day 8. Thereafter, it is administered via 2,000 mg IV every four weeks.

Maximum dose depends on treatment setting. An ofatumumab plus chlorambucil regimen for CLL has 12 maximum cycles. Ofatumumab in combination with fludarabine and cyclophosphamide for relapsed CLL has six maximum cycles. For extended treatment as a single agent, ofatumumab has a maximum treatment time of two years. For refractory CLL, the maximum number of doses is four when 2,000 mg is administered every 28 days (Novartis Pharmaceuticals Corp., 2016).

Premedication recommendations for ofatumumab include the following (Novartis Pharmaceuticals Corp., 2016):
• Untreated, relapsed, or extended-treatment CLL
  – Acetaminophen: 1,000 mg prior to each infusion
  – Antihistamine: Diphenhydramine 50 mg or cetirizine 10 mg (IV or PO)
  – Corticosteroid (e.g., prednisone): First and second infusions are 50 mg, and subsequent infusions are 0–50 mg.
• Refractory CLL
  – Acetaminophen: 1,000 mg prior to each infusion
  – Antihistamine: Diphenhydramine 50 mg or cetirizine 10 mg (IV or PO)
  – Corticosteroid (e.g., prednisone): Infusions 1, 2, and 9 are 50 mg; infusions 3–8 are 0–50 mg; and infusions 10–12 are 50–100 mg.

Ofatumumab has shown efficacy in heavily pretreated patients. In a pivotal international study, it was administered in 12 doses over a 28-week period to 138 patients with CLL refractory to fludarabine and alemtuzumab (Wierda et al., 2010). ORR was 58% in the fludarabine-refractory group and 47% in the alemtuzumab-refractory group. Median PFS (13.7 months vs. 5.7 months) and OS (15.4 months vs. 5.9 months) were stronger in the alemtuzumab group. Based on this study, FDA approved ofatumumab in combination with chlorambucil for previously untreated CLL in patients who are not candidates for fludarabine-based therapy. A follow-up study evaluated the effect of ofatumumab for patients refractory to rituximab therapy (Wierda, Padmanabhan, et al., 2011). ORRs were 43%, 44%, and 53% in rituximab-treated, rituximab-refractory, and rituximab-naïve patients, respectively. No significant differences in ofatumumab-related infusion reactions or hematologic/infectious complications were found.

Studies with ofatumumab have conflicting results. The European Research Initiative on CLL published a large retrospective, phase 4, noninterventional observational study of ofatumumab in heavily pre-treated patients with poor CLL prognosis. This study could not replicate prior results by Coiffier et al. (2008) and Wierda et al. (2010). ORR was 22%, less than half of that reported in the two prior studies.

In another study, monotherapy ofatumumab was found to be inferior to ibrutinib based on approval and safety profile, making its role questionable in the relapsed/refractory setting (Laurenti, Innocenti, Autore, Sica, & Efremov, 2016). Ofatumumab's low complete response rate as a single agent suggests it should be added to other agents (Laurenti et al., 2016). Additional studies have used ofatumumab with bendamustine, dexamethasone, chlorambucil, lenalidomide, ibrutinib, fludarabine/cyclophosphamide, and pentostatin/cyclophosphamide (Cortelezzi et al., 2014; Costa et al., 2015; Doubek et al., 2015; Shanafelt et al., 2013; Wierda, Kipps, et al., 2011).

Obinutuzumab

Obinutuzumab is a humanized type II anti-CD20 mAb approved for the treatment of CLL and follicular lymphoma. It is believed to be the most effective CD20 antibody for the management of CLL. Although obinutuzumab also targets CD20, its mechanism of action is distinct from rituximab. Obinutuzumab results in lower CDC but significantly higher ADCC and direct cell death as compared to rituximab and ofatumumab (Robak et al., 2016; Smolej, 2015).

Obinutuzumab is used in combination with chlorambucil for the treatment of patients with previously untreated CLL. It is also combined with bendamustine followed by monotherapy for patients with follicular lymphoma who have relapsed after, or are refractory to, a rituximab-containing regimen (Genentech, Inc., 2017b).

Obinutuzumab for CLL is administered at a 1,000 mg flat dose on days 1, 8, and 15 of cycle 1 and on day 1 of cycles 2–6. The first 1,000 mg dose is divided into two parts: 100 mg over four hours on day 1, and the remaining 900 mg on day 2. Premedication for CLL and follicular lymphoma include the following (Genentech, Inc., 2017b):

- First infusions for CLL (days 1 and 2) and follicular lymphoma (day 1)
  - Acetaminophen: 650–1,000 mg at least 30 minutes prior to each infusion
  - Antihistamine: Diphenhydramine 50 mg IV at least 30 minutes prior to each infusion
  - Corticosteroid: Dexamethasone 20 mg or methylprednisolone 80 mg IV at least 60 minutes prior to infusion
- Subsequent infusions for patients who have experienced infusion-related reactions (grade 1) or with a lymphocyte count greater than 25,000/mm^3

- Acetaminophen: 650–1,000 mg at least 30 minutes prior to each infusion (subsequent use in all patients, regardless of condition)
- Antihistamine: Diphenhydramine 50 mg IV at least 30 minutes prior to each infusion
- Corticosteroid: Dexamethasone 20 mg or methylprednisolone 80 mg IV at least 60 minutes prior to infusion

In the phase 1/2 GAUGUIN study, obinutuzumab monotherapy was given to 33 heavily pretreated patients with relapsed/refractory CLL. ORR was 62% in the phase 1 component and 15% in phase 2. All responses were partial. In phase 2, median PFS was 10.7 months (Cartron et al., 2014). In a randomized trial by Goede et al. (2015), patients received either chlorambucil alone, chlorambucil plus rituximab, or chlorambucil plus obinutuzumab. The obinutuzumab group showed increased response rates, including complete response of 20.7% versus 7.0% and prolonged PFS (26.7 months vs. 16.3 months), over the rituximab group.

Side Effects

Infusion Reactions

CD20-targeted mAb administration is commonly associated with infusion reactions, including fever, chills, rigors, and allergic (type IV) anaphylactoid spectrum reactions, such as urticaria, angioedema, and hypotension. Symptoms typically occur during infusions and are most frequent and severe during the first infusion. Reactions are more common in patients with hematologic malignancies than those with autoimmune diseases. With rituximab, risk is estimated at approximately 77% for the first infusion, with a 10% incidence in grade 3 or 4. Even after the fourth infusion, 30% of patients react to rituximab. This drops to 14% following the eighth infusion (Baldo, 2013). In a study of 103 patients with CLL treated with single-agent ofatumumab, infusion reaction incidence was 28%, with 4% incidence of grade 3 or 4 (Moreno et al., 2015). Most were mild to moderate and occurred during the first or second infusion. When ofatumumab is combined with chlorambucil, infusion reaction incidence is 67% (Novartis Pharmaceuticals Corp., 2016); however, in the GAUGUIN study, infusion reaction incidence was 96%, with 30% representing grade 3 reactions, which are higher percentages than typically seen (Cartron et al., 2014). Severe infusion-related reactions were higher with combination obinutuzumab plus chlorambucil than with chlorambucil plus rituximab; however, with added precautions, such as premedicating, dose splitting, and withholding antihypertensive medications, reactions were manageable and limited to the first infusion (Goede et al., 2015). Typically, infusion reactions associated with obinutuzumab occur during the first hour or shortly after the first infusion. Frequency decreases with subsequent infusions (Genentech, Inc., 2017b).

Acetaminophen, corticosteroid, and antihistamine use with these agents can decrease infusion reaction occurrence and slow infusion rates. The mechanism for infusions reactions is not clearly understood; however, complement activation and mast cell degranulation in the setting of rapid cell lysis are thought to related, as they occur during the first dose (Karmacharya et al., 2015). It is thought that mAb-target interaction may cause the release of cytokines, such as tumor necrosis factor-alpha(TNF-α) and interleukin-6 (IL-6), which can produce many of the symptoms seen in infusion reactions.

Cytokine Release Syndrome

Cytokine release syndrome (CRS) is a rare, potentially fatal reaction associated with mAb administration. The mildest form of CRS is manifested as an infusion reaction (Nair, Gheith, & Lamparella, 2016). The underlying mechanism of CRS is thought to be related to changes in serum cytokine levels caused by rapid infusion of an antibody. CRS usually occurs at least 90 minutes after the first infusion. CRS, including a 5- to 10-fold increase in liver enzymes, D-dimer elevation, lactate dehydrogenase, and prolongation of prothrombin time, can occur after rituximab administration (Kulkarni & Kasi, 2012). Higher tumor burden makes patients more prone to CRS progressing to systemic inflammatory response syndrome (SIRS). Severe SIRS and disseminated intravascular coagulation can occur within 24 hours of rituximab administration (Kulkarni & Kasi, 2012). In those with similar but less severe reactions, a reduced dose or pretreatment with steroids prior to infusion may reduce reaction severity in future infusions (Kulkarni & Kasi, 2012). Cytokine levels have been noted after obinutuzumab infusion.

Serum Sickness

Serum sickness is characterized by fever, urticarial or morbilliform rash demonstrating leukocytoclastic vasculitis, arthralgia/arthritis, gastrointestinal disturbances, lymphadenopathy, and proteinuria. The term *serum sickness* also describes a drug reaction that includes urticarial or morbilliform rash, fever, and arthralgia but shows no evidence of cutaneous or systemic vasculitis (Karmacharya et al., 2015).

Tumor Lysis Syndrome

Tumor lysis syndrome (TLS), including the need for hospitalization, has occurred in patients treated with CD20-targeted agents. Patients with high tumor burden and/or high circulating lymphocyte counts (greater than $25,000/mm^3$) are at greater risk for TLS. Prophylaxis includes antihyperuricemics and hydration beginning 12–24 hours prior to antibody infusion. Treatment for TLS includes aggressive IV hydration, antihyperuricemic agents, and electrolyte correction. Renal function should also be monitored (Genentech, Inc., 2017b; Novartis Pharmaceuticals Corp., 2016).

Cytopenias

Cytopenias have been reported with each of the CD20-targeted agents. Acute cytopenias associated with rituximab are uncommon. Rituximab-associated cytopenias are self-limited, uncomplicated, and usually occur a few hours after infusion. Nadir is reached within one day and resolves spontaneously within a few days. In the literature, 82% of rituximab-associated cytopenias were preceded by clinical presentation of CRS (Ram et al., 2009). Severe anemia, including autoimmune hemolytic anemia, has been reported in 1.1% of patients receiving rituximab monotherapy. Transient severe acute thrombocytopenia after rituximab administration is associated with CRS and complement. This condition reverses a few days after withdrawal of the antibody (Baldo, 2013; Ram et al., 2009). Early neutropenia has been reported in 4.2% of patients receiving rituximab (Baldo, 2013; McLaughlin et al., 1998). Late-onset neutropenia has been associated with rituximab and has an incidence of 3%–27%. It occurs 38–175 days after the last infusion and lasts 5–77 days (Wolach, Bairey, & Lahav, 2010). A higher incidence has been noted in patients with AIDS-related lymphoma and after autologous stem cell transplantation (ASCT) (Cairoli et al., 2004; Dunleavy et al., 2005). Late-onset neutropenia seems to be unique to rituximab. Its cause is not well understood. Direct toxicity of rituximab is considered unlikely, as CD20 is not expressed on granulocytes or stem cells. Some believe it may be related to an immune-mediated phenomenon (Wolach et al., 2010).

Hematologic toxicities associated with ofatumumab include neutropenia (20%–54%), thrombocytopenia (15%–31%), lymphopenia (10%–41%), anemia (8%–25%), and febrile neutropenia (8%–10%). Grade 4 neutropenia (35%) and thrombocytopenia (15%), febrile neutropenia (9%), grade 3 infections (13%), and autoimmune hemolytic anemia have been reported (Cartron et al., 2014; Moreno et al., 2015). When ofatumumab is combined with other agents (e.g., chlorambucil), myelosuppression is more pronounced.

Rare Toxicities

A rare toxicity with CD20-targeted mAbs is vasculitis, which can occur following the first infusion of rituximab and is primarily seen in patients with CLL (Baldo, 2013). Rituximab has also been implicated in a heterogeneous spectrum of lung disorders, including bronchiolitis obliterans organizing pneumonia (most common), interstitial pneumonitis, acute respiratory distress syndrome, and hypersensitivity pneumonitis (Baldo, 2013; Ergin, Fong, & Daw, 2012).

Progressive multifocal leukoencephalopathy (PML) has also been associated with each of the CD20-targeted mAbs (Genentech, Inc., 2017b; Moreno et al., 2015; Novartis Pharmaceuticals Corp., 2016). It is a viral disease with symptoms that resemble multiple sclerosis and is linked to John Cunningham (JC) virus. JC virus persists in about 50%–90% of adults but is reactivated in those who are immunocompromised or have received certain agents, such as rituximab (Bellizzi et al., 2013).

Delayed-onset hypogammaglobulinemia has been described in approximately 20% of patients who have received rituximab. Low IgM has also been seen in this population, and 4% have developed low IgG levels for approximately four months. B-cell depletion has also been reported with ofatumumab and obinutuzumab, though it is faster and more complete with the latter (Cartron et al., 2014; Coiffier et al., 2008). Rituximab has been found to reactivate hepatitis B, which is considered a CD20-targeted mAb class effect. Patients should be tested for prior exposure to hepatitis B prior to starting rituximab and given antiviral medications. If the patient has been previously exposed, viral loads should be evaluated throughout treatment.

Other toxicities include infection, diarrhea, constipation, fatigue, nausea, rash, urticaria, insomnia, headache, muscle spasm, and edema; however, incidence and grade of these toxicities are low and not a significant problem for patients. It is unclear if these toxicities are related to mAb agents, premedication, or disease.

SLAMF7-Targeted Antibodies

SLAM cell surface Ig receptors are involved in immune homeostasis. These receptors are not expressed on nonimmune cells. Specific SLAM family members are expressed throughout the development of B and T cells, including signaling lymphocytic activation molecule F7 (SLAMF7), which is found early in the development of B cells, lost as B cells mature, and restored in mature plasmacytes (Sherbenou, Mark, & Forsberg, 2017). SLAMF7 is highly expressed on multiple myeloma and NK cells but not in normal tissue (Wang, Sanchez, Siegel, & Wang, 2016). It potentially plays a role in myeloma cell adhesion to bone marrow stromal cells, which may contribute to myeloma cell survival and growth. It also plays a role in NK-cell activation (Taniwaki et al., 2018).

Elotuzumab (Empliciti™) is a humanized mAb directed against the cell surface glycoprotein CD319 (SLAMF7). Its mechanism of action includes disrupting multiple myeloma cell adhesion to bone marrow stromal cells, enhancing NK-cell cytotoxicity, and mediating ADCC. It is not thought to affect CDC (Jung, Lee, Vo, Kim, & Lee, 2017).

Elotuzumab is indicated in combination with lenalidomide and dexamethasone for the treatment of patients with multiple myeloma who have received one to three prior treatments (Bristol-Myers Squibb Co., 2017). It is administered as a recommended dose of 10 mg/kg IV every week for the first two cycles and every two weeks thereafter in combination with lenalidomide and low-dose dexamethasone. Treatment is continued until disease progression or unacceptable toxicity (Bristol-Myers Squibb Co., 2017). Premedication must be given 45–90 minutes prior to each dose and includes the following (Bristol-Myers Squibb Co., 2017):

- Acetaminophen: 650–1,000 mg PO
- Antihistamine: Diphenhydramine 25–50 mg (IV or PO); ranitidine (50 mg IV or 150 mg PO); famotidine 20 mg (IV or PO)
  Dexamethasone administration criteria include the following:
- On days that elotuzumab is administered:
  – Dexamethasone 28 mg PO 3–24 hours before elotuzumab
  – Dexamethasone 8 mg IV 45–90 minutes before elotuzumab
- On days that elotuzumab is not administered but dexamethasone is scheduled (days 8 and 22 of cycle 3 and all subsequent cycles): Dexamethasone 40 mg PO

In the phase 3 ELOQUENT-2 trial, elotuzumab plus lenalidomide and dexamethasone (E-Ld) was compared to lenalidomide plus dexamethasone (Ld) for multiple myeloma. Results showed E-Ld had a higher ORR (79% vs. 66%) and median PFS (19.4 months vs. 14.9 months) compared to Ld (Lonial et al., 2015). No significant increase in adverse events was noted with the addition of elotuzumab. Infusion reactions were noted in approximately 10% of patients treated with E-Ld, with 1% experiencing a grade 3 reaction. Common symptoms included fever, chills, and hypertension. Bradycardia and hypotension also developed during infusions. Most reactions occurred during the first infusion (70%) (Lonial et al., 2015). Infections were reported in 81.4% receiving E-Ld and 74.4% receiving Ld. Grade 3 and 4 infections were noted in 28% using E-Ld and 24.3% using Ld. Fatal infections were similar (2.5% E-Ld vs. 2.2% Ld). Opportunistic infections (22% vs. 12.9%), fungal infections (9.7% vs. 5.4%), and herpes zoster (13.5% vs. 6.9%) were higher in the E-Ld arm (Lonial et al., 2015).

Patients receiving elotuzumab should be monitored for second primary malignancies. In the ELOQUENT-2 trial of patients with multiple myeloma (N = 635), invasive second primary malignancies were observed in 9.1% treated with E-Ld and 5.7% with Ld. The rate of hematologic malignancies was the same between the arms (1.6%). Solid tumor (3.5% vs. 2.2%) and skin cancer (4.4% vs. 2.8%) occurrences were higher in the E-Ld arm (Lonial et al., 2015).

Elevations in liver enzymes (AST/ALT) greater than three times the upper limit of normal, total bilirubin greater than two times the upper limit of normal, and alkaline phosphatase less than two times the upper limit (consistent with hepatotoxicity) were reported in 2.5% and 0.6% of patients treated with E-Ld and Ld in the ELOQUENT-2 trial of patients with multiple myeloma (N = 635). Two of eight patients experiencing hepatotoxicity were not able to continue treatment. Patients receiving elotuzumab should have their liver enzymes monitored periodically. Elotuzumab should be withdrawn with grade 3 or higher elevation of enzymes. After liver function tests return to baseline, treatment continuation may be considered. Additional side effects associated with elotuzumab include chills, fatigue, pyrexia, cough, headache, anemia, nausea, and back pain.

Elotuzumab can be detected on the serum protein electrophoresis and immunofixation assays used for clinical monitoring of multiple myeloma. This can interfere with determination of complete response and possibly with evidence of relapse from complete response in patients with IgG kappa myeloma.

CD38-Targeted Monoclonal Antibodies

CD38 has been found in a variety of tissues, including epithelial cells of the gut, lung, prostate, and on certain neurons; osteoclasts; retinal cells; and smooth and striated muscle. It is also expressed on committed hematopoietic progenitor cells, erythrocytes, platelets, basophils, NK cells, and monocytes. CD38 is a cell-surface molecule expressed by malignant plasma cells and at low levels on normal lymphoid and myeloid cells (Lokhorst et al., 2015).

Daratumumab (Darzalex®) is an IgG1k mAb that binds to CD38 on myeloma cells and induces cell death through several immune-mediated mechanisms, including CDC, ADCC, ADCP, induction of apoptosis, and modulation of CD38 enzyme activity (Overdijk et al., 2015). In patients with relapsed/refractory multiple myeloma, it has been shown to have immune-modulating effects through reduction of CD38 immunosuppressive cells and an increase in CD8 cytotoxic T cells and CD4 helper T cells (Krejcik et al., 2016).

Daratumumab is indicated in the management of multiple myeloma with the following (Janssen Biotech, Inc., 2017):

• In combination with lenalidomide and dexamethasone, or bortezomib and dexamethasone, in patients who have received at least one prior therapy

- In combination with pomalidomide and dexamethasone in patients who have received at least two prior therapies, including lenalidomide and a proteasome inhibitor (PI)
- As monotherapy in patients who have received at least three prior therapies, including a PI and an immunomodulatory agent, or who are refractory to both a PI and an immunomodulatory agent

The recommended dose is 16 mg/kg using the patient's actual body weight, administered as an IV infusion (Janssen Biotech, Inc., 2017). Prior to receiving daratumumab, patients should receive premedication with corticosteroids, antipyretics, and antihistamines (Janssen Biotech, Inc., 2017). Daratumumab is administered as a monotherapy or in combination with lenalidomide or pomalidomide plus low-dose dexamethasone. The administration schedule for daratumumab includes the following:

- Weeks 1–8: Weekly (eight doses)
- Weeks 9–24: Every two weeks (eight doses)
- Week 25 and onward until disease progression: Every four weeks

The infusion rate of daraumumab is increased with each subsequent infusion (maximum 200 ml/hr):

- First infusion: Initially 50 ml/hr; increase by 50 ml/hr every hour.
- Second infusion: Initially 50 ml/hr; increase by 50 ml/hr every hour.
- Subsequent infusions: Initially 100 ml/hr; increase by 50 ml/hr every hour.

In the phase 1/2 GEN501 trial, a dose escalation design of 3+3 was used. The maximum tolerated dose was not reached with doses up to 24 mg/kg. In patients treated with a 16 mg/kg dose, ORR was 36%, median PFS was 5.6 months, and OS at 12 months was 77% (Lokhorst et al., 2015).

In the phase 2, open-label SIRIUS trial, patients with multiple myeloma who had received at least three prior lines of treatment were administered daratumumab. ORR was 29.2% for those treated at a dose of 16 mg/kg. At least a partial response was noted in 21% shown to be refractory to four drugs, including bortezomib, lenalidomide, pomalidomide, and carfilzomib. Median PFS was 3.7 months, and 12-month OS was 64.8% (Lonial et al., 2016).

Daratumumab has also been studied in combination with bortezomib and dexamethasone. In the phase 3 CASTOR trial, this regimen was compared to bortezomib plus dexamethasone alone in patients with relapsed/refractory multiple myeloma. The daratumumab arm had significantly higher OS (82.9% vs. 63.2%) and PFS. Of note, although PFS of bortezomib and dexamethasone alone was 7.2 months, PFS in the daratumumab arm was not reached. This regimen also caused higher rates of thrombocytopenia and neutropenia (Palumbo et al., 2016).

Infusion reactions are common during initial treatment with daratumumab and require premedication with steroids, acetaminophen, antihistamine, and montelukast. Daratumumab reacts with CD38 on red blood cells, and patients treated with daratumumab have had panagglutination during indirect Coombs testing. This complicates the process of crossmatching blood for transfusion; however, patient ABO and Rh blood typing is not affected. Positivity of an indirect Coombs test can persist for up to six months after the last daratumumab infusion. AABB (formerly American Association of Blood Banks) recommends that a transfusion service is informed before a patient starts daratumumab so that extensive baseline phenotyping and screening can be completed (Zhang & Xu, 2017).

During daratumumab treatment, there may be interference with serum protein electrophoresis and immunofixation. This makes the demonstration of a complete response difficult, especially in IgG multiple myeloma. A daratumumab-specific immunofixation reflex assay has been developed for disease assessment and monitoring; however, it may be more useful in clinical trials (Sherbenou et al., 2017).

Patients receiving daratumumab should also be assessed for neutropenia and signs of infection. Dose delays may be needed to allow for neutrophil recovery; however, dose reduction is not recommended. The use of growth factors should be considered. Thrombocytopenia that occurs with other drugs may be increased with daratumumab. A patient's complete blood count should be monitored periodically during treatment, and dose delays may be needed to allow platelet count recovery; however, dose reduction is not recommended. Platelet transfusions may be necessary (Janssen Biotech, Inc., 2017).

Interleukin-6–Targeted Monoclonal Antibodies

IL-6 is one of many proinflammatory cytokines (e.g., IL-1, IL-2, TNF-α). It is produced by T cells, B cells, monocytes, fibroblasts, and endothelial cells. Certain diseases, such as Castleman disease, have increased levels of inflammatory markers such as IL-6.

Siltuximab (Sylvant®) is a chimeric, human murine Ig mAb that binds to and neutralizes human IL-6. It has been approved for the management of idiopathic multicentric Castleman disease (Janssen Biotech, Inc., 2014). Siltuximab may improve or restore cytochrome P450 activity, and drugs metabolized by the cytochrome P450 pathway (e.g., warfarin) may have increased metabolism; therefore, drug levels of these agents should be monitored during siltuximab treatment.

Patients with Castleman disease have increased levels of multiple inflammatory markers. Castleman disease is a rare lymphoproliferative disorder that has an estimated 6,500 new cases per year in the United States. It has multiple histologic patterns and two distinct clinical forms—unicentric and multicentric (Sarosiek, Shah, & Munshi, 2016). The unicentric form is typically localized, presents without systemic symptoms, and is usually cured with resection of the affected lymph node. The multicentric form usually involves more than one lymph node area and requires systemic therapy. Despite its association with human herpesvirus 9, multicentric Castleman disease is often seen in patients with no viral etiology (Sarosiek et al., 2016). Symptoms can be constitutional (e.g., fever, fatigue, night sweats, anorexia, weight loss) or associated with organomegaly, diffuse lymphadenopathy, effusions, and edema. Patients may also have anemia, thrombocythemia, leukocytosis, hypoalbuminemia, polyclonal hypergammaglobulinemia, or increases in inflammatory markers (e.g., C-reactive protein [CRP], erythrocyte sedimentation rate, ferritin, fibrinogen, IL-6) (Janssen Biotech, Inc., 2014). Mild initial symptoms may progress to more severe pancytopenia, life-threatening infection, secondary malignancy, multiorgan failure, or death (Sarosiek et al., 2016). IL-6 levels cannot be used to measure drug efficacy; however, CRP can be used as a surrogate marker for serum IL-6 inhibition.

Siltuximab is administered via IV infusion of 11 mg/kg over 60 minutes every three weeks. Blood counts should be performed prior to each treatment to ensure adequate absolute neutrophil count, platelets, and hemoglobin levels. Patients with renal dysfunction and those with mild to moderate hepatic impairment do not require dose adjustments (Janssen Biotech, Inc., 2014).

Approval was based on a phase 3, randomized, double-blind, international trial published by van Rhee et al. (2015). In this study, 79 patients received either siltuximab every three weeks or placebo plus supportive care. The siltuximab arm showed a 34% durable response compared to 0% in the control group. Patients with plasmacytic subtype achieved the highest percentage (62%) of durable response. In contrast, 45% with mixed subtype and 0% with hyaline vascular subtype had a durable and symptomatic response to treatment. Baseline IL-6 levels did not correlate with response. Median time to radiologic response was 155 days, with a median duration of response of 383 days. Although the siltuximab arm received treatment longer, toxicities in both arms were similar and minimal (van Rhee et al., 2015). A total of seven patients experienced a mild infusion reaction, including one grade 3 anaphylactic reaction. Pruritus, rash, weight gain, upper respiratory tract infection, localized edema, and nausea were the common toxicities (greater than 30%). In the trial, four patients treated with siltuximab experienced low-grade infusion reactions, including one case of anaphylaxis. Fatigue and night sweats were the only grade 3 toxicities that occurred in more than 5% of patients. No evidence exists of cumulative toxicity in patients who have received siltuximab on a longer basis (van Rhee et al., 2015).

CD52-Targeted Antibodies

CD52 is an antigen involved in T-cell activation. It is highly expressed on both normal and malignant B and T lymphocytes and, to a lesser extent, on monocytes and eosinophils. CD52 must be present on the cell surface for alemtuzumab (Campath®) to be effective. In malignancies, CD52 is present in most B-cell NHLs. Jiang et al. (2009) reported high CD52 expression on angioimmunoblastic T-cell lymphoma, hepatosplenic T-cell lymphoma, T-prolymphocytic leukemia, peripheral T-cell lymphoma (not otherwise specified), and T-cell leukemia/lymphoma. The exact function of CD52 remains undefined (Teo et al., 2016).

Alemtuzumab is a recombinant humanized IgG1 mAb that targets CD52. It is active in advanced fludarabine-refractory CLL and has proven effective in patients with deletions of chromosome 17p and with p53 mutations; however, in patients with bulky lymph nodes with CLL, no benefit has been observed. Alemtuzumab is more effective on tumor cells in the blood and bone marrow than the lymph nodes; therefore, studies have focused on CLL malignancies.

Alemtuzumab was previously approved for use in CLL in 2001. It was withdrawn from the market in 2012 but is still available through the Campath Distribution Program for patients with CLL and for the management of multiple sclerosis (Robak et al., 2016).

The starting dose for alemtuzumab is 3 mg daily. The dose is kept at 3 mg until infusion reactions are no higher than a grade 2. This is followed by 10 mg daily until infusion reactions are up to grade 2. Thereafter, it is administered at 30 mg three times a week for up to 12 weeks. Although SC administration has shown high response rates, studies have not compared it to the approved IV administration (Warner & Arnason, 2012). Premedication includes corticosteroids (1,000 mg methylprednisolone or equivalent) immediately prior to infusion and for the first three days of each treatment course. Antihistamines and antipyretics should also be considered (Gemzyme Corp., 2017).

In the pivotal CAM211 trial, which led to initial alemtuzumab approval for CLL, 93 patients with relapsed/refractory CLL who had failed prior therapy with fludarabine and an alkylating agent were treated with a stepped-up dosing followed by 30 mg three times a week for 12 weeks. ORR was 33%, including 2% complete response and 31% partial responses. Median time to progression was 9.5 months for responders and 4.7 months overall (Keating et al., 2002).

Alemtuzumab is associated with toxicities, primarily bacterial and viral infections. Cytopenias and infections also occur because of profound cellular immune suppression. Reactivated herpes viruses are common opportunistic infections (15%–25%) (Robak et al., 2016). In the CM-307 trial, cytomegalovirus reactivation was seen in 52% of patients.

Anticytomegalovirus therapies can potentially cause bone marrow suppression and are not routinely administered in alemtuzumab therapy (Warner & Arnason, 2012).

Infections reported with alemtuzumab include aspergillosis, zygomycosis, listeria meningitis, and pneumocystis pneumonia (Keating et al., 2002). To combat opportunistic infections, patients should be on a prophylactic antiviral and an agent directed against *Pneumocystis jiroveci* for six months after treatment. Some continue prophylaxis until CD4 T-lymphocyte count recovers to greater than $200/mm^3$ (Warner & Arnason, 2012). Infusion reactions primarily occur during the first several alemtuzumab infusions. SC administration significantly reduces the intensity of these reactions.

Receptor Activator of Nuclear Factor Kappa-B Ligand

At times, cancer cells can secrete parathyroid hormone-related protein (PTHrP), which can lead to humoral hypercalcemia of malignancy. PTHrP production by cancer cells causes osteoblast precursors to express receptor activator of nuclear factor kappa-B ligand (RANKL), which binds to RANK receptor on osteoclast precursors. This interaction enables maturation of osteoclast precursors to active osteoclasts. This mediates bone resorption, releases calcium and phosphorus into circulation, and causes hypercalcemia (Thosani & Hu, 2015). Bone destruction (osteolysis) by cancer is mediated by osteoclasts. RANKL contributes to the development of osteoclasts by cancer cells. Disruption of RANKL can inhibit this development.

Denosumab (Xgeva®/Prolia®) is a human mAb that binds to RANKL and inhibits its function in the bone microenvironment (Amgen Inc., 2017a). While Xgeva and Prolia are both denosumab, they have different approvals for use. Xgeva is used for bone events associated with malignancy, whereas Prolia is for osteoporosis. It decreases bone resorption via osteoclast inhibition, therefore preventing bone turnover for approximately six months (Bekker et al., 2005). Denosumab is approved for the prevention of skeletal-related events (SREs) in patients with bone metastases from solid tumors and for the management of hypercalcemia associated with malignancy refractory to bisphosphonate therapy. It is also approved for the management of adults and skeletally mature adolescents with unresectable giant cell tumor of bone or where surgical resection is likely to result in severe morbidity (Amgen Inc., 2018).

Denosumab is administered at a dose of 120 mg SC once a month. Because of the risk of hypocalcemia, patients should be started on calcium and vitamin D supplementation prior to first administration (Amgen Inc., 2018; Huynh, Baker, Stewardson, & Johnson, 2016).

In a meta-analysis by Zheng et al. (2017), denosumab was superior to zoledronic acid (4 mg IV monthly) in delaying or preventing SREs in patients with advanced solid tumors. However, no difference in OS was found. Although their mechanisms of action are different, both agents improve quality and quantity of life by inhibiting bone resorption, fractures, and pain (Zheng et al., 2017). Since 2012, multiple reports have demonstrated the safety and effectiveness of denosumab in managing cancer-associated hypercalcemia. In an open-label, single-arm trial, 33 patients with hypercalcemia of malignancy (with or without bone metastases) refractory to IV bisphosphonate therapy were administered denosumab subcutaneously on days 1, 8, 15, and 29, then every four weeks thereafter. Approximately 64% of patients responded to treatment, and 36% achieved a complete response. The median time to response was 9 days, with a median duration of response of 104 days (Hu et al., 2014). This study led to FDA approval of denosumab for the treatment of bisphosphonate-refractory hypercalcemia of malignancy.

In a trial by Body et al. (2015), hypocalcemia incidence with denosumab use was approximately 12.4% in metastatic bone disease over a 34-month period. Because denosumab inhibits osteoclastic bone resorption (Huynh et al., 2016), the resulting imbalance of osteoclast and osteoblastic activity causes dose-dependent hypocalcemia (Bekker et al., 2005). This is corrected with a compensatory increase in parathyroid hormone, which increases calcium reabsorption in the distal tubule of the kidney and in the small intestine. Secondary hyperparathyroidism that can occur in advanced kidney dysfunction may impair the compensatory increase of parathyroid hormone, leading to an increased risk for hypocalcemia. Factors related to this risk include renal failure and male gender (Body et al., 2015). Denosumab is associated with a 1.8% incidence of osteonecrosis of the jaw, which is like that of bisphosphonates; however, denosumab may be preferred in patients with hypercalcemia and renal impairment because it does not have nephrotoxic effects, making dose adjustment based on renal function unneccssary (Thosani & Hu, 2015).

Other adverse events found in more than 20% of patients using denosumab include nausea, dyspnea, decreased appetite, headache, peripheral edema, vomiting, anemia, constipation, and diarrhea. Events found with a severity of grade 3 or higher include fatigue and infection. Grade 3 laboratory abnormalities include hypomagnesemia, hypokalemia, and hypophosphatemia.

Antibody–Drug Conjugates

Most mAbs have little antitumor activity, excluding those targeted to HER2, EGFR, VEGF and CD20 (Thomas, Teicher, & Hassan, 2016).

Regardless, the specificity of target antigens makes mAbs useful agents for the management of malignancies. Antibody–drug conjugates make use of antibodies specific to the cell-surface receptors on cancer cells and have specificity and potency not achievable with traditional drugs. The early drug–antibody conjugates included mouse mAbs, though success was limited by immunogenicity. To prevent this, murine antibodies have been replaced with humanized or fully human antibodies. The antibody target is important to consider when developing the conjugate. It must have an extracellular epitope amenable to antibody binding and be capable of internalization into target cells where the drug can be released. The target antigen should be expressed on the surface of the cell but have low expression elsewhere.

Antitumor activity can be accomplished by conjugating antibodies with effector molecules. The antibody binds to the receptor target on the surface of the cancer cell, is internalized, and the effector molecule is released from the antibody inside the cancer cell. Such effector molecules include cytotoxic agents, immunotoxins, and radiopharmaceuticals (Thomas et al., 2016). Most drugs used in antibody–drug conjugates are highly potent (100–1,000 times more potent than earlier agents) and target tubulin or DNA; however, only a small amount of these drugs reach the intracellular target (Thomas et al., 2016). Immunotoxins are recombinant proteins that have an antibody or antibody fragment that targets the tumor antigen. The antibody is linked to toxins such as diphtheria toxin or *Pseudomonas* exotoxin. Immunotoxins have been less effective in solid tumors because they induce an immune response that restricts their activity. The only immunotoxin approved by FDA was denileukin diftitox for the treatment of CD25-positive cutaneous T-cell lymphoma, but it was removed from the U.S. market in 2014. Immunotoxins that are inherently less immunogenic have shown promise in preclinical trials (Hassan, Alewine, & Pastan, 2016; Thomas et al., 2016).

Other antibody–drug conjugates have achieved and maintained FDA approval. For example, ado-trastuzumab emtansine was FDA approved in 2013 for the management of metastatic breast cancer, gemtuzumab ozogamicin in 2000 for the management of acute myeloid leukemia (AML), and brentuximab vedotin in 2011 for the treatment of systemic anaplastic large-cell lymphoma and refractory Hodgkin lymphoma. It should be noted that gemtuzumab ozogamicin was withdrawn from the market in 2010 because it did not meet efficacy targets in postmarketing clinical trials; however, it was reapproved in 2017.

Brentuximab Vedotin

Brentuximab vedotin (Adcetris®) targets CD30 with an anti-CD30 chimeric antibody (Seattle Genetics, Inc., 2017). This antibody is conjugated with the microtubule disrupting agent monomethyl auristatin E (MMAE) by a linker that attaches cytotoxic agents covalently to the antibody. After it binds to CD30, brentuximab vedotin is internalized rapidly and transported to lysosomes, where the peptide linker is cleaved. MMAE is then released into the cell, binding to tubulin and prompting cell cycle arrest between the gap 2 phase and mitosis, leading to cell apoptosis (Katz, Janik, & Younes, 2011). As the cells die, a small amount of MMAE is released into the tumor microenvironment, which can lead to the killing of neighbor cells (Alperovich & Younes, 2016).

Brentuximab vedotin is administered as 1.8 mg/kg IV over 30 minutes every 21 days until disease progression or unacceptable toxicity (Seattle Genetics, Inc., 2017). It is approved for the management of relapsed/refractory CD30-positive Hodgkin lymphoma after ASCT or after two previous therapies when ASCT or multiagent chemotherapy are not treatment options. It is also approved for the management of relapsed/refractory systemic anaplastic large-cell lymphoma.

Drug approval was based on two single-arm studies. For Hodgkin lymphoma, 77 patients who had relapsed after ASCT were subsequently treated with brentuximab vedotin. Objective response rate was 75%, and complete response rate was 34%. The median duration of response was 6.7 months and 20.5 months, respectively (Younes et al., 2012). The second trial included 58 patients with systemic anaplastic large-cell lymphoma. Objective response was 86%, and complete response rate was 57%. The median duration of response was 12.6 months and 13.2 months, respectively (Pro et al., 2012). Responses to brentuximab vedotin are rapid and typically occur within the first three to four cycles (Zinzani, Sasse, Radford, Gautam, & Bonthapally, 2016).

The most common toxicities associated with brentuximab vedotin include neutropenia, peripheral sensory neuropathy, fatigue, nausea, anemia, upper respiratory tract infection, diarrhea, pyrexia, rash, thrombocytopenia, cough, and vomiting. Any grade neuropathy occurred in 28%–31% of patients, with grade 3 or 4 occurring in 2%–3% (Salihoglu et al., 2015). Serious adverse events reported with brentuximab vedotin include Stevens-Johnson syndrome, TLS, and progressive multifocal leukoencephalopathy (de Claro et al., 2012).

Ado-Trastuzumab Emtansine

Ado-trastuzumab emtansine is an antibody–drug conjugate of trastuzumab and mertansine (DM1). Mertansine is conjugated covalently to the antibody by a stable linker and acts on microtubules. After binding to HER2, ado-trastuzumab emtansine is internalized, and with subsequent proteolytic digestion, it releases DM1 within the cells. It blocks HER2-mediated signal transduction, facilitates ADCC, and inhibits

HER2 extracellular domain shedding (Amiri-Kordestani et al., 2014; Lambert & Chari, 2014).

Ado-trastuzumab emtansine was FDA approved in 2013 for the treatment of patients with HER2-positive metastatic breast cancer who previously received trastuzumab and a taxane, separately or in combination. NCCN (2018) guidelines recommend ado-trastuzumab emtansine as the preferred agent for trastuzumab-exposed HER2-positive recurrent breast cancer or metastatic breast cancer.

Ado-trastuzumab emtansine is administered as 3.6 mg/kg IV every three weeks until disease progression or unacceptable toxicity occurs. Initial administration is over 90 minutes, while subsequent administration are over 30 minutes. Initial and subsequent doses are administered without premedications. Patients should be monitored for infusion-related reactions for an amount of time equal to infusion duration (Genentech, Inc., 2016a).

Drug approval was based on a phase 3 trial that included 991 patients with HER2-positive metastatic breast cancer. These patients were randomly assigned to receive either ado-trastuzumab emtansine or lapatinib plus capecitabine. Results showed higher median PFS (9.6 months vs. 6.4 months) and OS (30.9 months vs. 25.1 months) in the ado-trastuzumab arm (Krop et al., 2014).

The effectiveness of ado-trastuzumab emtansine was also evaluated in patients with advanced HER2-positive breast cancer previously treated with two or more HER2-directed regimens, including lapatinib, trastuzumab, and taxane therapies. In this phase 3 trial, median PFS was improved with ado-trastuzumab emtansine compared to investigator's choice (6.2 months vs. 3.3 months) (Krop et al., 2014).

No trials have evaluated the potential for drug–drug interactions with ado-trastuzumab emtansine. However, because the cytotoxic component is metabolized by CYP3A4 and CYP3A5, the potential exists for interactions between ado-trastuzumab emtansine and medications that are strong CYP3A4 inhibitors. Concomitant administration of CYP3A4 inhibitors with ado-trastuzumab emtansine should be avoided to reduce the risk of increasing DM1 levels and subsequent toxicities (Genentech, Inc., 2016a).

The most common toxicities with ado-trastuzumab emtansine include nausea, thrombocytopenia, musculoskeletal pain, fatigue, headache, increased transaminases, constipation, diarrhea, epistaxis, and peripheral neuropathy. Rare but serious adverse events include hepatotoxicity, which can lead to liver failure and reduced LVEF (Krop et al., 2014; Verma et al., 2012). Grade 3 or 4 toxicities include diarrhea, abdominal pain, asthenia, cellulitis, pulmonary embolism, dyspnea, thrombocytopenia, increased transaminases, anemia, hypokalemia, fatigue, neutropenia, leukopenia, hemorrhage, and pneumonitis. LVD and infusion-related reactions have also been reported. Dose reductions, dose delays, or drug discontinuation is recommended with the occurrence of hepatotoxicity, hyperbilirubinemia, LVD, thrombocytopenia, peripheral neuropathy, pulmonary toxicity, and infusion reactions (Genentech, Inc., 2016a).

Gemtuzumab Ozogamicin

Gemtuzumab ozogamicin (GO) (Mylotarg®) is a humanized mAb drug conjugate that targets CD33 (Wyeth Pharmaceuticals Inc., 2017b). The conjugate, a semisynthetic derivative of calicheamicin, is attached to the mAb by an acid-labile linker. The linker connects the cytotoxic agent to the mAb and maintains the conjugated antibody with the drug in circulation (Thomas et al., 2016). Although the linker is stable in circulation, when it is internalized, it quickly releases toxin, leading to double-strand DNA breaks and cell death (Appelbaum & Bernstein, 2017). AML precursors are mainly or entirely CD33 positive.

GO is approved for the treatment of newly diagnosed CD33-positive AML in adults and for relapsed/refractory CD33-positive AML in adults and pediatric patients aged two years and older. It is also approved in newly diagnosed de novo AML (combination regimen), newly diagnosed AML (single-agent regimen), and relapsed/refractory AML (single-agent regimen) (Wyeth Pharmaceuticals Inc., 2017b). Newly diagnosed de novo AML includes an induction cycle of 3 mg/m^2 (up to one 4.5 mg vial) on days 1, 4, and 7 in combination with daunorubicin plus cytarabine and a consolidation cycle of 3 mg/m^2 (up to one 4.5 mg vial) on day 1 in combination with daunorubicin and cytarabine. Newly diagnosed AML as a single-agent regimen includes a 6 mg/m^2 infusion on day 1 and 3 mg/m^2 on day 8. For patients without evidence of disease progression following induction, eight additional courses are recommended of 2 mg/m^2 on day 1 every four weeks. Relapsed/refractory AML as a single-agent regimen includes administration of 3 mg/m^2 on days 1, 4, and 7. Premedication includes a corticosteroid, antihistamine, and acetaminophen one hour prior to GO administration (Amadori et al., 2016).

In a pivotal multicenter, open-label, randomized trial, patients were randomized to receive either GO (3 mg/m^2 on days 1, 4, and 7), daunorubicin (60 mg/m^2 on days 1–3), and cytarabine (200 mg/m^2 as a continuous infusion days 1–7) or daunorubicin plus cytarabine alone as induction and consolidation of patients with previously untreated de novo AML (Castaigne et al., 2012). Although complete response rates were similar (70.4% vs. 69.9%), three-year event-free survival was significantly higher in the GO arm (39.8% vs. 13.6%).

A meta-analysis of 3,325 patients from five trials concluded that GO significantly reduced the risk of relapse and improved relapse-free survival and OS at five years. Survival benefit was most apparent in patients who had favorable-risk cytogenetics and those with intermediate-risk disease (Hills et al., 2014).

The most frequent (1% or greater) side effects from GO that led to permanent discontinuation included thrombocytopenia, veno-occlusive disease (VOD), and septic shock (Wyeth Pharmaceuticals Inc., 2017b). GO causes acute infusion-related toxicities; however, these are transient and usually respond to standard interventions. Life-threatening or fatal infusion reactions can occur during or within 24 hours following GO infusion. Signs and symptoms of infusion reactions may include fever, chills, hypotension, tachycardia, hypoxia, and respiratory failure.

GO eliminates early myeloid precursors, making bone marrow suppression evident when GO is used as a single agent. When GO is used in combination chemotherapy, myeloid recovery following induction is not delayed; however, platelet recovery is prolonged by an additional four days (Appelbaum & Bernstein, 2017).

GO can cause fatal or life-threatening hemorrhage due to prolonged thrombocytopenia. When combined with chemotherapy, all-grade bleeding events were reported in 90% of patients, with 21% experiencing grade 3 or 4 bleeding. Thrombocytopenia with platelet counts less than 50,000/mm^3 persisting more than 42 days occurred in 19% of patients in the induction phase (Wyeth Pharmaceuticals Inc., 2017b).

VOD occurs with GO; however, this risk is low if GO is administered at 3 mg/m^2 or lower in patients receiving frontline therapy. Risk increases at higher doses and in heavily pretreated patients (Appelbaum & Bernstein, 2017).

Inotuzumab Ozogamicin

Inotuzumab ozogamicin (InO) (Besponsa™) is a humanized anti-CD22 mAb conjugated to the cytotoxic antibody calicheamicin (Wyeth Pharmaceuticals Inc., 2017a). CD22 is a cell surface glycoprotein that facilitates signal transduction. It is expressed in more than 90% of patients with B-cell acute lymphoblastic leukemia (ALL). After the conjugate binds to CD22, it is rapidly internalized, and calicheamicin is released. The calicheamicin binds to the minor groove of DNA and induces double-strand cleavage and apoptosis (Kantarjian et al., 2016).

InO is indicated for the treatment of adults with relapsed/refractory B-cell precursor ALL (Wyeth Pharmaceuticals Inc., 2017a). An administration cycle for InO is 21 days. The recommended total dose for all patients is 1.8 mg/m^2 per cycle. This is administered as three divided doses on day 1 (0.8 mg/m^2), day 8 (0.5 mg/m^2), and day 15 (0.5 mg/m^2). This cycle may be extended to four weeks if the patient achieves complete remission or complete remission with incomplete hematologic recovery (CRi). An extension may also be needed for toxicity recovery. Subsequent cycles are similar in dose and schedule; however, these cycles last four weeks. Patients who do not achieve a complete remission or CRi within three cycles should discontinue treatment.

For patients proceeding to hematopoietic stem cell transplantation (HSCT), the recommended duration of treatment with InO is two cycles. A third cycle may be considered for patients who do not achieve complete remission or CRi and have negative minimal residual disease after two cycles. This is because of the increased risk of VOD. For patients not proceeding to HSCT, a maximum of six InO cycles may be administered.

For patients with circulating lymphoblasts, cytoreduction with a combination of hydroxyurea, steroids, and/or vincristine to a peripheral blast count of less than or equal to $10,000/mm^3$ is recommended prior to the first InO dose (Wyeth Pharmaceuticals Inc., 2017a).

Premedication with a corticosteroid, antipyretic, and antihistamine is recommended prior to InO infusions. Patients should be observed during and for at least one hour after the infusion for symptoms of infusion-related reactions (Wyeth Pharmaceuticals Inc., 2017a).

In the open-label, phase 3 INO-VATE ALL trial, patients aged 18 years or older with ALL were randomized to receive either InO or the investigator's choice of the following standard therapy regimens: FLAG (fludarabine, cytarabine, and granulocyte macrophage–colony-stimulating factor [GM-CSF]) for up to four 28-day cycles; cytarabine plus mitoxantrone for up to four cycles of 15–20 days; or high-dose cytarabine in one 12-dose cycle. Patients who achieved complete remission could undergo HSCT. Complete remission was significantly higher in the InO group than in the standard group (80.7% vs. 29.4%). The duration of remission was longer in the InO group (4.6 months vs. 3.1 months). PFS was significantly longer in the InO group (5 months vs. 1.8 months) (Kantarjian et al., 2016). Hepatotoxicity, including severe, life-threatening, and sometimes fatal hepatic VOD, was observed in 14% receiving InO. This occurred during treatment, following treatment, and following HSCT after treatment. VOD was reported up to 56 days after the last dose. The median time from subsequent HSCT to VOD onset was 15 days (3–57 days). The risk of VOD was greater in patients who underwent HSCT after InO treatment, used HSCT conditioning regimens containing two alkylating agents, or had a total bilirubin level greater than or equal to the upper limit of normal before HSCT. Other risk factors for VOD include ongoing or prior liver disease, prior HSCT, increased age, later salvage lines, and a greater number of InO treatment cycles. Patients should be monitored closely for signs and symptoms of VOD, including hyperbilirubinemia, hepatomegaly, rapid weight gain, and ascites (Kantarjian et al., 2016).

Myelosuppression was also reported in the INO-VATE ALL trial, with 51% of patients experiencing thrombocytopenia (14% grade 3) and 49% experiencing neutropenia (20% grade 3). Febrile neutropenia and infections occurred in 26% and 48% of patients, respectively. Along with bacterial, viral, and fungal infections, reported fatal infections included pneumonia, neutropenic sepsis, sepsis, septic shock, and *Pseudomonas* sepsis. Hemorrhagic events occurred in 33% of patients. Patients should have blood counts monitored prior to each dose of InO. They should also be monitored for signs and symptoms of infection, bleeding, and other effects of myelosuppression. Prophylactic anti-infective agents should be considered (Kantarjian et al., 2016).

Infusion reactions were noted in patients receiving InO and usually occurred after cycle 1. These typically resolved spontaneously or with medical intervention. Prolongation of QT interval was noted in approximately 3% of patients during the INO-VATE ALL trial; however, no patients were noted to have a QTc greater than 500 ms (Kantarjian et al., 2016). Electrocardiograms and electrolytes should be obtained at baseline and monitored during treatment. Patients should be monitored more frequently when concomitantly using other medications known to prolong QT interval (Wyeth Pharmaceuticals Inc., 2017a).

Antibody–Radiopharmaceutical Conjugates

Radioimmunotherapy (RIT) involves an antibody that targets a specific antigen conjugated with a radioisotope. The antibody should ideally target tumor-specific antigens, such as CD20 for lymphomas, but spare normal cells. RIT primarily targets B-cell lymphomas. CD20 is an attractive target because it is expressed in more than 90% of B-cell NHL but is not present in plasma cells or stem cells. An advantage of RIT is that lymphoma cells are inherently radiosensitive. In addition, RIT can kill surrounding tumor cells within the path of the isotope by crossfire effect, which can help kill tumor cells in bulky or poorly vascularized tumors or in those that express low or absent levels of CD20. Solid tumors are more resistant to radiation and less accessible to large molecules such as antibodies; therefore, the clinical efficacy of RIT with solid tumors remains limited (Kraeber-Bodéré et al., 2014). Previously, two RITs were available for the management of NHL, iodine-131 (^{131}I) tositumomab and yttrium-90 (^{90}Y) ibritumomab tiuxetan, but ^{131}I-tositumomab was recently withdrawn from the market because of a decline in use. Particle emissions of these agents have a limited path length with a selective antibody; therefore, surrounding normal tissue is exposed to less radiation than tumor cells. RIT delivers continuous radiation directly to malignant tissue with a lower peak dose than conventional external beam radiation therapy. Because of this continuous exposure, malignant cells are usually unable to perform DNA damage repair (Skarbnik & Smith, 2012).

Ibritumomab tiuxetan (Zevalin®) is a CD20-targeted mAb conjugated with the radionuclide ^{90}Y. It emits beta particles that penetrate only short distances through tissue. Imaging was required to determine proper biodistribution but is no longer necessary in the United States. Dosimetry is not needed because the incidence of abnormal biodistribution is less than 1% (Skarbnik & Smith, 2012). No significant radiation precautions are necessary following ibritumomab tiuxetan administration. Standard universal precautions should be sufficient to prevent radiation exposure to personnel working with patients who have received ibritumomab tiuxetan.

^{90}Y-ibritumomab tiuxetan is approved in the United States for the treatment of recurrent/refractory NHL and as a consolidation for patients with follicular lymphoma who have responded to first-line therapy (Witzig et al., 2011). Patients must have adequate bone marrow reserve with adequate normal cellularity and less than 25% involvement of the bone marrow space with lymphoma to receive RIT. Adequate bone marrow sampling is necessary and may lead to the need for bilateral core biopsies. A platelet count of 150,000/mm^3 is required for full dosing, but patients with platelet counts of 100,000–149,000/mm^3 are eligible for treatment at a reduced dose. Treatment with ^{90}Y-ibritumomab tiuxetan first includes infusion of CD20-targeted cold antibody (rituximab), which clears circulating normal or malignant B cells that express CD20 and blocks CD20 sites in the spleen. A second "cold" dose of anti-CD20 antibody is given approximately one week later, prior to the therapeutic dose of RIT. This dose binds peripheral sites of tumor masses, facilitating the penetration of the radiolabeled antibody. RIT is administered by either a nuclear medicine or radiation oncology specialist.

On day 1, the rituximab infusion should be administered as a 250 mg/m^2 IV infusion at an initial rate of 50 mg/hr. In the absence of infusion reactions, escalate the infusion rate in 50 mg/hr increments every 30 minutes to a maximum of 400 mg/hr. On days 7–9, this increment is increased to 100 mg/hr. After rituximab is infused, the patient is transferred to the appropriate specialist to administer the ^{90}Y-ibritumomab tiuxetan component.

The ^{90}Y-ibritumomab tiuxetan is administered at a dose range of 0.4–32 mCi/kg provided that the platelet count is greater than 150,000/mm^3. If the platelet count is 100,000–149,000/mm^3, the patient is administered a reduced 0.3 mCi/kg dose. The ^{90}Y-ibritumomab tiuxetan is administered through a free-flowing IV line within four hours following completion of rituximab infusion. A 0.22 mcm low-protein-binding in-line filter should be used between the syringe and the infusion port.

After injection, the line should be flushed with at least 10 ml of normal saline. Infusion must be immediately stopped and restarted in another limb if any signs or symptoms of extravasation are present. Premedication includes acetaminophen (50 mg PO) and diphenhydramine (50 mg PO prior to rituximab infusion) on days 1, 7, 8, and 9.

Several studies have documented the efficacy of RIT in the management of NHL. In an analysis of five clinical trials using either tositumomab or ^{131}I-tositumomab in 250 patients with relapsed/refractory low-grade follicular and transformed low-grade NHL, ORR was 47%–68% with a complete response rate of 20%–38% (Fisher et al., 2005).

A phase 3 multicenter trial evaluated the efficacy of consolidation with ^{90}Y-ibritumomab tiuxetan in 414 patients with advanced follicular lymphoma who responded to induction therapy. Consolidation with RIT significantly improved median PFS from 13.3 months to 36.5 months. Approximately 77% of patients who achieved partial response from induction therapy converted to complete response after consolidation with RIT (Morschhauser et al., 2008).

RIT has also been used in patients with NHL. A prospective, multi-center, phase 2 trial evaluated the efficacy and safety of ^{90}Y-ibritumomab tiuxetan in 104 patients with relapsed or primary refractory diffuse large B-cell lymphoma who were ineligible for stem cell transplantation. The ORR of patients previously treated with chemotherapy was 52% for those with refractory disease and 53% for those who relapsed after achieving a complete response. ORR was 19% for patients previously treated with chemoimmunotherapy (Morschhauser et al., 2007).

RIT is not widely used in either the community setting or within comprehensive cancer centers. In a study of RIT utilization, community-based physicians treated fewer patients with RIT, used RIT later in the course of therapy, and had financial and administrative concerns, including time constraints, high costs, radiation safety, and difficulty in performing dosimetry. In centers where these issues were less of a concern, collaboration developed between departments involved in this treatment (e.g., medical oncologist, infusion centers, nuclear medicine/radiation oncology department) (Hadid et al., 2016).

The most common toxicity for ^{90}Y-ibritumomab tiuxetan is delayed myelosuppression. Thrombocytopenia and neutropenia usually begin to appear two to three weeks following therapeutic dose of RIT, remain low for several weeks, and recover to baseline levels after two or three months. Patient blood count is monitored weekly for approximately three months and can be discontinued once returned to baseline. Nonhematologic toxicities are uncommon and usually mild (Skarbnik & Smith, 2012). Secondary malignancies may result following ^{90}Y-ibritumomab tiuxetan treatment. Myelodysplastic syndrome and/or AML have been reported in 5.2% of patients with relapsed/refractory NHL (Rizzieri, 2016). Additional side effects related to the rituximab administered prior to ^{90}Y-ibritumomab tiuxetan can also occur. Patients must wash their hands thoroughly after using the toilet for three days following treatment. In addition, for the first week after treatment, they should use condoms during sexual relations (Wagner et al., 2002).

Bispecific T-Cell Engager Antibodies

BiTEs are bispecific antibodies that have dual-binding specificities. BiTE antibodies are linked by a single polypeptide, forming the BiTE molecule. This double binding leads to T-cell–mediated lysis of normal and malignant B cells. The small size of the BiTE molecule allows cancer and cytotoxic cells to be in proximity, which allows lysis to occur (Topp et al., 2015).

Blinatumomab (Blincyto®) is a first-in-class BiTE. It is a murine anti-human mAb that targets CD3 and CD19. Blinatumomab simultaneously binds CD3-positive T cells and CD19-positive B lymphocytes, which leads to T-cell–mediated lysis of CD19-positive normal and malignant B cells. CD19 is the earliest B-cell lineage–restricted antigen expressed on the surface of B lymphocytes. It is expressed with high frequency on B-cell lineage–derived leukemia and lymphoma. CD3 is a component of the T-cell receptor expressed on the surface of cytotoxic T lymphocytes. Blinatumomab does not rely on ADCC and CDC but rather directly activates T cells, thus avoiding the mechanism of resistance some malignancies develop against other immunotherapeutic agents (Folan, Rexwinkle, Autry, & Bryan, 2016).

Blinatumomab is approved for the management of relapsed/refractory Philadelphia chromosome–negative, precursor B-cell ALL. It is given as a flat-dose continuous infusion for 28 days followed by a two-week break. During cycle 1, the dose is escalated from 9 mcg/day for the first seven days to 28 mcg/day afterward. On subsequent cycles, blinatumomab is administered at 28 mcg/day. During the first nine days of cycle 1 and the first two days of cycle 2, hospitalization with close monitoring for reactions is recommended. If infusion needs to be stopped for longer than four hours, reinitiation should occur under close supervision or within the hospital.

A premedication of dexamethasone 20 mg should be administered one hour prior to the first dose of each cycle, prior to dose escalation on day 8 of cycle 1, and prior to reinitiation after any time infusion is stopped for more than four hours. Dose adjustments and alterations to the infusion schedule are based on grading of toxicities. For any grade 3 toxicity, blinatumomab infusion should be held until the toxicity resolves to at least a grade 1. Once the infusion is restarted, a 9 mcg/day dose should be used for the first seven days, and if it is tolerated, the dose should be escalated to 28 mcg/day. However, if toxicity recurs at this dose, blinatumomab should be discontinued permanently.

Central nervous system (CNS) prophylaxis with concomitant intrathecal chemotherapy should be considered in patients receiving blinatumomab, as it has very limited activity in the CNS. However, this combination has not been studied (Folan et al., 2016).

Blinatumomab has been shown to be effective against relapsed/refractory B-cell malignancies, including NHL and B-cell ALL. Blinatumomab received FDA approval in 2014 for the treatment of relapsed/refractory Philadelphia chromosome–negative, precursor B-cell ALL based on the results of a multicenter, international, open-label, single-arm phase 2 trial (Topp et al., 2015). In this study of 189 patients, 34% relapsed after an allogeneic HSCT, and 51% received at least one salvage regimen but no prior allogeneic stem cell transplant. The complete remission or hematologic complete remission (CRh) rate was 43%, which occurred during the first two cycles. At a median follow-up of 8.9 months, 45% of these patients were alive and still in remission. The OS for all patients was 6.1 months. Prior history of an allogeneic stem cell transplant did not affect complete remission or CRh. Minimal residual disease was noted in 82% of those who achieved either a complete remission or CRh.

The most common grade 3 or 4 toxicities associated with blinatumomab included febrile neutropenia, anemia, and neutropenia (Topp et al., 2015). Fatal adverse events were noted in 15% of patients, with the majority related to infection. Approximately 99% of patients experienced an adverse event of any grade, most commonly pyrexia, headache, febrile neutropenia, peripheral edema, nausea, hypokalemia, constipation, and anemia. CRS occurred in 2% of patients and manifested as fever, asthenia, headache, nausea, transaminitis, hyperbilirubinemia, or hypotension; however, CRS incidence was lower in this study, most likely because of dose escalation and dexamethasone, which was required in patients with high tumor burden (Topp et al., 2015).

Rare manifestations have been seen with blinatumomab, including disseminated intravascular coagulation and secondary hemophagocytic lymphohistiocytosis (HLH)/macrophage activation syndrome (Lee et al., 2014). HLH is characterized by fever, splenomegaly with hyperferritinemia, coagulopathy, hypertriglyceridemia, and cytopenia. It has been linked to IL-6 and is managed with tocilizumab (Klinger et al., 2012).

Neurologic toxicities were reported in 52% of trial patients. Most neurologic side effects were grade 1 or 2 and manifested by tremor, dizziness, confusion, encephalopathy, ataxia, and somnolence. These events occurred early in treatment (87% in cycle 1). The median time to onset of symptoms was seven days. Grade 3 (11%) and 4 (2%) neurologic toxicities were reported in 13% of patients. Seizures have also been reported. If a patient experiences more than one seizure, blinatumomab should be discontinued permanently. CNS events are thought to be caused by local release of cytokines activated by T cells at the neuroendothelium (Nagorsen, Kufer, Baeuerle, & Bargou, 2012).

Hypersensitivity Reactions

Hypersensitivity is a term used to indicate "adverse signs and symptoms that are initiated by an antigenic stimulus tolerated by a 'normal' person and that have an immune basis or component" (Baldo, 2013, p. 2). Sometimes it describes reactions that have no immune basis; however, these reactions are not easy to classify, and their mechanisms are yet to be determined (Baldo, 2013). In this instance, *hypersensitivity* is used in a more global sense. The mAbs are known to have the potential to cause hypersensitivity reactions but vary in incidence.

Premedications are used to minimize a patient's risk for an infusion reaction. The determination for premedications is based on the incidence of infusion reactions. Agents that may be used as premedications include acetaminophen, H_1 and H_2 blockers, and dexamethasone. Montelukast, a drug used often in the allergy specialty, blocks mast cell mediators released during hypersensitivity reactions. It is frequently administered with acetylsalicylic acid and offers the most benefit for skin and respiratory symptoms. Montelukast should be administered 60 minutes prior to the initiation of an infusion (Castells Guitart, 2014).

Some mAbs have specific premedication schedule recommendations, most notably CD20-targeted mAbs. Package inserts outline the recommended premedications and infusion rates for each drug to minimize infusion reaction frequency and severity. Nurses administering these agents should consult the package insert to ensure safety measures.

Once a patient begins to exhibit an infusion reaction, drug infusion should be stopped and normal saline started. Additional H_1 and H_2 blockers or dexamethasone may be administered. In patients experiencing respiratory symptoms, oxygen or bronchodilators may be administered. Epinephrine may be needed if the patient experiences hypotension or airway-obstructive symptoms. The patient should be monitored until all symptoms of the reaction resolve (Bonamichi-Santos & Castells, 2018; Dawson, Moran, Guindon, & Wan, 2016; Picard & Galvão, 2017; Tham, Cheng, Tay, Alcasabas, & Shek, 2015). Thereafter, a decision concerning the safety of rechallenging the patient with the drug can be made. To expedite treatment for the infusion reaction, nurses should execute agent administration standards (while waiting for the physician or advanced practitioner to provide input into patient management).

Skin testing is included in the Oncology Nursing Society's *Chemotherapy and Immunotherapy Guidelines and Recommendations for Practice* (Olsen, LeFebvre, & Brassil, in press); however, it is mostly suggested for platin agents (e.g., carboplatin), and no information regarding skin testing for mAbs could be found in this review of the literature.

Desensitization is also a potential option for patients experiencing an infusion reaction to an anticancer agent. This includes administration of incremental doses of drug in succession to allow the temporary tolerance to drug antigens (Tham et al., 2015). The purpose of desensitization is to render mast cells unresponsive to further antigen stimulation. Although full desensitization is not widely used for mAbs, it has been reported in the literature (Brennan, Bouza, Hsu, Sloane, & Castells, 2009). Decreased rate of administration of mAbs is used more frequently and often assists in the prevention of infusion reactions.

Adoptive Cell Transfer

The term *adoptive cell transfer* (ACT) refers to the passive administration of antitumor T cells. ACT is a specific variant of cell-based immunotherapy that involves the collection of circulating or tumor-infiltrating lymphocytes (TILs); their selection, modification, expansion, and activation ex vivo; and their readministration to patients, usually after lymphodepleting preconditioning and in combination with immunostimulatory agents. Large numbers of antitumor T cells can be grown in vitro and selected for those with a high avidity against a desired antigen. In ACT, T cells are harvested from the patient's blood or tumor. They are then stimulated to grow and expand in an in vitro culture system. After sufficient in vitro expansion, the cells are reinfused into the host. At this time, the hope is that these cells will mediate tumor destruction (Perica, Varela, Oelke, & Schneck, 2015). Current examples of ACT include the use of TILs and chimeric antigen receptor (CAR) T cells. At this time, TILs remain investigational; however, in 2017, two specific CAR T-cell therapy agents were approved by FDA.

Adoptive immunotherapy has beneficial properties useful for cancer treatment. T-cell responses are specific and can therefore distinguish between healthy and cancer tissue. T-cell responses are also robust and can traffic to the site of the antigen, suggesting a mechanism for eradication of distant metastases. These responses have memory and maintain therapeutic effect for many years after initial treatment.

Chimeric Antigen Receptor T Cells

CAR T cells are synthetic molecules of an extracellular antigen-binding domain that are fused via a spacer region to intracellular signaling domains capable of activating T cells. To develop CAR T cells, primary T cells are collected from a specific patient's peripheral blood. These cells need to be activated, with the help of primary and costimulatory signals, before they are redirected with CAR genes. During this activation, special beads coated with anti-CD3 and anti-CD28 antibodies are used. The anti-CD3 antibody provides the primary signal, and the anti-CD28 antibody provides the costimulatory signal. Cytokines can be added into a culture system to enhance the activation efficiency. The activated T cells are then genetically modified. Viral and nonviral systems are used to deliver CAR genes to T cells. Following effective transfection, expansion of CAR T cells is needed before administration through the bloodstream (Han et al., 2017).

CAR T cells have been shown to have a therapeutic effect on hematologic malignancies. Most studies using CARs to treat hematologic malignancies have targeted CD19. Complete remission rate is more than 90% with relapsed/refractory B-cell ALL, 23%–50% with CLL, and 47%–100% with B-cell NHL (Shank et al., 2017). The antitumor effect from CAR T cells is improved with conditioning chemotherapy administered prior to infusion. Conditioning intensification to achieve myeloablation with chemotherapy and total body irradiation prior to the CAR T-cell infusion increases responses dramatically (Shank et al., 2017). Additional clinical trials are underway using CARs to treat hematologic malignancies with the use of other antigens. Strategies to use CAR T cells to treat solid tumors have been difficult because of multiple obstacles, including CRS and "on-target, off-tumor" side effects (Zhang & Xu, 2017). These toxicities are especially important because no unique tumor antigens exist that can generate highly specific CAR T cells for treating solid tumors. The activation and effector functions of T cells are impaired by inhibitory molecular pathways, including cytotoxic T-lymphocyte antigen 4 and programmed cell death protein 1. In addition, there may be inefficient homing of the redirected T cells to tumor sites that can lower the therapeutic efficacy of this treatment for solid tumors (Han et al., 2017).

CAR T cells can cause side effects via several mechanisms, including damage to the targeted TAA, cross-reaction with a protein not expressed on tumor cells, allergic reactions, and TLS. The most prominent toxicity is CRS. CAR T cells can damage tissues that express the antigen recognized by CAR. For example, patients with renal cell cancer who received CAR T cells that targeted carbonic anhydrase 9 experienced grade 3 and 4 increases ALT, AST, and total bilirubin (Lamers et al., 2006). CRS is a common and potentially life-threatening toxicity that occurs because of T-cell activation and production of endogenous cytokines associated with CAR T-cell therapy. Activation of CAR T cells can lead to the production of several cytokines, such as IL-6, interferon gamma, and interferon alfa (Zhang & Xu, 2017).

The levels of several cytokines are markedly elevated in the serum of patients after receiving genetically engineered T cells. Following the infusion of CAR T cells, patients have cytokine levels several hundred times higher than at baseline. This typically causes a clinical syndrome, including fever and flu-like symptoms, tachycardia, arrhythmias, hypotension, decreased cardiac ejection fraction, pulmonary edema, hypoxia, dyspnea, pneumonitis, elevations in serum transaminases and bilirubin, diarrhea, colitis, nausea, abdominal pain, acute renal injury, cytopenia, infection, and elevated creatine kinase. This can also lead to multiorgan failure or death (Brudno & Kochenderfer, 2016; Shank et al., 2017).

CRS time of onset varies with the type of CAR T cells. The mechanism of these symptoms remains unknown. A grading system for CRS has been published by Lee et al. (2014). Monitoring patients at risk for severe CRS can include serial monitoring of CRP. Patients with a CRP level of greater than 20 mg/dl were noted to be at the highest risk for developing clinical complications secondary to severe CRS (Davila et al., 2014).

CRS toxicity can be controlled by reducing the dosage of active T cells; however, the number of T cells is difficult to control. Patients who develop CRS are often likely to respond to treatment. The severity of CRS may correlate with tumor burden. CRS can be controlled by cytokine-blocking agents such as corticosteroids; however, because immunosuppression could compromise antitumor efficacy, anticytokine therapy should be reserved for grade 3 or 4 CRS or for patients with grade 2 CRS who are older or have extensive comorbidities (Shank et al., 2017).

Tocilizumab (Actemra®) is a humanized mAb that blocks the IL-6 receptor and decreases production of proinflammatory mediators. It has been associated with rapid resolution of respiratory distress and hypotension in patients with severe CRS after CAR T-cell therapy. Tocilizumab is not thought to adversely affect the efficacy of CAR T-cell therapy (Shank et al., 2017). Clinical trials are underway to investigate the optimal timing of anti–IL-6 treatment.

CAR T-cell–related encephalopathy syndrome is the second most common toxicity associated with CAR T-cell therapy. It can occur in the presence of CRS or after CRS (Neelapu et al., 2018). Detectable levels of CD19 CAR T cells have been noted in the cerebrospinal fluid of treated patients, suggesting CAR T cells penetrate the CNS. Most neurologic symptoms occurred within eight weeks after the CAR T-cell infusion and included headache, encephalopathy, delirium, anxiety, tremor, disturbances in consciousness, disorientation, confusion, agitation, seizures, mutism, and aphasia.

Somnolence, confusion, encephalopathy, and dysphasia should be monitored in patients receiving CAR T-cell infusion to appropriately manage symptoms. Prophylactic antiepileptic therapy should be started in patients at risk of seizures. Systemic and intrathecal corticosteroids should be considered in patients with severe or life-threatening neurologic symptoms. The use of tocilizumab is controversial because it does not cross the blood–brain barrier (Shank et al., 2017).

Nearly all patients who receive CAR T-cell treatment will develop a fever, with 80%–100% developing grade 3 or higher (Brentjens et al., 2011; Grupp et al., 2013; Kochenderfer et al., 2015). Although fever and hypotension are symptoms noted with CRS, patients developing a fever should also be evaluated for infection. Empiric antibiotics may be administered until infection is ruled out (Shank et al., 2017). Nonsteroidal anti-inflammatory drugs (NSAIDs) inhibit interferon gamma and TNF-α, cytokines associated with T-cell activation. NSAIDs can cause renal dysfunction and inhibit platelets, which could confuse the presentation of other toxicities (Shank et al., 2017). Fever management should include the use of acetaminophen over NSAIDs.

On-target side effects are pharmacodynamic and occur when an inhibited target is on normal tissue and affected by a drug. Off-target side effects are the result of effects from other targets or the structure of the drug. B-cell aplasia is an on-target result of CD19-directed therapies. Normal B cells express CD19; therefore, B-cell depletion can occur, resulting in hypogammaglobulinemia following a CD19-targeted CAR T-cell infusion. This can persist for up to 13 months, and the patient will have an increased risk of infection. The presence of B-cell aplasia has been used as a surrogate to determine the persistence and effectiveness of CD19-directed CAR T cells. Exogenous Ig is usually needed for infection prophylaxis. In a patient with metastatic renal cell carcinoma, grade 2–4 liver enzyme alterations can occur after receiving modified CAR T cells against the carbonic anhydrase 9 antigen (Zhang & Xu, 2017). Patients with metastatic colorectal cancer who receive CAR T cells can develop severe colitis. CAR T-cell therapies can also cause TLS.

Neutropenia can occur even in patients who do not receive a conditioning regimen. GM-CSF prophylaxis may be initiated 24 hours after completion of a conditioning regimen and continued until neutrophil recovery. Prophylactic antimicrobial antibiotics may also be considered (Shank et al., 2017).

TLS has been reported in patients who have received CAR T-cell therapy. Patients should be assessed for the risk of TLS and considered for prophylactic IV hydration and antihyperuricemics such as allopurinol. Patients may experience signs of TLS despite prophylactic allopurinol initiated the day prior to infusion. These patients may require rasburicase. Frequent monitoring of creatinine, uric acid, potassium, phosphorus, and calcium should be initiated with a conditioning regimen in patients at risk for TLS (Shank et al., 2017).

Nausea and vomiting incidence depends on regimen used. Although antiemetic regimens frequently include corticosteroids, these should not be used because of the potential inhibition of CAR T cells. Once CAR T cells are infused, avoid antiemetics with sedating properties so mental status changes can be more clearly assessed (Shank et al., 2017).

Summary

Passive immunotherapy provides a useful method of targeting cancers. These agents are useful in patients with malignancies in which the immune system may not be intact. As more is discovered about the functioning of the immune system, the best mechanisms for various agents hopefully will be determined. From there, information about the best ways to use available immunotherapy agents can enable the best responses for patients with malignancy. Nurses hold an important role in the care of patients receiving these agents. They are key to safe drug administration, identification of potential side effects, and management of toxicities.

References

Alperovich, A., & Younes, A. (2016). Targeting CD30 using brentuximab vedotin in the treatment of Hodgkin lymphoma. *Cancer Journal, 22,* 23–26. https://doi.org/10.1097/PPO.0000000000000168

Amadori, S., Suciu, S., Selleslag, D., Aversa, F., Gaidano, G., Musso, M., … Baron, F. (2016). Gemtuzumab ozogamicin versus best supportive care in older patients with newly diagnosed acute myeloid leukemia unsuitable for intensive chemotherapy: Results of the randomized phase III EORTC-GIMEMA AML-19 trial. *Journal of Clinical Oncology, 34,* 972–979. https://doi.org/10.1200/JCO.2015.64.0060

American Medical Association. (n.d.). Monoclonal antibodies. Retrieved from https://www.ama-assn.org/about/monoclonal-antibodies

Amgen Inc. (2017a). *Prolia® (denosumab)* [Package insert]. Thousand Oaks, CA: Author.

Amgen Inc. (2017b). *Vectibix® (panitumumab)* [Package insert]. Thousand Oaks, CA: Author.

Amgen Inc. (2018). *Xgeva® (denosumab)* [Package insert]. Thousand Oaks, CA: Author.

Amiri-Kordestani, L., Blumenthal, G.M., Xu, Q.C., Zhang, L., Tang, S.W., Ha, L., … Cortazar, P. (2014). FDA approval: Ado-trastuzumab emtansine for the treatment of patients with HER2-positive metastatic breast cancer. *Clinical Cancer Research, 20,* 4436–4441. https://doi.org/10.1158/1078-0432.CCR-14-0012

Appelbaum, F.R., & Bernstein, I.D. (2017). Gemtuzumab ozogamicin for acute myeloid leukemia. *Blood, 130,* 2373–2376. https://doi.org/10.1182/blood-2017-09-797712

Armenian, S.H., Lacchetti, C., Barac, A., Carver, J., Constine, L., Denduluri, N., … Lenihan, D. (2017). Prevention and monitoring of cardiac dysfunction in survivors of adult cancers: American Society of Clinical Oncology Clinical Practice Guideline. *Journal of Clinical Oncology, 35,* 893–911. https://doi.org/10.1200/JCO.2016.70.5400

Aw, D.C., Tan, E.H., Chin, T.M., Lim, H.L., Lee, H.Y., & Soo, R.A. (2017). Management of epidermal growth factor receptor tyrosine kinase inhibitor-related cutaneous and gastrointestinal toxicities. *Asian Pacific Journal of Clinical Oncology, 14,* 23–31. https://doi .org/10.1111/ajco.12687

Baas, J.M., Krens, L.L., Guchelaar, H.-J., Ouwerkerk, J., de Jong, F.A., Lavrijsen, A.P.M., & Gelderblom, H. (2012). Recommendations on the management of EGFR inhibitor-induced skin toxicity: A systemic review. *Cancer Treatment Reviews, 38,* 505–514. https:// doi.org/10.1016/j.ctrv.2011.09.004

Baldo, B. (2013). Adverse events to monoclonal antibodies used for cancer therapy: Focus on hypersensitivity responses. *Oncoimmunology, 2,* e26333. https://doi.org/10.4161/onci .26333

Bang, Y.-J., Van Cutsem, E., Feyereislova, A., Chung, H.C., Shen, L., Sawaki, A., … Kang, Y.-K. (2010). Trastuzumab in combination with chemotherapy versus chemotherapy alone for treatment of HER2-positive advanced gastric or gastro-oesophageal junction cancer (ToGA): A phase 3, open-label, randomised controlled trial. *Lancet, 376,* 687–697. https:// doi.org/10.1016/S0140-6736(10)61121-X

Barroso-Sousa, R., Santana, I.A., Testa, L., de Melo Gagliato, D., & Mano, M. (2013). Biological therapies in breast cancer: Common toxicities and management strategies. *Breast, 22,* 1009–1018. https://doi.org/10.1016/j.breast.2013.09.009

Baselga, J., Cortés, J., Kim, S.-B., Im, S.-A., Hegg, R., Im, Y.-H., … Swain, S.M. (2012). Pertuzumab plus trastuzumab plus docetaxel for metastatic breast cancer. *New England Journal of Medicine, 366,* 109–119. https://doi.org/10.1056/NEJMoa1113216

Baselga, J., Gelmon, K.A., Verma, S., Wardley, A., Conte, P., Miles, D., … Gianni, L. (2010). Phase II trial of pertuzumab and trastuzumab in patients with human epidermal growth factor receptor 2-positive metastatic breast cancer that progressed during prior trastuzumab therapy. *Journal of Clinical Oncology, 28,* 1138–1144. https://doi.org/10.1200 /JCO.2009.24.2024

Bekker, P.J., Holloway, D.L., Rasmussen, A.S., Murphy, R., Martin, S.W., Leese, P.T., … DePaoli, A.M. (2005). A single-dose placebo-controlled study of AMG 162, a fully human monoclonal antibody to RANKL, in postmenopausal women. *Journal of Bone and Mineral Research, 20,* 2275–2282. https://doi.org/10.1359/jbmr.2005.20.12.2274

Bellizzi, A., Anzivino, E., Rodio, D.M., Palamara, A.T., Nencioni, L., & Pietropaolo, V. (2013). New insights on human polyomavirus JC and pathogenesis of progressive multifocal leukoencephalopathy. *Clinical Development in Immunology, 2013,* 839719. https://doi.org /10.1155/2013/839719

Body, J.-J., Bone, H.G., de Boer, R.H., Stopeck, A., Poznak, C.V., Damião, R., … Kostenuik, P.J. (2015). Hypocalcaemia in patients with metastatic bone disease treated with denosumab. *European Journal of Cancer, 51,* 1812–1821. https://doi.org/10.1016/j.ejca.2015.05.016

Bonamichi-Santos, R., & Castells, M. (2018). Diagnosis and management of drug hypersensitivity and anaphylaxis in cancer and chronic inflammatory diseases: Reactions to taxanes and monoclonal antibodies. *Clinical Reviews in Allergy and Immunology, 54,* 375–385. https://doi.org/10.1007/s12016-016-8556-5

Brennan, P.J., Bouza, T.R., Hsu, F.I., Sloane, D.E., & Castells, M.C. (2009). Hypersensitivity reactions to mAbs: 105 desensitizations in 23 patients, from evaluation to treatment. *Journal of Allergy and Clinical Immunology, 124,* 1259–1266. https://doi.org/10.1016/j.jaci.2009.09.009

Brentjens, R.J., Rivière, I., Park, J.H., Davila, M.L., Wang, X., Stefanski, J., … Sadelain, M. (2011). Safety and persistence of adoptively transferred autologous CD19-targeted T cells in patients with relapsed or chemotherapy refractory B-cell leukemias. *Blood, 18,* 4817–4828. https://doi.org/10.1182/blood-2011-04-348540

Bristol-Myers Squibb Co. (2012). *Erbitux® (cetuximab)* [Package insert]. Princeton, NJ: Author.

Bristol-Myers Squibb Co. (2017). *Empliciti™ (elotuzumab)* [Package insert]. Princeton, NJ: Author.

Brody, J., Kohrt, H., Marabelle, A., & Levy, R. (2011). Active and passive immunotherapy for lymphoma: Proving principles and improving results. *Journal of Clinical Oncology, 29,* 1864–1875. https://doi.org/10.1200/JCO.2010.33.4623

Brudno, J.N., & Kochenderfer, J.N. (2016). Toxicities of chimeric antigen receptor T cells: Recognition and management. *Blood, 127*, 3321–3330. https://doi.org/10.1182/blood -2016-04-703751

Burger, R.A., Sill, M.W., Monk, B.J., Greer, B.E., & Sorosky, J.I. (2007). Phase II trial of bevacizumab in persistent or recurrent epithelial ovarian cancer or primary peritoneal cancer: A Gynecologic Oncology Group Study. *Journal of Clinical Oncology, 25*, 5165–5171. https://doi.org/10.1200/JCO.2007.11.5345

Cairoli, R., Grillo, G., Tedeschi, A., D'Avanzo, G., Marenco, P., & Morra, E. (2004). High incidence of neutropenia in patients treated with rituximab after autologous stem cell transplantation. *Haematologica, 89*, 361–363.

Carlson, J., Cox, K., Bedwell, K., & Ku, M. (2015). Rituximab for subcutaneous delivery: Clinical management principles from a nursing perspective. *International Journal of Nursing Practice, 21*(Suppl. 3), 1–13. https://doi.org/10.1111/ijn.12413

Cartron, G., de Guibert, S., Dilhuydy, M.-S., Morschhauser, G., Leblond, V., Dupuis, J., ... Hallek, M. (2014). Obinutuzumab (GA-101) in relapsed/refractory chronic lymphocytic leukemia: Final data from the phase 1/2 GAUGUIN study. *Blood, 124*, 2196–2202. https:// doi.org/10.1182/blood-2014-07-586610

Castaigne, S., Paulas, C., Terré, C., Raffoux, E., Bordessoule, D., Bastie, J.-N., ... Dombret, H. (2012). Effect of gemtuzumab ozogamicin on survival of adult patients with de-novo acute myeloid leukaemia (ALFA-0701): A randomised, open-label, phase 3 study. *Lancet, 379*, 1508–1516. https://doi.org/10.1016/S0140-6736(12)60485-1

Castells Guitart, M.C. (2014). Rapid drug desensitization for hypersensitivity reactions to chemotherapy and monoclonal antibodies in the 21st century. *Journal of Investigational Allergology and Clinical Immunology, 24*, 72–79.

Chen, Z., & Ai, D. (2016). Cardiotoxicity associated with targeted cancer therapies (Review). *Molecular and Clinical Oncology, 4*, 675–681. https://doi.org/10.3892/mco.2016.800

Cohen, M.H., Shen, Y.L., Keegan, P., & Pazdur, R. (2009). FDA drug approval summary: Bevacizumab (Avastin®) as treatment of recurrent glioblastoma multiforme. *Oncologist, 14*, 1131–1138. https://doi.org/10.1634/theoncologist.2009-0121

Coiffier, B., Haioun, C., Ketterer, N., Engert, A., Tilly, H., Ma, D., ... Reyes, F. (1998). Rituximab (anti-CD20 monoclonal antibody) for the treatment of patients with relapsing or refractory aggressive lymphoma: A multicenter phase II study. *Blood, 92*, 1927–1932.

Coiffier, B., Lepretre, S., Pedersen, L.M., Gadeberg, O., Fredriksen, H., van Oers, M.H.J., ... Robak, T. (2008). Safety and efficacy ofatumumab, a fully human monoclonal anti-CD20 antibody, in patients with relapsed or refractory B-cell chronic lymphocytic leukemia: A phase 1-2 study. *Blood, 111*, 1094–1100. https://doi.org/10.1182/blood-2007-09-111781

Coiffier, B., Thieblemont, C., Van Den Neste, E., Lepeu, G., Plantier, I., Castaigne, S., ... Tilly, H. (2010). Long-term outcome of patients in the LNH-98.5 trial, the first randomized study comparing rituximab-CHOP to standard CHOP chemotherapy in DLBCL patients: A study by the Groupe d'Etudes des Lymphomes de l'Adulte. *Blood, 116*, 2040–2045. https://doi.org/10.1182/blood-2010-03-276246

Cortelezzi, A., Sciumè, M., Liberati, A.M., Vincenti, D., Cuneo, A., Reda, G., ... Foà, R. (2014). Bendamustine in combination with ofatumumab in relapsed or refractory chronic lymphocytic leukemia: A GIMEMA multicenter phase II trial. *Leukemia, 28*, 642–648. https://doi.org/10.1038/leu.2013.334

Costa, L.J., Fanning, S.R., Stephenson, J., Jr., Afrin, L.B., Kistner-Griffin, E., Bentz, T.A., & Stuart, R.K. (2015). Sequential ofatumumab and lenalidomide for the treatment of relapsed and refractory chronic lymphocytic leukemia and small lymphocytic lymphoma. *Leukemia and Lymphoma, 56*, 645–649. https://doi.org/10.3109/10428194.2014 .935369

Davidson, M., Smyth, E., & Cunningham, D. (2016). Clinical role of ramucirumab alone or in combination with paclitaxel for gastric and gastro-esophageal junction adenocarcinoma. *OncoTargets and Therapy, 6*, 4539–4548. https://doi.org/10.2147/OTT.S84153

Davila, M.L., Rivière, I., Wang, X., Bartido, S., Park, J., Curran, K., ... Brentjens, S. (2014). Efficacy and toxicity management of 19–28z CAR T cell therapy in B cell acute lymphoblastic leukemia. *Science Translational Medicine, 224,* 224ra25. https://doi.org/10.1126/scitranslmed.3008226

Dawson, K., Moran, M., Guindon, K., & Wan, H. (2016). Managing infusion-related reactions for patients with chronic lymphocytic leukemia receiving obinutuzumab [Online exclusive]. *Clinical Journal of Oncology Nursing, 20,* E41–E48. https://doi.org/10.1188/16.CJON.E41-E48

Day, A., Abramson, A.K., Patel, M., Warren, R.B., & Menter, M.A. (2014). The spectrum of oculocutaneous disease. Part II. Neoplastic and drug-related causes of oculocutaneous disease. *Journal of the American Academy of Dermatology, 70,* 821.e1–821.e19. https://doi.org/10.1016/j.jaad.2013.12.019

de Claro, R.A., McGinn, K., Kwitkowski, V., Bullock, J., Khandelwal, A., Habtemariam, B., ... Pazdur, R. (2012). U.S. Food and Drug Administration approval summary: Brentuximab vedotin for the treatment of relapsed Hodgkin lymphoma or relapsed systemic anaplastic large-cell lymphoma. *Clinical Cancer Research, 18,* 5845–5849. https://doi.org/10.1158/1078-0432.CCR-12-1803

Doubek, M., Brychtova, Y., Panovska, A., Sebejova, L., Stehlikova, O., Chovancova, J., ... Mayer, J. (2015). Ofatumumab added to dexamethasone in patients with relapsed or refractory chronic lymphocytic leukemia: Results from a phase II study. *American Journal of Hematology, 90,* 417–421. https://doi.org/10.1002/ajh.23964

Douillard, J.-Y., Siena, S., Cassidy, J., Tabernero, J., Burkes, R., Barugel, M., ... Gansert, J. (2010). Randomized, phase III trial of panitumumab with infusional fluorouracil, leucovorin, and oxaliplatin (FOLFOX4) versus FOLFOX4 alone as first-line treatment in patients with previously untreated metastatic colorectal cancer: The PRIME study. *Journal of Clinical Oncology, 28,* 4697–4705. https://doi.org/10.1200/JCO.2009.27.4860

Du, F., Yuan, P., Zhu, W., Wang, J., Ma, F., Fan, Y., & Xu, B. (2014). Is it safe to give anthracyclines concurrently with trastuzumab in neo-adjuvant or metastatic settings for HER2-positive breast cancer? A meta-analysis of randomized controlled trials. *Medical Oncology, 31,* 340. https://doi.org/10.1007/s12032-014-0340-x

Dunleavy, K., Hakim, F., Kim, H.K., Janik, J.E., Grant, N., Nakayama, T., ... Wilson, W.H. (2005). B-cell recovery following rituximab-based therapy is associated with perturbations in stromal derived factor-1 and granulocyte homeostasis. *Blood, 106,* 795–802. https://doi.org/10.1182/blood-2004-08-3198

Dy, G.K., & Adjei, A.A. (2013). Understanding, recognizing, and managing toxicities of targeted anticancer therapies. *CA: A Cancer Journal for Clinicians, 63,* 249–279. https://doi.org/10.3322/caac.21184

Eilers, R.E., Jr., Gandhi, M., Patel, J.D., Mulcahy, M.F., Agulnik, M., Hensing, T., & Lacouture, M.E. (2010). Dermatologic infections in cancer patients treated with epidermal growth factor receptor inhibitor therapy. *Journal of the National Cancer Institute, 102,* 47–53. https://doi.org/10.1093/jnci/djp439

Eli Lilly and Co. (2017a). *Cyramza® (ramucirumab)* [Package insert]. Indianapolis, IN: Author.

Eli Lilly and Co. (2017b). *Lartruvo® (olaratumab)* [Package insert]. Indianapolis, IN: Author.

Enokida, T., Suzuki, S., Wakasugi, T., Yamazaki, T., Okano, S., & Tahara, M. (2016). Incidence and risk factors of hypomagnesemia in head and neck cancer patients treated with cetuximab. *Frontiers in Oncology, 6,* 1–6. https://doi.org/10.3389/fonc.2016.00196

Ergin, A.B., Fong, N., & Daw, H.A. (2012). Rituximab-induced bronchiolitis obliterans organizing pneumonia. *Case Reports in Medicine, 2012,* 680431. https://doi.org/10.1155/2012/680431

Ewer, M.S., & Ewer, S.M. (2016). Trastuzumab cardiotoxicity: The age-old balance of risk and benefit. *British Journal of Cancer, 115,* 1441–1442. https://doi.org/10.1038/bjc.2016.381

Fisher, R.I., Kaminski, M.S., Wahl, R.L., Knox, S.J., Zelenetz, A.D., Vose, J.M., ... Coleman, M. (2005). Tositumomab and iodine-131 tositumomab produces durable complete remissions in a subset of heavily pretreated patients with low-grade and transformed non-Hodgkin's lymphomas. *Journal of Clinical Oncology, 23,* 7565–7573. https://doi.org/10.1200/JCO.2004.00.9217

Folan, S.A., Rexwinkle, A., Autry, J., & Bryan, J.C. (2016). Blinatumomab: Bridging the gap in adult relapsed/refractory B-cell acute lymphoblastic leukemia. *Clinical Lymphoma, Myeloma and Leukemia, 16*(Suppl.), S2–S5. https://doi.org/10.1016/j.clml.2016.02.001

Foldi, J., Mougalian, S., Silber, A., Lannin, D., Killelea, B., Chagpar, A., ... Pusztai, L. (2018). Single-arm, neoadjuvant, phase II trial of pertuzumab and trastuzumab administered concomitantly with weekly paclitaxel followed by 5-fluorouracil, epirubicin, and cyclophosphamide (FEC) for stage I-III HER2-positive breast cancer. *Breast Cancer Research and Treatment, 169,* 333–340. https://doi.org/10.1007/s10549-017-4653-2

Fountzilas, G., Razis, E., Tsavdaridis, D., Karina, M., Labropoulos, S., Christodoulou, C., ... Skarlos, D. (2003). Continuation of trastuzumab beyond disease progression is feasible and safe in patients with metastatic breast cancer: A retrospective analysis of 80 cases by the Hellenic Cooperative Oncology Group. *Clinical Breast Cancer, 4,* 120–125. https://doi.org/10.3816/CBC.2003.n.017

Fuchs, C.S., Tomasek, J., Yong, C.J., Dumitru, F., Passalacqua, R., Goswan, C., ... Tabernero, J. (2014). Ramucirumab monotherapy for previously treated advanced gastric or gastro-oesophageal junction adenocarcinoma (REGARD): An international, randomised, multicentre, placebo-controlled, phase 3 trial. *Lancet, 383,* 31–39. https://doi.org/10.1016/S0140-6736(13)61719-5

Galluzzi, L., Vacchelli, E., Bravo-San Pedro, J.-M., Buqué, A., Senovilla, L., Baracco, E., ... Kroemer, G. (2014). Classification of current anticancer immunotherapies. *Oncotarget, 5,* 12472–12508. https://doi.org/10.18632/oncotarget.2998

Garnock-Jones, K.P., Keating, G.M., & Scott, L.J. (2010). Spotlight on trastuzumab as adjuvant treatment in human epidermal growth factor receptor 2 (HER2)-positive early breast cancer. *BioDrugs, 24,* 207–209. https://doi.org/10.2165/11204680-000000000-00000

Gelmon, K.A., Mackey, J., Verma, S., Gertler, S.Z., Bangemann, N., Klimo, P., ... Dias, R. (2004). Use of trastuzumab beyond disease progression: Observations from a retrospective review of case histories. *Clinical Breast Cancer, 5,* 52–58. https://doi.org/10.3816/CBC.2004.n.010

Gemzyme Corp. (2017). *Lemtrada® (alemtuzumab)* [Package insert]. Cambridge, MA: Author.

Genentech, Inc. (2016a). *Kadcyla® (ado-trastuzumab emtansine)* [Package insert]. South San Francisco, CA: Author.

Genentech, Inc. (2016b). *Rituxan® (rituximab)* [Package insert]. South San Francisco, CA: Author.

Genentech, Inc. (2017a). *Avastin® (bevacizumab)* [Package insert]. South San Francisco, CA: Author.

Genentech, Inc. (2017b). *Gazyva® (obinutuzumab)* [Package insert]. South San Francisco, CA: Author.

Genentech, Inc. (2017c). *Herceptin® (trastuzumab)* [Package insert]. South San Francisco, CA: Author.

Genentech, Inc. (2017d). *Perjeta® (pertuzumab)* [Package insert]. South San Francisco, CA: Author.

Genentech, Inc. (2017e). *Rituxan Hycela® (rituximab and hyaluronidase human)* [Package insert]. South San Francisco, CA: Author.

George, B.A., Zhou, X.J., & Toto, R. (2007). Nephrotic syndrome after bevacizumab: Case report and literature review. *American Journal of Kidney Disease, 49,* e23–e29.

Gianni, L., Pienkowski, T., Im, Y.-K., Roman, L., Tseng, L.-M., Liu, M.-C., ... Valagussa, P. (2012). Efficacy and safety of neoadjuvant pertuzumab and trastuzumab in women with locally advanced, inflammatory, or early HER2-positive breast cancer (NeoSphere): A randomised multicentre, open-label phase 2 trial. *Lancet Oncology, 13,* 25–32. https://doi.org/10.1016/S1470-2045(11)70336-9

Giantonio, B.J., Catalano, P.J., Meropol, N.J., O'Dwyer, P.J., Mitchell, E.P., Alberts, S.R., ... Benson, A.B., III. (2007). Bevacizumab in combination with oxaliplatin, fluorouracil, and leucovorin (FOLFOX4) for previously treated metastatic colorectal cancer: Results from the Eastern Cooperative Oncology Group Study E3200. *Journal of Clinical Oncology, 25,* 1539–1544. https://doi.org/10.1200/JCO.2006.09.6305

Goede, V., Fischer, K., Engelke, A., Schlag, R., Lepretre, S., Montero, L.F.C., ... Hallek, M. (2015). Obinutuzumab as frontline treatment of chronic lymphocytic leukemia: Updated results of the CLL11 study. *Leukemia, 29*, 1602–1604. https://doi.org/10.1038/leu.2015.14

Gradishar, W.J. (2013). Emerging approaches for treating HER2-positive metastatic breast cancer beyond trastuzumab. *Annals of Oncology, 24*, 2492–2500. https://doi.org/10.1093/annonc/mdt217

Grupp, S.A., Kalos, M., Barrett, D., Aplenc, R., Porter, D.L., Rheingold, S.R., ... June, C.H. (2013). Chimeric antigen receptor–modified T cells for acute lymphoid leukemia. *New England Journal of Medicine, 368*, 1509–1518. https://doi.org/10.1056/NEJMoa1215134

Hadid, T., Raufi, A., Kafri, Z., Mandziara, M., Kalabat, J., Szpunar, S., ... Al-Katib, A. (2016). Safety and efficacy of radioimmunotherapy (RIT) in treatment of non-Hodgkin's lymphoma in the community setting. *Nuclear Medicine and Biology, 43*, 227–231. https://doi.org/10.1016/j.nucmedbio.2015.12.004

Hamo, C.E., Bloom, M.W., Cardinale, D., Ky, B., Nohria, A., Baer, L., ... Butler, J. (2016). Cancer therapy–Related cardiac dysfunction and heart failure. Part 2: Prevention, treatment, guidelines, and future directions. *Circulation: Heart Failure, 9*, e002843. https://doi.org/10.1161/CIRCHEARTFAILURE.115.002843

Han, S., Latchoumanin, O., Wu, G., Zhou, G., Hebbard, L., George, J., & Qiao, L. (2017). Recent clinical trials utilizing chimeric antigen receptor T cells therapies against solid tumors. *Cancer Letters, 390*, 188–200. http://doi.org/10.1016/j.canlet.2016.12.037

Hapani, S., Chu, D., & Wu, S. (2009). Risk of gastrointestinal perforation in patients with cancer treated with bevacizumab: A meta-analysis. *Lancet Oncology, 10*, 559–568. https://doi.org/10.1016/S1470-2045(09)70112-3

Hassan, R., Alewine, C., & Pastan, I. (2016). New life for immunotoxin cancer therapy. *Clinical Cancer Research, 22*, 1055–1058. https://doi.org/10.1158/1078-0432.CCR-15-1623

Hills, R.K., Castaigne, S., Appelbaum, F.R., Delaunay, J., Petersdorf, S., Othus, M., ... Burnett, A.K. (2014). Addition of gemtuzumab ozogamicin to induction chemotherapy in adult patients with acute myeloid leukaemia: A meta-analysis of individual patient data from randomised controlled trials. *Lancet Oncology, 15*, 986–996. https://doi.org/10.1016/S1470-2045(14)70281-5

Holubec, L., Polivka, J., Jr., Safanda, M., Karas, M., & Liska, V. (2016). The role of cetuximab in the induction of anticancer immune response in colorectal cancer treatment. *Anticancer Research, 36*, 4421–4426. https://doi.org/10.21873/anticanres.10985

Hu, M.I., Glezerman, I.G., Leboulleux, S., Insogna, K., Gucalp, R., Misiorowski, W., ... Jain R.K. (2014). Denosumab for treatment of hypercalcemia of malignancy. *Journal of Clinical Endocrinology and Metabolism, 99*, 3144–3152. https://doi.org/10.1210/jc.2014-1001

Hurwitz, H., Fehrenbacher, L., Novotny, W., Cartwright, T., Hainsworth, J., Heim, W., ... Kabbinavar, F. (2004). Bevacizumab plus irinotecan, fluorouracil, and leucovorin for metastatic colorectal cancer. *New England Journal of Medicine, 350*, 2335–2342. https://doi.org/10.1056/NEJMoa032691

Huynh, A.L.H., Baker, S.T., Stewardson, A.J., & Johnson, D.F. (2016). Denosumab-associated hypocalcaemia: Incidence, severity and patient characteristics in a tertiary hospital setting. *Pharmacoepidemiology and Drug Safety, 25*, 1274–1278. https://doi.org/10.1002/pds.4045

Ishizuna, K., Ninomiya, J., Ogawa, T., & Tsuji, E. (2014). Hepatotoxicity induced by trastuzumab used for breast cancer adjuvant therapy: A case report. *Journal of Medical Case Reports, 8*, 417. https://doi.org/10.1186/1752-1947-8-417

Janssen Biotech, Inc. (2014). *Sylvant® (siltuximab)* [Package insert]. Horsham, PA: Author.

Janssen Biotech, Inc. (2017). *Darzalex® (daratumumab)* [Package insert]. Horsham, PA: Author.

Jatoi, A., Rowland, K., Sloan, J.A., Gross, H.M., Fishkin, P.A., Kahanic, S.P., ... Loprinzi, C.L. (2008). Tetracycline to prevent epidermal growth factor receptor inhibitor-induced skin rashes: Results of a placebo-controlled trial from the North Central Cancer Treatment Group (N03CB). *Cancer, 113*, 847–853. https://doi.org/10.1002/cncr.23621

Jawa, Z., Perez, R.M., Garlie, L., Singh, M., Qamar, R., Khandheria, B.K., ... Shi, Y. (2016). Risk factors of trastuzumab-induced cardiotoxicity in breast cancer: A meta-analysis. *Medicine, 95*, e5195. https://doi.org/10.1097/MD.0000000000005195

Jiang, L., Yuan, C.M., Hubacheck, J., Janik, J.E., Wilson, W., Morris, J.C., … Stetler-Stevenson, M. (2009). Variable CD52 expression in mature T cell and NK cell malignancies: Implications for alemtuzumab therapy. *British Journal of Haematology, 145,* 173–179. https://doi .org/10.1111/j.1365-2141.2009.07606.x

Jung, S.-H., Lee, H.-J., Vo, M.-C., Kim, H.-J., & Lee, J.-J. (2017). Immunotherapy for the treatment of multiple myeloma. *Critical Reviews in Oncology/Hematology, 111,* 87–93. https:// doi.org/10.1016/j.critrevonc.2017.01.011

Kantarjian, H.M., DeAngelo, D.J., Stelljes, M., Martinelli, G., Liedtke, M., Stock, W., … Advani, A.S. (2016). Inotuzumab ozogamicin versus standard therapy for acute lymphoblastic leukemia. *New England Journal of Medicine, 375,* 740–753. https://doi.org/10.1056 /NEJMoa1509277

Karmacharya, P., Poudel, D.R., Pathak, R., Donato, A.A., Ghimire, S., Giri, S., … Bingham, C.O., III. (2015). Rituximab-induced serum sickness: A systematic review. *Seminars in Arthritis and Rheumatism, 45,* 334–340. https://doi.org/10.1016/j.semarthrit.2015.06.014

Katz, J., Janik, J.E., & Younes, A. (2011). Brentuximab vedotin (SGN-35). *Clinical Cancer Research, 17,* 6428–6436. https://doi.org/10.1158/1078-0432.CCR-11-0488

Keating, M.J., Flinn, I., Jain, V., Binet, J.-L., Hillmen, P., Byrd, J., … Rai, K.R. (2002). Therapeutic role of alemtuzumab (Campath-1H) in patients who have failed fludarabine: Results of a large international study. *Blood, 99,* 3554–3561. https://doi.org/10.1182 /blood.V99.10.3554

Klinger, M., Brandl, C., Zugmaier, G., Hijazi, Y., Bargou, R., Topp, M.S., … Kufer, P. (2012). Immunopharmacologic response of patients with B-lineage acute lymphoblastic leukemia to continuous infusion of T cell-engaging CD19/CD3-bispecific BiTE antibody blinatumomab. *Blood, 119,* 6226–6233. https://doi.org/10.1182/blood-2012-01-400515

Kochenderfer, J.N., Dudley, M.E., Kassim, S.H., Somerville, R.P.T., Carpenter, R.O., Stetler-Stevenson, M., … Rosenberg, S.A. (2015). Chemotherapy-refractory diffuse large B-cell lymphoma and indolent B-cell malignancies can be effectively treated with autologous T cells expressing an anti-CD19 chimeric antigen receptor. *Journal of Clinical Oncology, 33,* 540–549. https://doi.org/10.1200/JCO.2014.56.2025

Kraeber-Bodéré, F., Bodet-Milin, C., Rousseau, C., Eugène, T., Pallardy, A., Frampas, E., … Chérel, M. (2014). Radioimmunoconjugates for the treatment of cancer. *Seminars in Oncology, 41,* 613–622. https://doi.org/10.1053/j.seminoncol.2014.07.004

Krejcik, J., Casneuf, T., Nijhof, I.S., Verbist, B., Bald, J., Plesner, T., … Sasser, A.K. (2016). Daratumumab depletes CD38+ immune regulatory cells, promotes T-cell expansion, and skews T-cell repertoire in multiple myeloma. *Blood, 128,* 384–394. https://doi.org/10 .1182/blood-2015-12-687749

Krop, I.E., Kim, S.-B., González-Martín, A., LoRusso, P.M., Ferrero, J.-M., Smitt, M., … Wildiers, H. (2014). Trastuzumab emtansine versus treatment of physician's choice for pretreated HER2-positive advanced breast cancer (TH3RESA): A randomized, open-label, phase 3 trial. *Lancet Oncology, 15,* 689–699. https://doi.org/10.1016/S1470-2045(14) 70178-0

Kulkarni, H.S., & Kasi, P.M. (2012). Rituximab and cytokine release syndrome. *Case Reports in Oncology, 5,* 134–140. https://doi.org/10.1159/000337577

Kyllo, R.L., & Anadkat, M.J. (2014). Dermatologic adverse events to chemotherapeutic agents, part 1: Cytotoxics, epidermal growth factor receptors, multikinase inhibitors, and proteasome inhibitors. *Seminars in Cutaneous Medicine and Surgery, 33,* 28–39. https://doi .org/10.12788/j.sder.0060

Lacouture, M.E., Mitchell, E.P., Piperdi, B., Pillai, M.V., Shearer, H., Iannotti, N., … Yassine, M. (2010). Skin toxicity evaluation protocol with panitumumab (STEPP), a phase II, open-label, randomized trial evaluating the impact of a pre-emptive skin treatment regimen on skin toxicities and quality of life in patients with metastatic colorectal cancer. *Journal of Clinical Oncology, 28,* 1351–1357. https://doi.org/10.1200/JCO.2008.21.7828

Lambert, J.M., & Chari, R.V.J. (2014). Ado-trastuzumab emtansine (T-DM1): An antibody–drug conjugate (ADC) for HER2-positive breast cancer. *Journal of Medicinal Chemistry, 57,* 6949–6964. https://doi.org/10.1021/jm500766w

Lamers, C.H.J., Sleijfer, S., Vulto, A.G., Kruit, W.H.J., Kliffen, M., Debets, R., ... Oosterwijk, E. (2006). Treatment of metastatic renal cell carcinoma with autologous T-lymphocytes genetically retargeted against carbonic anhydrase IX: First clinical experience [Abstract]. *Journal of Clinical Oncology, 24*, e20–e22. https://doi.org/10.1200/JCO.2006.05.9964

Laurenti, L., Innocenti, I., Autore, F., Sica, S., & Efremov, D. (2016). New developments in the management of chronic lymphocytic leukemia: Role of ofatumumab. *Oncotargets and Therapy, 8*, 421–429. https://doi.org/10.2147/OTT.S72845

Lee, C.S., Alwan, L.M., Sun, X., McLean, K.A., & Urban, R.R. (2016). Routine proteinuria monitoring for bevacizumab in patients with gynecologic malignancies. *Journal of Oncology Pharmacy Practice, 22*, 771–776. https://doi.org/10.1177/1078155215609987

Lee, D.W., Gardner, R., Porter, D.L., Louis, C.U., Ahmed, N., Jensen, M., ... Mackall, C.L. (2014). Current concepts in the diagnosis and management of cytokine release syndrome. *Blood, 124*, 188–195. https://doi.org/10.1182/blood-2014-05-552729

Liu, A.Y., Robinson, R.R., Murray, E.D., Jr., Ledbetter, J.A., Hellström, I., & Hellström, K.E. (1987). Production of a mouse-human chimeric monoclonal antibody to CD20 with potent Fc-dependent biologic activity. *Journal of Immunology, 15*, 3521–3526.

Lokhorst, H.M., Plesner, T., Laubach, J.P., Nahi, H., Gimsing, P., Hansson, M., ... Richardson, P.G. (2015). Targeting CD38 with daratumumab monotherapy in multiple myeloma. *New England Journal of Medicine, 373*, 1207–1219. https://doi.org/10.1056/NEJMoa1506348

Lonial, S., Dimopoulos, M., Palumbo, A., White, D., Grosicki, S., Spicka, I., ... Richardson, P. (2015). Elotuzumab therapy for relapsed or refractory multiple myeloma. *New England Journal of Medicine, 373*, 621–631. https://doi.org/10.1056/NEJMoa1505654

Lonial, S., Weiss, B.M., Usmani, S.Z., Singhal, S., Chari, A., Bahlis, N.J., ... Voorhees, P.M. (2016). Daratumumab monotherapy in patients with treatment–refractory multiple myeloma (SIRIUS): An open-label, randomised, phase 2 trial. *Lancet, 387*, 1551–1560. https://doi.org/10.1016/S0140-6736(15)01120-4

MacDonald, D., Crosbie, T., Christofides, A., Assaily, W., & Wiernikowski, J. (2017). A Canadian perspective on the subcutaneous administration of rituximab in non-Hodgkin lymphoma. *Current Oncology, 24*, 33–39. https://doi.org/10.3747/co.24.3470

Mahipal, A., & Grothey, A. (2016). Role of biologics in first-line treatment of colorectal cancer. *Journal of Oncology Practice, 12*, 1219–1228. https://doi.org/10.1200/JOP.2016.018382

Maloney, D.G., Liles, T.M., Czerwinski, D.K., Waldichuk, C., Rosenberg, J., Grillo-Lopez, A., & Levy, R. (1994). Phase I clinical trial using escalating single-dose infusion of chimeric anti-CD20 monoclonal antibody (IDEC-C2B8) in patients with recurrent B-cell lymphoma. *Blood, 84*, 2457–2466.

Maughan, T.S., Adams, R.A., Smith, C.G., Meade, A.M., Seymour, M.T., Wilson, R.H., ... Cheadle, J.P. (2011). Addition of cetuximab to oxaliplatin-based first-line combination chemotherapy for treatment of advanced colorectal cancer: Results of randomised phase 3 MRC COIN trial. *Lancet, 377*, 2103–2114. https://doi.org/10.1016/S0140-6736(11) 60613-2

Maximiano, S., Magalhães, P., Guerreiro, M.P., & Morgado, M. (2016). Trastuzumab in the treatment of breast cancer. *BioDrugs, 30*, 75–86. https://doi.org/10.1007/s40259-016 -0162-9

McLaughlin, P., Grillo-López, A.J., Link, B.K., Levy, R., Czuczman, M.S., Williams, M.E., ... Dallaire, B.K. (1998). Rituximab chimeric anti-CD20 monoclonal antibody therapy of relapsed indolent lymphoma: Half of patients respond to a four-dose treatment program. *Journal of Clinical Oncology, 16*, 2825–2833. https://doi.org/10.1200/JCO.1998.16.8.2825

Melichar, B., Procházková-Studentová, H., & Vitásková, D. (2012). Bevacizumab in combination with IFN-α in metastatic renal cell carcinoma: The AVOREN trial. *Expert Review of Anticancer Therapy, 12*, 1253–1262. https://doi.org/10.1586/era.12.103

Moreno, C., Montillo, M., Panayiotidis, P., Dimou, M., Bloor, A., Dupuis, J., ... Montserrat, E. (2015). Ofatumumab in poor-prognosis chronic lymphocytic leukemia: A phase IV, non-interventional, observational study from the European Research Initiative on Chronic Lymphocytic Leukemia. *Haematologica, 100*, 511–516. https://doi.org/10.3324 /haematol.2014.118158

Morschhauser, F., Illidge, T., Huglo, D., Martinelli, G., Paganelli, G., Zinzani, P.L., … Marcus, R. (2007). Efficacy and safety of yttrium-90 ibritumomab tiuxetan in patients with relapsed or refractory diffuse large B-cell lymphoma not appropriate for autologous stem-cell transplantation. *Blood, 110,* 54–58. https://doi.org/10.1182/blood-2007-01-068056

Morschhauser, F., Radford, J., Van Hoof, A., Vitolo, U., Soubeyran, P., Tilly, H., … Hagenbeek, A. (2008). Phase III trial of consolidation therapy with yttrium-90-ibritumomab tiuxetan compared with no additional therapy after first remission in advanced follicular lymphoma. *Journal of Clinical Oncology, 26,* 5156–5164. https://doi.org/10.1200/JCO.2008.17.2015

Moya-Horno, I., & Cortés, J. (2015). The expanding role of pertuzumab in the treatment of HER2-positive breast cancer. *Breast Cancer: Targets and Therapy, 7,* 125–132. https://doi.org/10.2147/BCTT.S61579

Nagorsen, D., Kufer, P., Baeuerle, P.A., & Bargou, R. (2012). Blinatumomab: A historical perspective. *Pharmacology and Therapeutics, 136,* 334–342. https://doi.org/10.1016/j.pharmthera.2012.07.013

Nair, R., Gheith, S., & Lamparella, N. (2016). Rituximab-induced splenic rupture and cytokine release. *American Journal of Case Reports, 17,* 165–169. https://doi.org/10.12659/AJCR.896671

Nalluri, S.R., Chu, D., Keresztes, R., Zhu, X., & Wu, S. (2008). Risk of venous thromboembolism with the angiogenesis inhibitor bevacizumab in cancer patients: A meta-analysis. *JAMA, 300,* 2277–2285. https://doi.org/10.1001/jama.2008.656

National Comprehensive Cancer Network. (2017). *NCCN Clinical Practice Guidelines in Oncology (NCCN Guidelines®): Colon cancer* [v.1.2017]. Retrieved from https://www.nccn.org/patients/guidelines/colon/files/assets/common/downloads/files/colon.pdf

National Comprehensive Cancer Network. (2018). *NCCN Clinical Practice Guidelines in Oncology (NCCN Guidelines®): Breast cancer* [v.4.2017]. Retrieved from https://www.nccn.org/professionals/physician_gls/pdf/breast.pdf

Neelapu, S.S., Tummala, S., Kebriaei, P., Wierda, W., Gutierrez, C., Locke, F.L., … Shpall, E.J. (2018). Chimeric antigen receptor T-cell therapy—Assessment and management of toxicities. *Nature Reviews Clinical Oncology, 15,* 47–62. https://doi.org/10.1038/nrclinonc.2017.148

Novartis Pharmaceuticals Corp. (2016). *Arzerra® (ofatumumab)* [Package insert]. East Hanover, NJ: Author.

Novartis Pharmaceuticals Corp. (2017). *Kymriah® (tisagenlecleucel)* [Package insert]. East Hanover, NJ: Author.

O'Brien, S.M., Kantarjian, H., Thomas, D.A., Giles, F.J., Freireich, E.J., Cortes, J., … Keating, M.J. (2001). Rituximab dose-escalation trial in chronic lymphocytic leukemia. *Journal of Clinical Oncology, 19,* 2165–2170. https://doi.org/10.1200/JCO.2001.19.8.2165

Ohtsu, A., Shah, M.A., Van Cutsem, E., Rha, S.Y., Sawaki, A., Park, S.R., … Kang, Y.-K. (2011). Bevacizumab in combination with chemotherapy as first-line therapy in advanced gastric cancer: A randomized, double-blind, placebo-controlled phase III study. *Journal of Clinical Oncology, 29,* 3968–3976. https://doi.org/10.1200/JCO.2011.36.2236

Olsen, M., LeFebvre, K.B., & Brassil, K.J. (Eds.). (in press). *Chemotherapy and immunotherapy guidelines and recommendations for practice.* Pittsburgh, PA: Oncology Nursing Society.

Overdijk, M.B., Verploegen, S., Bögels, M., van Egmond, M., Lammerts van Bueren, J.J., Mutis, T., … Parren, P.W.H.I. (2015). Antibody-mediated phagocytosis contributes to the anti-tumor activity of the therapeutic antibody daratumumab in lymphoma and multiple myeloma. *Mabs, 7,* 311–320. https://doi.org/10.1080/19420862.2015.1007813

Palumbo, A., Chanan-Khan, A., Weisel, K., Nooka, A.K., Masszi, T., Beksac, M., … Sonneveld, P. (2016). Daratumumab, bortezomib, and dexamethasone for multiple myeloma. *New England Journal of Medicine, 375,* 754–766. https://doi.org/10.1056/NEJMoa1606038

Pavanello, F., Zucca, E., & Ghielmini, M. (2017). Rituximab: 13 open questions after 20 years of clinical use. *Cancer Treatment Reviews, 53,* 38–46. https://doi.org/10.1016/j.ctrv.2016.11.015

Perez, E.A., Romond, E.H., Suman, V.J., Jeong, J.-H., Davidson, N.E., Geyer, C.E., Jr., … Wolmark, N. (2011). Four-year follow-up of trastuzumab plus adjuvant chemotherapy for operable human epidermal growth factor receptor 2-positive breast cancer: Joint analysis of data from NCCTG N9831 and NSABP B-31. *Journal of Clinical Oncology, 29*, 3366–3373. https://doi.org/10.1200/JCO.2011.35.0868

Perez, E.A., Romond, E.H., Suman, V.J., Jeong, J.-H., Sledge, G., Geyer, C.E., Jr., … Wolmark, N. (2014). Trastuzumab plus adjuvant chemotherapy for human epidermal growth factor receptor 2-positive breast cancer: Planned joint analysis of overall survival from NSABP B-31 and NCCTG N9831. *Journal of Clinical Oncology, 32*, 3744–3752. https://doi.org/10.1200/JCO.2014.55.5730

Perica, K., Varela, J.C., Oelke, M., & Schneck, J. (2015). Adoptive T cell immunotherapy for cancer [Abstract]. *Rambam Maimonides Medical Journal, 6*, e0004. https://doi.org/10.5041/RMMJ.10179

Petrelli, F., & Barni, S. (2012). Meta-analysis of concomitant compared to sequential adjuvant trastuzumab in breast cancer: The sooner the better. *Medical Oncology, 29*, 503–510. https://doi.org/10.1007/s12032-011-9897-9

Peuvrel, L., & Dréno, B. (2014). Dermatological toxicity associated with targeted therapies in cancer: Optimal management. *American Journal of Clinical Dermatology, 15*, 425–444. https://doi.org/10.1007/s40257-014-0088-2

Picard, M., & Galvão, V.R. (2017). Current knowledge and management of hypersensitivity reactions to monoclonal antibodies. *Journal of Allergy and Clinical Immunology: In Practice, 5*, 600–609. https://doi.org/10.1016/j.jaip.2016.12.001

Plana, J.C., Galderisi, M., Barac, A., Ewer, M.S., Ky, B., Scherrer-Crosbie, M., … Lancellotti, P. (2014). Expert consensus for multimodality imaging evaluation of adult patients during and after cancer therapy: A report of the American Society of Echocardiography and the European Association of Cardiovascular Imaging. European Heart Journal of Cardiovascular Imaging. *Journal of the American Society of Echocardiography, 27*, 911–939. https://doi.org/10.1016/j.echo.2014.07.012

Polito, A. (2010). Pulmonary reactions to novel chemotherapeutic agents and biomolecules. In P. Camus & E.C. Rosenow III (Eds.), *Drug-induced and iatrogenic respiratory disease* (pp. 146–160). London, England: Hodder Arnold.

Ponikowski, P., Voors, A.A., Anker, S.D., Bueno, H., Cleland, J., Coats, A.J.S., … van der Meer, P. (2016). 2016 ESC Guidelines for the diagnosis and treatment of acute and chronic heart failure. The task force for the diagnosis and treatment of acute and chronic heart failure of the European Society of Cardiology (ESC). Developed with the special contribution of the Heart Failure Association (HFA) of the ESC. *European Heart Journal, 37*, 2129–2200. https://doi.org/10.1093/eurheartj/ehw128

Pro, B., Advani, R., Brice, P., Bartlett, N.L., Rosenblatt, J.D., Illidge, T., … Shustov, A. (2012). Brentuximab vedotin (SGN-35) in patients with relapsed or refractory systemic anaplastic large-cell lymphoma: Results of a phase II study. *Journal of Clinical Oncology, 30*, 2190–2196. https://doi.org/10.1200/JCO.2011.38.0402

Pugliese, S., Neal, J.W., & Kwong, B.Y. (2015). Management of dermatologic complications of lung cancer therapies. *Current Treatment Options in Oncology, 16*, 50. https://doi.org/10.1007/s11864-015-0368-y

Ram, R., Bonstein, L., Grafter-Gvili, A., Ben-Bassat, I., Shpilberg, O., & Raanani, P. (2009). Rituximab-associated acute thrombocytopenia: An under-diagnosed phenomenon. *American Journal of Hematology, 84*, 247–250. https://doi.org/10.1002/ajh.21372

Richardson, D.L., Backes, F.J., Hurt, J.D., Seamon, L.G., Copeland, L.J., Fowler, J.M., … O'Malley, D.M. (2010). Which factors predict bowel complications in patients with recurrent epithelial ovarian cancer being treated with bevacizumab? *Gynecologic Oncology, 118*, 47–51. https://doi.org/10.1016/j.ygyno.2010.01.011

Rizzieri, D. (2016). Zevalin® (ibritumomab tiuxetan): After more than a decade of treatment experience, what have we learned? *Critical Reviews in Oncology/Hematology, 105*, 5–17. https://doi.org/10.1016/j.critrevonc.2016.07.008

Robak, T. (2008). Ofatumumab, a human monoclonal antibody for lymphoid malignancies and autoimmune disorders. *Current Opinion in Molecular Therapy, 10*, 294–309.

Robak, T., Blonski, J.Z., & Robak, P. (2016). Antibody therapy alone and in combination with targeted drugs in chronic lymphocytic leukemia. *Seminars in Oncology, 43*, 280–290. https://doi.org/10.1053/j.seminoncol.2016.02.010

Roviello, G., Bachelot, T., Hudis, C.A., Curigliano, G., Reynolds, A.R., Petrioli, R., & Generali, D. (2017). The role of bevacizumab in solid tumours: A literature based meta-analysis of randomised trials. *European Journal of Cancer, 75,* 245–258. https://doi.org/10.1016 /j.ejca.2017.01.026

Rummel, M., Kim, T.M., Jensen, P., Pereira, W.V., Re, F., Mendoza, M., … Grigg, A. (2016). Subcutaneous versus intravenous rituximab administration in first-line diffuse large B-cell lymphoma and follicular lymphoma: Prefmab study of patient preference and satisfaction in 19 countries [Abstract]. Retrieved from https://learningcenter.ehaweb.org /eha/2016/21st/132505/mathias.rummel.subcutaneous.versus.intravenous.rituximab .administration.in.html?f=m3e968

Rummel, M., Kim, T.M., Plenteda, C., Capochiani, E., Mendoza, M., Smith, R., … Grigg, A. (2015). PrefMab: Final analysis of patient satisfaction with subcutaneous versus intravenous rituximab in previously untreated CD20+ diffuse large B-cell lymphoma or follicular lymphoma [Abstract]. *Value in Health, 126,* A469. https://doi.org/10.1016 /j.jval.2015.09.1237

Salihoglu, A., Elverdi, T., Karadogan, I., Paydas, S., Ozdemir, E., Erdem, G., … Ferhanoglu, B. (2015). Brentuximab vedotin for relapsed or refractory Hodgkin lymphoma: Experience in Turkey. *Annals of Hematology, 94,* 415–420. https://doi.org/10.1007/s00277-014-2215-9

Sandler, A., Gray, R., Perry, M.C., Brahmer, J., Schiller, J.H., Dowlati, A., … Johnson, D.H. (2006). Paclitaxel–carboplatin alone or with bevacizumab for non–small-cell lung cancer. *New England Journal of Medicine, 355,* 2542–2550. https://doi.org/10.1056/NEJMoa061884

Sarosiek, S., Shah, R., & Munshi, N.C. (2016). Review of siltuximab in the treatment of multicentric Castleman's disease. *Therapeutic Advances in Hematology, 7,* 360–366.

Scappaticci, F.A., Skillings, J.R., Holden, S.N., Gerber, H.-P., Miller, K., Kabbinavar, F., … Hurwitz, H. (2007). Arterial thromboembolic events in patients with metastatic carcinoma treated with chemotherapy and bevacizumab. *Journal of the National Cancer Institute, 99,* 1232–1239. https://doi.org/10.1093/jnci/djm086

Schneeweiss, A., Chia, S., Hickish, T., Harvey, V., Eniu, A., Hegg, R., … Cortés, J. (2013). Pertuzumab plus trastuzumab in combination with standard neoadjuvant anthracycline-containing and anthracycline-free chemotherapy regimens in patients with HER2-positive early breast cancer: A randomized phase II cardiac safety study (TRYPHAENA). *Annals in Oncology, 24,* 2278–2284. https://doi.org/10.1093/annonc/mdt182

Schwartzberg, L.S., Rivera, F., Karthaus, M., Fasola, G., Canon, J.-L., Hecht, J.R., … Go, W.Y. (2014). PEAK: A randomized, multicenter phase II study of panitumumab plus modified fluorouracil, leucovorin, and oxaliplatin (mFOLFOX6) or bevacizumab plus mFOLFOX6 in patients with previously untreated, unresectable, wild-type KRAS exon 2 metastatic colorectal cancer. *Journal of Clinical Oncology, 32,* 2240–2247. https://doi.org /10.1200/JCO.2013.53.2473

Seattle Genetics, Inc. (2017). *Adcetris® (brentuximab vedotin)* [Package insert]. Bothell, WA: Author.

Shanafelt, T., Lanasa, M.C., Call, T.G., Beaven, A.W., Leis, J.F., LaPlant, B., … Zent, C.S. (2013). Ofatumumab-based chemoimmunotherapy is effective and well tolerated in patients with previously untreated chronic lymphocytic leukemia (CLL). *Cancer, 119,* 3788–3796. https://doi.org/10.1002/cncr.28292

Shank, B.R., Do, B., Sevin, A., Chen, S.E., Neelapu, S.S., & Horowitz, S.B. (2017). Chimeric antigen receptor T cells in hematologic malignancies. *Pharmacology, 37,* 334–345. https:// doi.org/10.1002/phar.1900

Shen, L., Li, J., Xu, J., Pan, H., Dai, G., Qin, S., … Piao, Y. (2015). Bevacizumab plus capecitabine and cisplatin in Chinese patients with inoperable locally advanced or metastatic gastric or gastroesophageal junction cancer: Randomized, double-blind, phase III study (AVATAR study). *Gastric Cancer, 18,* 168–176. https://doi.org/10.1007 /s10120-014-0351-5

Sherbenou, D.W., Mark, T.M., & Forsberg, P. (2017). Monoclonal antibodies in multiple myeloma: A new wave of the future. *Clinical Lymphoma, Myeloma and Leukemia, 17,* 545–554. https://doi.org/10.1016/j.clml.2017.06.030

Shord, S.S., Bressler, L.R., Tierney, L.A., Cuellar, S., & George, A. (2009). Understanding and managing the possible adverse effects associated with bevacizumab. *American Journal of Health-System Pharmacy, 66*, 999–1013. https://doi.org/10.2146/ajhp080455

Simpkins, F., Belinson, J.L., & Rose, P.G. (2007). Avoiding bevacizumab related gastrointestinal toxicity for recurrent ovarian cancer by careful patients screening. *Gynecologic Oncology, 107*, 118–123. https://doi.org/10.1016/j.ygyno.2007.06.004

Skarbnik, A.P., & Smith, M.R. (2012). Radioimmunotherapy in mantle cell lymphoma. *Best Practice and Research Clinical Haematology, 25*, 201–210. https://doi.org/10.1016/j.beha.2012.04.004

Smolej, L. (2015). Targeted treatment for chronic lymphocytic leukemia: Clinical potential of obinutuzumab. *Pharmacogenomics and Personalized Medicine, 8*, 1–7. https://doi.org/10.2147/PGPM.S55501s

Swain, S.M., Kim, S.-B., Cortés, J., Ro, J., Semiglazov, V., Campone, M., ... Baselga, J. (2013). Pertuzumab, trastuzumab, and docetaxel for HER2-positive metastatic breast cancer (CLEOPATRA study): Overall survival results from a randomised, double-blind, placebo-controlled, phase 3 study. *Lancet Oncology, 14*, 461–471. https://doi.org/10.1016/S1470-2045(13)70130-X

Taniwaki, M., Yoshida, M., Matsumoto, Y., Shimura, K., Kuroda, J., & Kaneko, H. (2018). Elotuzumab for the treatment of relapsed or refractory multiple myeloma, with special reference to its modes of action and SLAMF7 signaling. *Mediterranean Journal of Hematology and Infectious Diseases, 10*, e2018014.

Tap, W.D., Jones, R.L., Van Tine, B.A., Chmielowski, B., Elias, A.D., Adkins, D., ... Schwartz, G.K. (2016). Olaratumab and doxorubicin versus doxorubicin alone for treatment of soft-tissue sarcoma: An open-label phase 1b and randomised phase 2 trial. *Lancet, 388*, 488–497. https://doi.org/10.1016/S0140-6736(16)30587-6

Tejpar, S., Piessevaux, H., Claes, K., Piront, P., Hoenderop, J.G.J., Verslype, C., & Van Cutsem, E. (2007). Magnesium wasting associated with epidermal-growth-factor receptor-targeting antibodies in colorectal cancer: A prospective study. *Lancet Oncology, 8*, 387–394. https://doi.org/10.1016/S1470-2045(07)70108-0

Teo, E.C.-Y., Chew, Y., & Phipps, C. (2016). A review of monoclonal antibody therapies in lymphoma. *Critical Reviews in Oncology/Hematology, 97*, 72–84. https://doi.org/10.1016/j.critrevonc.2015.08.014

Tham, E.H., Cheng, Y.K., Tay, M.H., Alcasabas, A.P., & Shek, L.P.-C. (2015). Evaluation and management of hypersensitivity reactions to chemotherapy agents. *Postgraduate Medical Journal, 91*, 145–150. https://doi.org/10.1136/postgradmedj-2014-132686

Thomas, A., Teicher, B.A., & Hassan, R. (2016). Antibody–drug conjugates for cancer therapy. *Lancet Oncology, 17*, e254–e262. https://doi.org/10.1016/S1470-2045(16)30030-4

Thompson, L.M., Eckmann, K., Boster, B.L., Hess, K.R., Michaud, L.B., Esteva, F.J., ... Barnett, C.M. (2014). Incidence, risk factors, and management of infusion related reactions in breast cancer patients receiving trastuzumab. *Oncologist, 19*, 228–234. https://doi.org/10.1634/theoncologist.2013-0286

Thosani, S., & Hu, M.I. (2015). Denosumab: A new agent in the management of hypercalcemia of malignancy. *Future Oncology, 11*, 2865–2871. https://doi.org/10.2217/fon.15.232

Tian, R., Yan, H., Zhang, F., Sun, P., Zheng, X., Zhu, Y., ... He, J. (2016). Incidence and relative risk of hemorrhagic events associated with ramucirumab in cancer patients: A systematic review and meta-analysis. *Oncotarget, 7*, 66182–66191. https://doi.org/10.18632/oncotarget.11097

Topp, M.S., Gökbuget, N., Stein, A.S., Zugmaier, G., O'Brien, S., Bargou, R.C., ... Kantarjian, H.M. (2015). Safety and activity of blinatumomab for adult patients with relapsed or refractory B-precursor acute lymphoblastic leukaemia: A multicentre, single-arm, phase 2 study. *Lancet Oncology, 16*, 57–66. https://doi.org/10.1016/S1470-2045(14)71170-2

Tripathy, D., Slamon, D.J., Cobleigh, M., Arnold, A., Saleh, M., Mortimer, J.E., ... Stewart, S.J. (2004). Safety of treatment of metastatic breast cancer with trastuzumab beyond disease progression. *Journal of Clinical Oncology, 22,* 1063–1070. https://doi.org/10.1200 /JCO.2004.06.557

Valachis, A., Nearchou, A., Polyzos, N.P., & Lind, P. (2013). Cardiac toxicity in breast cancer patients treated with dual HER2 blockade. *International Journal of Cancer, 133,* 2245–2252. https://doi.org/10.1002/ijc.28234

Valentine, J., Belum, V.R., Duran, J., Ciccolini, K., Schindler, K., Wu, S., & Lacouture, M.E. (2015). Incidence and risk of xerosis with targeted anticancer therapies. *Journal of the American Academy of Dermatology, 72,* 656–667. https://doi.org/10.1016/j.jaad.2014.12.010

Van Cutsem, E., Köhne, C.-H., Hitre, E., Zaluski, J., Chang Chien, C.-R., Makhson, A., ... Rougier, P. (2009). Cetuximab and chemotherapy as initial treatment for metastatic colorectal cancer. *New England Journal of Medicine, 360,* 1408–1417. https://doi.org/10 .1056/NEJMoa0805019

van Rhee, F., Casper, C., Voorhees, P.M., Fayad, L.E., van de Velde, H., Vermeulen, J., ... Kurzrock, R. (2015). A phase 2, open-label, multicenter study on the long-term safety of siltuximab (an anti-interleukin-6 monoclonal antibody) in patients with multicentric Castleman disease. *Oncotarget, 6,* 30408–30419. https://doi.org/10.18632/oncotarget.4655

Vennepureddy, A., Singh, P., Rastogi, R., Atallah, J.P., & Terjanian, T. (2017). Evolution of ramucirumab in the treatment of cancer–A review of literature. *Journal of Oncology Pharmacy Practice, 23,* 1–15. https://doi.org/10.1177/1078155216655474

Verma, S., Miles, D., Gianni, L., Krop, I.E., Welslau, M., Baselga, J., ... Blackwell, K. (2012). Trastuzumab emtansine for HER2-positive advanced breast cancer. *New England Journal of Medicine, 367,* 1783–1791. https://doi.org/10.1056/NEJMoa1209124

Vidal, L., Gafter-Gvili, A., Gurion, R., Raanani, P., Dreyling, M., & Shpilberg, O. (2012). Bendamustine for patients with indolent B cell lymphoid malignancies including chronic lymphocytic leukaemia. *Cochrane Database of Systematic Reviews, 2012*(4). https://doi.org /10.1002/14651858.CD009045

Vincenzi, B., Badalamenti, G., Napolitano, A., Ceruso, M.S., Pantano, F., Grignani, G., ... Tonini, G. (2017). Olaratumab: PDGFR-α inhibition as a novel tool in the treatment of advanced soft tissue sarcomas. *Critical Reviews in Oncology/Hematology, 118,* 1–6. https:// doi.org/10.1016/j.critrevonc.2017.06.006

Wagner, H.N., Jr., Wiseman, G.A., Marcus, C.S., Nabi, H.A., Nagle, C.E., Fink-Bennett, D.M., ... Conti, P.S. (2002). Administration guidelines for radioimmunotherapy of non-Hodgkin's lymphoma with (90)Y-labeled anti-CD20 monoclonal antibody. *Journal of Nuclear Medicine, 43,* 267–272.

Wang, Y., Sanchez, L., Siegel, D.S., & Wang, M.L. (2016). Elotuzumab for the treatment of multiple myeloma. *Journal of Hematology and Oncology, 9,* 55. https://doi.org/10.1186 /s13045-016-0284-z

Warner, J.L., & Arnason, J.E. (2012). Alemtuzumab use in relapsed and refractory chronic lymphocytic leukemia: A history and discussion of future rational use. *Therapeutic Advances in Hematology, 3,* 375–389. https://doi.org/10.1177/2040620712458949

Wen, F., & Li, Q. (2016). Treatment dilemmas of cetuximab combined with chemotherapy for metastatic colorectal cancer. *World Journal of Gastroenterology, 22,* 5332–5341. https:// doi.org/10.3748/wjg.v22.i23.5332

Wierda, W.G., Kipps, T.J., Dürig, J., Griskevicius, L., Stilgenbauer, S., Mayer, J., ... Russell, C.A. (2011). Chemoimmunotherapy with O-FC in previously untreated patients with chronic lymphocytic leukemia. *Blood, 117,* 6450–6458. https://doi.org/10.1182/blood -2010-12-323980

Wierda, W.G., Kipps, T.J., Mayer, J., Stilgenbauer, S., Williams, C.D., Hellmann, A., ... Österborg, A. (2010). Ofatumumab as single-agent CD20 immunotherapy in fludarabine-refractory chronic lymphocytic leukemia. *Journal of Clinical Oncology, 28,* 1749–1755. https://doi.org/10.1200/JCO.2009.25.3187

Wierda, W.G., Padmanabhan, S., Chan, G.W., Gupta, I.V., Lisby, S., & Österborg, A. (2011). Ofatumumab is active in patients with fludarabine-refractory CLL irrespective of prior rituximab: Results from the phase 2 international study. *Blood, 118,* 5126–5129. https:// doi.org/10.1182/blood-2011-04-348656

Wilke, H., Muro, K., Van Cutsem, E., Oh, S.-C., Bodoky, G., Shimada, Y., ... Ohtsu, A. (2014). Ramucirumab plus paclitaxel versus placebo plus paclitaxel in patients with previously treated advanced gastric or gastro-oesophageal junction adenocarcinoma (RAINBOW): A double-blind, randomised phase 3 trial. *Lancet Oncology, 15,* 1224–1235. https://doi .org/10.1016/S1470-2045(14)70420-6

Witzig, T.E., Fishkin, P., Gordon, L.I., Gregory, S.A., Jacobs, S., Macklis, R., ... Zelenetz, A.D. (2011). Treatment recommendations for radioimmunotherapy in follicular lymphoma: A consensus conference report. *Leukemia and Lymphoma, 52,* 1188–1199. https://doi.org /10.3109/10428194.2011.570396

Wolach, O., Bairey, O., & Lahav, M. (2010). Late-onset neutropenia after rituximab treatment: Case series and comprehensive review of the literature. *Medicine, 89,* 308–318. https:// doi.org/10.1097/MD.0b013e3181f2caef

Wu, Y.S., Shui, L., Shen, D., & Chen, X. (2016). Bevacizumab combined with chemotherapy for ovarian cancer: An updated systematic review and meta-analysis of randomized controlled trials. *Oncotarget, 8,* 10703–10713. https://doi.org/10.18632/oncotarget.12926

Wyeth Pharmaceuticals Inc. (2017a). *Besponsa™ (inotuzumab ozogamicin)* [Package insert]. Philadelphia, PA: Author.

Wyeth Pharmaceuticals Inc. (2017b). *Mylotarg® (gemtuzumab ozogamicin)* [Package insert]. Philadelphia, PA: Author.

Yang, X.D., Jia, X.C., Corvalan, J.R., Wang, P., Davis, C.G., & Jakobovits, A. (1999). Eradication of established tumors by a fully human monoclonal antibody to the epidermal growth factor receptor without concomitant chemotherapy. *Cancer Research, 59,* 1236–1243.

Yazdi, M.H., Faramarzi, M.A., Nikfar, S., & Abdollahi, M. (2015). A comprehensive review of clinical trials on EGFR inhibitors such as cetuximab and panitumumab as monotherapy and in combination for treatment of metastatic colorectal cancer. *Avicenna Journal of Medical Biotechnology, 7,* 134–144.

Younes, A., Gopal, A.K., Smith, S.E., Ansell, S.M., Rosenblatt, J.D., Savage, K.J., ... Chen, R. (2012). Results of a pivotal phase II study of brentuximab vedotin for patients with relapsed or refractory Hodgkin's lymphoma. *Journal of Clinical Oncology, 30,* 2183–2189. https://doi.org/10.1200/JCO.2011.38.0410

Zhang, E., & Xu, H. (2017). A new insight in chimeric antigen receptor-engineered T cells for cancer immunotherapy. *Journal of Hematology and Oncology, 10,* 1. https://doi.org/10 .1186/s13045-016-0379-6

Zheng, G.Z., Chang, B., Lin, F.X., Xie, D., Hu, Q.X., Yu, G.Y., ... Li, X.D. (2017). Meta-analysis comparing denosumab and zoledronic acid for treatment of bone metastases in patients with advanced solid tumours. *European Journal of Cancer Care, 26,* e12541. https://doi. org/10.1111/ecc.12541

Zinzani, P.L., Sasse, S., Radford, J., Gautam, A., & Bonthapally, V. (2016). Brentuximab vedotin in relapsed/refractory Hodgkin lymphoma: An updated review of published data from the named patient program. *Critical Reviews in Oncology/Hematology, 104,* 65–70. https://doi.org/10.1016/j.critrevonc.2016.04.019

c h a p t e r   n i n e

Combination Therapies

Lisa Kottschade, APRN, MSN, CNP

Introduction

The role of immunotherapy in the treatment of cancer has expanded exponentially in the past decade. A significant paradigm shift has occurred in the treatment of malignancy with the approval of several key checkpoint inhibitors by the U.S. Food and Drug Administration (FDA). In this new era of combination therapy, unrealized opportunities in treatment are becoming a reality. This chapter will explore this exciting new area, as well as the historical use of chemoimmunotherapy (CIT) and radioimmunotherapy (RIT) in the treatment of a variety of cancers.

Chemoimmunotherapy

The term *chemoimmunotherapy* is defined as "chemotherapy combined with immunotherapy" (National Cancer Institute [NCI], n.d.). Traditional chemotherapy includes agents specifically designed to slow or kill cancer cells. Immunotherapy includes agents designed to work with and enhance the body's immune system to kill cells. Traditionally, chemotherapy has been described as *immunosuppressive*, or having the ability to reduce immune system responses (NCI, n.d.). However, recent data show that this term may be a bit of an overstatement. Growing evidence supports that standard chemotherapy may exert its immunomodulation through a variety of mechanisms. Historically, most chemotherapy drugs work through the induction of apoptosis, or programmed cell death. Although the exact mechanism of tumor immunomodulation is not completely understood, studies have suggested several methods based on the type of chemotherapy used. Chemotherapy is thought to promote tumor immunity through immunogenic cell death and through the ancillary effects on malignant and normal host cells within the tumor microenvironment (Chen & Emens, 2013).

Tumors may induce immunogenic cell death through Toll-like receptor 4 (TLR-4) or P2X purinoceptor 7 (P2RX7) (Chen & Emens, 2013). Loss-of-function polymorphisms in both TLR-4 and P2RX7 have been associated with a higher risk of breast cancer relapse in patients treated with adjuvant anthracycline-based chemotherapy regimens (Chen & Emens, 2013). This was also seen in patients undergoing oxaliplatin-based chemotherapy for advanced colon cancer. Patients with a TLR loss-of-function polymorphism had shorter progression-free survival (PFS) and overall survival compared to those who carried the normal TLR-4 allele (Chen & Emens, 2013).

Ancillary methods that may promote antitumor immunity include intrinsic tumor cell immunogenicity, modulation of a variety of immunoregulatory cells (e.g., regulatory T cells, other CD4+ T cells, myeloid-derived suppressor cells, dendritic cells), and the induction of homeostatic proliferation (Chen & Emens, 2013). With the high influx of immunotherapy agents hitting the market, most notably checkpoint blockade inhibitors, chemotherapy can exploit several unique pathways to induce antitumor immunity. For example, some chemotherapy drugs appear to induce the expression of molecules such as B7-1 on the tumor cell surface, enabling them to present tumor antigens to induce immune activation (Chen & Emens, 2013). Other chemotherapy drugs can decrease the expression of B7-H1 (programmed cell death-ligand 1 [PD-L1]) and B7-H4, both of which are expressed on the cell surfaces of tumors. This prevents infiltrating T cells from being deactivated (Chen & Emens, 2013).

Over the years, researchers have conducted numerous studies to improve outcomes with combination CIT. Traditional chemotherapy has been combined with tumor-derived vaccines, cytokines (e.g., interleukin-2 [IL-2]), checkpoint inhibitors, and other immune-modifying agents. This chapter will focus on some of the most common and significant regimens.

R-CHOP

One of the most well-known regimens is rituximab combined with CHOP (cyclophosphamide, doxorubicin, vincristine, and prednisone), or R-CHOP. Rituximab (Rituxan®) is a chimeric monoclonal antibody that targets CD20 on B cells. It depletes B cells via several mechanisms, including complement-mediated cell death, signaling apoptosis, and directed antibody-dependent cellular cytotoxicity (Dotan, Aggarwal, & Smith, 2010).

The treatment landscape for lymphoma was significantly changed when rituximab was FDA approved in 1997 as a single agent for the treatment of B-cell lymphoma. With the introduction of R-CHOP, phase 3 data showed a statistically significant improvement in both newly diagnosed and relapsed/refractory indolent follicular lymphoma (Hiddemann et al., 2005; van Oers et al., 2006). In newly diagnosed patients, overall response rate (90% to 96%; p < 0.05) and overall survival (90% to 95%) significantly improved (Hiddemann et al., 2005). In refractory/relapsed follicular lymphoma, overall response rate (72% to 85%; p < 0.05) and median PFS (20 months to 33 months) significantly improved (van Oers et al., 2006). Based on these and other favorable results, rituximab received FDA approval in 2006 as a frontline treatment in combination with CHOP and other anthracycline-based chemotherapy regimens for patients with CD20-positive diffuse large B-cell non-Hodgkin lymphoma (NHL) (Czuczman, Weaver, Alkuzweny, Berlfein, & Grillo-López, 2004; Hiddemann et al., 2005). Current National Comprehensive Cancer Network® (NCCN®, 2018a) guidelines also list R-CHOP as a frontline therapy. R-CVP (rituximab with cyclophosphamide, vincristine, and prednisone) regimens and CIT regimens containing bendamustine and rituximab are additional frontline therapies for follicular lymphoma (Czuczman et al., 2004; Flinn et al., 2014; Marcus et al., 2008; NCCN, 2018a; Rummel et al., 2013). Table 9-1 summarizes common CIT regimens, including typical dosing and administration schedules.

Typical side effects are those expected with traditional chemotherapy, including cytopenias, nausea and vomiting, peripheral neuropathy, hair loss, and diarrhea. With respect to rituximab, patients can experience infusion-related reactions, including hypotension, bronchospasm, angioedema (necessitating premedication), fever, chills/rigors, cytopenia, and gastrointestinal issues (i.e., nausea and vomiting, abdominal pain, diarrhea). Reactivation of hepatitis B virus is also possible; therefore, surface antigen testing should be performed in high-risk patients prior to therapy and approximately every three months while on therapy. Carriers should be closely monitored for symptoms of reactivation. Patients with large tumor burden should be closely monitored for tumor lysis syndrome. Frequent monitoring of electrolytes, creatinine, blood urea nitrogen, and lactate dehydrogenase is critical during the first 48–72 hours. Patients are usually started on allopurinol for the prevention of hyperuricemia. Rituximab should never be administered as an IV push or bolus, as this can increase the risk of severe adverse events.

Biochemotherapy

Another well-known example of CIT is what has traditionally been termed in the melanoma world as *biochemotherapy*. Metastatic melanoma

TABLE 9-1 Common Chemoimmunotherapy Regimens

Regimen	Agents and Typical Dosing	Schedule
R-CVP (lymphoma)	Rituximab: 375 mg/m²/day IV Cyclophosphamide: 1,000 mg/m²/day IV Vincristine: 1.4 mg/m²/day IV (max dose of 2 mg) Prednisone: 100 mg/m²/day PO	All drugs on day 1 of 21-day cycle Prednisone days 1–5 Repeat for 6–8 cycles
Rituximab/bendamustine (NHL/mantle cell lymphoma)	Rituximab: 375 mg/m²/day IV Bendamustine: 90 mg/m²/day IV	Day 1 of 28 Days 1 and 2 of 28 Repeat for 6 cycles
R-CHOP (lymphoma)	Rituximab: 375 mg/m²/day IV Cyclophosphamide: 750 mg/m²/day IV Doxorubicin: 50 mg/m²/day IV push Vincristine: 1.4 mg/m²/day IV (max dose of 2 mg) Prednisone: 100 mg/m²/day PO	All drugs on day 1 of 21-day cycle Prednisone days 1–5 Repeat for 6–8 cycles

NHL—non-Hodgkin lymphoma; R-CHOP—rituximab with cyclophosphamide, doxorubicin, vincristine, and prednisone; R-CVP—rituximab with cyclophosphamide, vincristine, and prednisone

Note. Based on information from Czuczman et al., 2004; Flinn et al., 2014; Marcus et al., 2008; National Comprehensive Cancer Network, 2018a, 2018b; Rummel et al., 2013.

has historically carried a poor prognosis, and until the recent approval of checkpoint inhibitors and targeted therapies, it was almost universally fatal, carrying a median survival of nine months (Balch et al., 2009). It is believed that immune system dysfunction allows this melanoma to grow. Given the relative lack of efficacy of the single-agent chemotherapy dacarbazine, which remains the only FDA-approved chemotherapeutic agent for metastatic melanoma as of this writing, researchers sought to combine interferon (IFN) alfa-2b (Intron A®) and IL-2 (Proleukin®), agents considered to be biologically and clinically active in melanoma with various chemotherapy agents.

Multiple randomized clinical trials have compared various biochemotherapy regimens in metastatic melanoma to traditional chemotherapy regimens using either single-agent dacarbazine, single-agent temozolomide, or combination CVD (cisplatin, vinblastine, and dacarbazine). A meta-analysis of 18 trials conducted between 1996 and 2006 looked at the impact of biochemotherapy versus traditional chemotherapy in 2,621 patients with metastatic melanoma (Ives, Stowe, Lorigan,

& Wheatley, 2007). Eleven trials involved chemotherapy with or without IFN, and the remaining seven trials included patients undergoing chemotherapy with or without IFN and IL-2 (Ives et al., 2007). Although response rates (complete response, partial response, and overall response) were statistically improved in the biochemotherapy regimens across studies, no statistically significant improvements in overall survival were reported (Ives et al., 2007).

Garbe, Eigentler, Keilholz, Hauschild, and Kirkwood (2011) conducted a systematic review of the therapies used in metastatic melanoma, including multiple CIT trials. Although this review showed improved response rates, data on overall survival rates were less significant. One included study was a randomized phase 3 trial led by the Eastern Cooperative Oncology Group that compared CVD alone versus CVD in combination with IL-2 and IFN as frontline therapy for patients with metastatic melanoma. Results revealed a slightly higher response rate (19.5% vs. 13.8%; p = 0.140) and significantly longer median PFS in the combination arm (4.8 months vs. 2.9 months; p = 0.015); however, no improvements in overall survival were noted (Garbe et al., 2011). Based on these data, as well as the increased toxicity noted in the combination arm, the authors concluded that this regimen could not be regularly recommended for patients with metastatic melanoma.

Biochemotherapy remains in NCCN guidelines as a category 2B (possible systemic therapy) regimen for patients with metastatic melanoma (NCCN, 2018b). In addition, IL-2–containing regimens require administration at specialty centers familiar with management of patients undergoing this type of therapy.

Typical side effects of biochemotherapy include cytopenias, nausea and vomiting, and cytokine release syndrome in IL-2–containing regimens (e.g., capillary leak syndrome, heart failure, respiratory distress, fever). High-dose IL-2 administration requires hospitalization and is usually administered in the intensive care unit.

Radioimmunotherapy

NCI defines *radioimmunotherapy* as "a type of radiation therapy in which a radioactive substance is linked to a monoclonal antibody and injected into the body" (NCI, n.d.). Multiple studies have demonstrated the value of RIT for patients with NHL (Bodet-Milin et al., 2013; Illidge et al., 2014; Kraeber-Bodéré et al., 2014; Morschhauser et al., 2008; Witzig et al., 2007). Currently, the only FDA-approved RIT is ibritumomab tiuxetan (Zevalin®) (Spectrum Pharmaceuticals, Inc., 2013). A second agent, tositumomab and iodine-131 tositumomab (Bexxar®), which was FDA approved and sold in the United States and

Canada as a treatment for NHL, was withdrawn from the market in 2014.

Ibritumomab tiuxetan is a CD20-directed radiotherapeutic agent used in the treatment of NHL. Specifically, it binds to the CD20 antigen (human B-lymphocyte–restricted differentiation antigen, Bp35) (Spectrum Pharmaceuticals, Inc., 2013). The CD20 antigen is expressed on pre-B and mature B lymphocytes and on more than 90% of B-cell NHL, making it an interesting treatment for this patient population (Spectrum Pharmaceuticals, Inc., 2013). Ibritumomab tiuxetan binding was observed in vitro on lymphoid cells of the bone marrow, lymph node, thymus, red and white pulp of the spleen, and lymphoid follicles of the tonsil, as well as on the lymphoid nodules of other organs, such as the large and small intestines (Spectrum Pharmaceuticals, Inc., 2013).

Ibritumomab tiuxetan is given in conjunction with rituximab for relapsed/refractory, low-grade or follicular B-cell NHL. Initial FDA approval was granted in 2002 after the completion of a pivotal phase 3 trial comparing the combination of ibritumomab tiuxetan and rituximab versus rituximab alone. This trial enrolled 143 patients with either relapsed/refractory low-grade, follicular, or transformed B-cell NHL and showed that the combination therapy was superior to rituximab alone (Witzig et al., 2002). This confirmed earlier single-arm phase 1/2 studies that noted the efficacy of ibritumomab tiuxetan (Knox et al., 1996; Witzig et al., 1999).

Ibritumomab tiuxetan is administered via IV injection over approximately 10 minutes (Spectrum Pharmaceuticals, Inc., 2013). A typical schedule for relapsed/refractory NHL includes administration of rituximab on day 1 of the cycle, followed by a second dose of rituximab on days 7, 8, or 9 with ibritumomab tiuxetan administered within four hours (Spectrum Pharmaceuticals, Inc., 2013). For patients with untreated NHL, ibritumomab tiuxetan should be administered at least 6 weeks, but no longer than 12 weeks, following the last dose of frontline chemotherapy (Spectrum Pharmaceuticals, Inc., 2013).

Common side effects from ibritumomab tiuxetan include severe and prolonged cytopenias, cutaneous and mucocutaneous reactions, infusion reactions, secondary leukemias and myelodysplastic syndrome, infections, and fatigue. Patients should not receive ibritumomab tiuxetan infusion if platelet counts are less than $100,000/mm^3$. Infusion should be stopped with any signs or symptoms of an infusion reaction, as fatal reactions have been reported. In addition, severe and even fatal cutaneous reactions have been seen, including Stevens-Johnson syndrome, toxic epidermal necrolysis, and erythema multiforme. The agent should be discontinued with any severe dermatologic reaction.

Combination Immunotherapy

The success of checkpoint inhibitors has improved survival in several malignancies, none more so than melanoma (Ansell et al., 2015; Antonia et al., 2016; Borghaei et al., 2015; Hellmann et al., 2017; Herbst et al., 2016; Hodi et al., 2010, 2016; Larkin, Chiarion-Sileni, et al., 2015; Larkin, Hodi, & Wolchok, 2015; Motzer et al., 2015; Reck et al., 2016; Robert et al., 2015). The first checkpoint inhibitor, ipilimumab (Yervoy®), was FDA approved in 2011 for the treatment of metastatic melanoma. The next generation of this class of agents includes drugs FDA approved for several malignancies, such as pembrolizumab (Keytruda®) and nivolumab (Opdivo®), which were approved in 2014; atezolizumab (Tecentriq®), approved in 2016; and avelumab (Bavencio®), approved in 2017. Because of the success of these drugs as single agents, many clinical trials were launched with the idea that dual checkpoint blockade would further improve outcomes.

Anti–PD-1 Agents

Ipilimumab exhibits its activity by blocking cytotoxic T-lymphocyte antigen 4 (CTLA-4), therefore upregulating antitumor immunity of T cells. Ipilimumab was the first single agent shown to improve survival in melanoma (Hodi et al., 2010). Pembrolizumab and nivolumab are anti–PD-1 (programmed cell death protein 1) agents. These agents work by blocking PD-1 from binding with PD-L1 and PD-L2 (programmed cell death-ligand 2) at the tumor, thus allowing activated T cells to attack cancer cells.

Pembrolizumab and nivolumab were first approved as second-line (after ipilimumab and/or *BRAF* inhibitor therapy), single-agent therapies for the treatment of metastatic melanoma in 2014. In 2015, pembrolizumab was approved as a first-line therapy after trial data showed superiority over ipilimumab alone (Robert et al., 2015). This class of agents has also been approved in numerous other malignancies, including non-small cell lung cancer, squamous cell carcinoma of the head and neck, and renal cell carcinoma (Ansell et al., 2015; Borghaei et al., 2015; Ferris et al., 2016; Herbst et al., 2016; Motzer et al., 2015; Reck et al., 2016; Seiwert et al., 2016).

Dual Checkpoint Blockade

Dual checkpoint blockade with anti–CTLA-4 and anti–PD-1 agents has been investigated as a frontline treatment for metastatic melanoma (Hodi et al., 2016; Larkin, Chiarion-Sileni, et al., 2015; Larkin, Hodi, & Wolchok, 2015). The hypothesis behind dual checkpoint blockade is a "one-two punch." Ipilimumab exerts its effects on the immune system during the priming phase, while nivolumab exerts its clinical effects during the proliferation phase.

After the CheckMate 067 and 069 trials, combination ipilimumab and nivolumab was FDA approved as frontline therapy for *BRAF* wild-type metastatic melanoma in 2015, with expanded labeling in 2016 to include frontline approval in *BRAF* mutant metastatic melanoma. CheckMate 067 was a randomized, double-blind, placebo-controlled phase 3 trial in patients with newly diagnosed, treatment-naïve metastatic melanoma. Patients were randomly assigned to one of three regimens: (a) nivolumab at 3 mg/kg every two weeks with matching ipilimumab placebo; (b) nivolumab at 1 mg/kg and ipilimumab at 3 mg/kg every three weeks for four doses, followed by nivolumab at 3 mg/kg with matching ipilimumab placebo every two weeks; and (c) ipilimumab at 3 mg/kg every three weeks with matching nivolumab placebo for four doses.

Patients were stratified by tumor PD-L1 status, *BRAF* mutation status, and M stage (M0, M1a, M1b, M1c). Patients were treated until progression or toxicity. This study concluded that combination ipilimumab and nivolumab showed statistically significant improvement in median PFS (p < 0.001) versus ipilimumab alone (11.5 months vs. 2.9 months) (Larkin, Chiarion-Sileni, et al., 2015). Improvement in PFS was statistically significant (p < 0.001) in the combination arm (11.5 months) versus the nivolumab arm alone (6.9 months) (Larkin, Chiarion-Sileni, et al., 2015). Among patients whose tumors showed PD-L1 positivity, median PFS was the same between the nivolumab and nivolumab/ipilimumab groups at 14 months (Larkin, Chiarion-Sileni, et al., 2015). Overall survival from this study has not yet been reported.

Survival data are available from the CheckMate 069 study, which was a phase 2, randomized, double-blind trial comparing combination nivolumab and ipilimumab to ipilimumab and placebo in patients with previously untreated metastatic melanoma. Approximately 142 patients enrolled, with 95 randomly assigned to the combination arm and 47 to the placebo arm. After a median follow-up of 24.5 months, the two-year overall survival rate in the combination arm was 63.8% versus 53.6% in the placebo arm. Median overall survival was not reached in either arm (Hodi et al., 2016). These combination regimens are seeing further research in the adjuvant setting in the hopes of decreasing recurrence rates after initial tumor resection.

The currently approved regimen for patients with metastatic melanoma comprises ipilimumab 3 mg/kg IV in combination with nivolumab 1 mg /kg IV on day 1 of a 21-day cycle for a total of four cycles. This is commonly called the *induction phase*. Patients who are responding and tolerating the treatment without significant side effects will go to the maintenance portion, or nivolumab 3 mg/kg IV every two weeks as a single agent. The side effect profile for this regimen is significantly different than that of chemotherapy and is a direct result of the upregulation of the patient's own immune system. Side effects are managed in a much different manner from traditional chemotherapy and must be recognized and treated early, as failure to do so can result in serious and potentially fatal toxicity. Unlike with chemotherapy and targeted therapy, simple drug withdrawal is not always effective at mitigating side effects, and immunosuppression in the form of steroids is often necessary.

The most common side effects experienced by patients on checkpoint inhibitor therapy include rash (dermatitis), diarrhea, colitis, (potentially leading to bowel perforation), autoimmune hepatitis, thyroiditis, hypophysitis, adrenal insufficiency, fatigue, peripheral neuropathy, pancreatitis, pneumonitis, and uveitis. Rare and potentially life-threatening side effects include myocarditis, pericarditis, myasthenia gravis, Guillain-Barré syndrome (acute demyelinating polyradiculoneuropathy), Stevens-Johnson syndrome, toxic epidermal necrolysis, myositis, and encephalitis. These side effects can occur anytime during the treatment course, including after the first dose and six months after the last dose. The side effect profile appears to be significantly higher in combination regimens (as high as 95% in grade 1–2 and 50% in grade 3–4). This should be taken into consideration during patient selection (Hodi et al., 2016; Larkin, Chiarion-Sileni, et al., 2015). Ongoing studies are evaluating different dosing strategies of combination ipilimumab and nivolumab in metastatic melanoma to decrease the incidence of toxicity and maintain the high response rates seen in the CheckMate 067 trial. Currently, combination therapy is being studied in non-small cell and small cell lung cancer, renal cell carcinoma, and glioblastoma, with likely expansion into other malignancies (Antonia et al., 2016; Hammers et al., 2015; Hellmann et al., 2017; Sampson et al., 2015).

Summary

With the explosion of immunotherapeutic treatments in the past 20 years, specifically checkpoint inhibitors, researchers have unlocked new and exciting treatment pathways in hematology and solid tumor oncology. The mechanism of action of a checkpoint inhibitor is unique in that it harnesses the body's own immune system and helps it adapt to fight the cancer. This allows applicability and efficacy across many cancers, including hematologic malignancies, and presents unique opportunities for exploration of additional combinations with traditional tumor-specific chemotherapies. With these combinations, researchers are hoping to provide patients with long-term remissions and disease control. Further research can build upon the foundation of chemotherapeutic-based regimens that offer significant tumor debulking but are usually of limited duration and long-term tolerability because of cumulative side effects.

References

Ansell, S.M., Lesokhin, A.M., Borrello, I., Halwani, A., Scott, E.C., Gutierrez, M., ... Armand, P. (2015). PD-1 blockade with nivolumab in relapsed or refractory Hodgkin's lymphoma. *New England Journal of Medicine, 372,* 311–319. https://doi.org/10.1056/NEJMoa1411087

Antonia, S.J., López-Martin, J.A., Bendell, J., Ott, P.A., Taylor, M., Eder, J.P., ... Calvo, E. (2016). Nivolumab alone and nivolumab plus ipilimumab in recurrent small-cell lung cancer (CheckMate 032): A multicentre, open-label, phase 1/2 trial. *Lancet Oncology, 17,* 883–895. https://doi.org/10.1016/S1470-2045(16)30098-5

Balch, C.M., Gershenwald, J.E., Soong, S.-J., Thompson, J.F., Atkins, M.B., Byrd, D.R., ... Sondak, V.K. (2009). Final version of 2009 AJCC melanoma staging and classification. *Journal of Clinical Oncology, 27,* 6199–6206. https://doi.org/10.1200/JCO.2009.23.4799

Bodet-Milin, C., Ferrer, L., Pallardy, A., Eugène, T., Rauscher, A., Faivre-Chauvet, A., & Kraeber-Bodéré, F. (2013). Radioimmunotherapy of B-cell non-Hodgkin's lymphoma. *Frontiers in Oncology, 3,* 177. https://doi.org/10.3389/fonc.2013.00177

Borghaei, H., Paz-Ares, L., Horn, L., Spigel, D.R., Steins, M., Ready, N.E., ... Brahmer, J.R. (2015). Nivolumab versus docetaxel in advanced nonsquamous non–small-cell lung cancer. *New England Journal of Medicine, 373,* 1627–1639. https://doi.org/10.1056/NEJMoa1507643

Chen, G., & Emens, L.A. (2013). Chemoimmunotherapy: Reengineering tumor immunity. *Cancer Immunology, Immunotherapy, 62,* 203–216. https://doi.org/10.1007/s00262-012-1388-0

Czuczman, M.S., Weaver, R., Alkuzweny, B., Berlfein, J., & Grillo-López, A.J. (2004). Prolonged clinical and molecular remission in patients with low-grade or follicular non-Hodgkin's lymphoma treated with rituximab plus CHOP chemotherapy: 9-year follow-up. *Journal of Clinical Oncology, 22,* 4711–4716. https://doi.org/10.1200/JCO.2004.04.020

Dotan, E., Aggarwal, C., & Smith, M.R. (2010). Impact of rituximab (Rituxan) on the treatment of B-cell non-Hodgkin's lymphoma. *P&T Journal, 35,* 148–157.

Ferris, R.L., Blumenschein, G., Jr., Fayette, J., Guigay, J., Colevas, A.D., Licitra, L., ... Gillison, M.L. (2016). Nivolumab for recurrent squamous-cell carcinoma of the head and neck. *New England Journal of Medicine, 375,* 1856–1867. https://doi.org/10.1056/NEJMoa1602252

Flinn, I.W., van der Jagt, R., Kahl, B.S., Wood, P., Hawkins, T.E., MacDonald, D., ... Burke, J.M. (2014). Randomized trial of bendamustine-rituximab or R-CHOP/R-CVP in first-line treatment of indolent NHL or MCL: The BRIGHT study. *Blood, 123,* 2944–2952. https://doi.org/10.1182/blood-2013-11-531327

Garbe, C., Eigentler, T.K., Keilholz, U., Hauschild, A., & Kirkwood, J.M. (2011). Systematic review of medical treatment in melanoma: Current status and future prospects. *Oncologist, 16,* 5–24. https://doi.org/10.1634/theoncologist.2010-0190

Hammers, H.J., Plimack, E.R., Infante, J.R., Rini, B.I., McDermott, D.F., Ernstoff, M., ... Amin, A. (2015). Expanded cohort results from CheckMate 016: A phase I study of nivolumab in combination with ipilimumab in metastatic renal cell carcinoma (mRCC). *Journal of Clinical Oncology, 33*(Suppl. 15), 4516.

Hellmann, M.D., Rizvi, N.A., Goldman, J.W., Gettinger, S.N., Borghaei, H., Brahmer, J.R., ... Antonia, S.J. (2017). Nivolumab plus ipilimumab as first-line treatment for advanced non-small-cell lung cancer (CheckMate 012): Results of an open-label, phase 1, multicohort study. *Lancet Oncology, 18,* 31–41. https://doi.org/10.1016/S1470-2045(16)30624-6

Herbst, R.S., Baas, P., Kim, D.-W., Felip, E., Pérez-Gracia, J.L., Han, J.-Y., … Garon, E.B. (2016). Pembrolizumab versus docetaxel for previously treated, PD-L1-positive, advanced non-small-cell lung cancer (KEYNOTE-010): A randomised controlled trial. *Lancet, 387,* 1540–1550. https://doi.org/10.1016/S0140-6736(15)01281-7

Hiddemann, W., Kneba, M., Dreyling, M., Schmitz, N., Lengfelder, E., Schmits, R., … Unterhalt, M. (2005). Frontline therapy with rituximab added to the combination of cyclophosphamide, doxorubicin, vincristine, and prednisone (CHOP) significantly improves the outcome for patients with advanced-stage follicular lymphoma compared with therapy with CHOP alone: Results of a prospective randomized study of the German Low-Grade Lymphoma Study Group. *Blood, 106,* 3725–3732. https://doi.org/10.1182/blood-2005-01-0016

Hodi, F.S., Chesney, J., Pavlick, A.C., Robert, C., Grossmann, K.F., McDermott, D.F., … Postow, M.A. (2016). Combined nivolumab and ipilimumab versus ipilimumab alone in patients with advanced melanoma: 2-year overall survival outcomes in a multicentre, randomised, controlled, phase 2 trial. *Lancet Oncology, 17,* 1558–1568. https://doi.org/10.1016/S1470-2045(16)30366-7

Hodi, F.S., O'Day, S.J., McDermott, D.F., Weber, R.W., Sosman, J.A., Haanen, J.B., … Urba, W.J. (2010). Improved survival with ipilimumab in patients with metastatic melanoma. *New England Journal of Medicine, 363,* 711–723. https://doi.org/10.1056/NEJMoa1003466

Illidge, T.M., Mayes, S., Pettengell, R., Bates, A.T., Bayne, M., Radford, J.A., … Morschhauser, F. (2014). Fractionated ⁹⁰Y-ibritumomab tiuxetan radioimmunotherapy as an initial therapy of follicular lymphoma: An international phase II study in patients requiring treatment according to GELF/BNLI criteria. *Journal of Clinical Oncology, 32,* 212–218. https://doi.org/10.1200/JCO.2013.50.3110

Ives, N.J., Stowe, R.L., Lorigan, P., & Wheatley, K. (2007). Chemotherapy compared with biochemotherapy for the treatment of metastatic melanoma: A meta-analysis of 18 trials involving 2,621 patients. *Journal of Clinical Oncology, 25,* 5426–5434. https://doi.org/10.1200/JCO.2007.12.0253

Knox, S.J., Goris, M.L., Trisler, K., Negrin, R., Davis, T., Liles, T.M., … Levy, R. (1996). Yttrium-90-labeled anti-CD20 monoclonal antibody therapy of recurrent B-cell lymphoma. *Clinical Cancer Research, 2,* 457–470.

Kraeber-Bodéré, F., Bodet-Milin, C., Rousseau, C., Eugène, T., Pallardy, A., Frampas, E., … Chérel, M. (2014). Radioimmunoconjugates for the treatment of cancer. *Seminars in Oncology, 41,* 613–622. https://doi.org/10.1053/j.seminoncol.2014.07.004

Larkin, J., Chiarion-Sileni, V., Gonzalez, R., Grob, J.J., Cowey, C.L., Lao, C.D., … Wolchok, J.D. (2015). Combined nivolumab and ipilimumab or monotherapy in untreated melanoma. *New England Journal of Medicine, 373,* 23–34. https://doi.org/10.1056/NEJMoa1504030

Larkin, J., Hodi, F.S., & Wolchok, J.D. (2015). Combined nivolumab and ipilimumab or monotherapy in untreated melanoma [Comment Letter]. *New England Journal of Medicine, 373,* 1270–1271. https://doi.org/10.1056/NEJMc1509660

Marcus, R., Imrie, K., Solal-Celigny, P., Catalano, J.V., Dmoszynska, A., Raposo, J.C., … Stein, G. (2008). Phase III study of R-CVP compared with cyclophosphamide, vincristine, and prednisone alone in patients with previously untreated advanced follicular lymphoma. *Journal of Clinical Oncology, 26,* 4579–4586. https://doi.org/10.1200/JCO.2007.13.5376

Morschhauser, F., Radford, J., Van Hoof, A., Vitolo, U., Soubeyran, P., Tilly, H., … Hagenbeek, A. (2008). Phase III trial of consolidation therapy with yttrium-90–ibritumomab tiuxetan compared with no additional therapy after first remission in advanced follicular lymphoma. *Journal of Clinical Oncology, 26,* 5156–5164. https://doi.org/10.1200/JCO.2008.17.2015

Motzer, R.J., Escudier, B., McDermott, D.F., George, S., Hammers, H.J., Srinivas, S., … Sharma, P. (2015). Nivolumab versus everolimus in advanced renal-cell carcinoma. *New England Journal of Medicine, 373,* 1803–1813. https://doi.org/10.1056/NEJMoa1510665

National Cancer Institute. (n.d.). NCI dictionary of cancer terms. Retrieved from https://www.cancer.gov/publications/dictionaries/cancer-terms

National Comprehensive Cancer Network. (2018a). *NCCN Clinical Practice Guidelines in Oncology (NCCN Guidelines®): B-cell lymphomas* [v.4.2018]. Retrieved from https://www.nccn.org/professionals/physician_gls/pdf/b-cell.pdf

National Comprehensive Cancer Network. (2018b). *NCCN Clinical Practice Guidelines in Oncology (NCCN Guidelines®): Melanoma* [v.2.2018]. Retrieved from https://www.nccn.org/professionals/physician_gls/pdf/melanoma.pdf

Reck, M., Rodríguez-Abreu, D., Robinson, A.G., Hui, R., Csőszi, T., Fülöp, A., ... Brahmer, J.R. (2016). Pembrolizumab versus chemotherapy for PD-L1–positive non–small-cell lung cancer. *New England Journal of Medicine, 375,* 1823–1833. https://doi.org/10.1056/NEJMoa1606774

Robert, C., Schachter, J., Long, G.V., Arance, A., Grob, J.J., Mortier, L., ... Ribas, A. (2015). Pembrolizumab versus ipilimumab in advanced melanoma. *New England Journal of Medicine, 372,* 2521–2532. https://doi.org/10.1056/NEJMoa1503093

Rummel, M.J., Niederle, N., Maschmeyer, G., Banat, G.A., von Grünhagen, U., Losem, C., ... Brugger, W. (2013). Bendamustine plus rituximab versus CHOP plus rituximab as first-line treatment for patients with indolent and mantle-cell lymphomas: An open-label, multicentre, randomised, phase 3 non-inferiority trial. *Lancet, 381,* 1203–1210. https://doi.org/10.1016/S0140-6736(12)61763-2

Sampson, J.H., Vlahovic, G., Sahebjam, S., Omuro, A.M.P., Baehring, J.M., Hafler, D.A., ... Reardon, D.A. (2015). Preliminary safety and activity of nivolumab and its combination with ipilimumab in recurrent glioblastoma (GBM): CHECKMATE-143. *Journal of Clinical Oncology, 33*(Suppl. 15), 3010.

Seiwert, T.Y., Burtness, B., Mehra, R., Weiss, J., Berger, R., Eder, J.P., ... Chow, L.Q. (2016). Safety and clinical activity of pembrolizumab for treatment of recurrent or metastatic squamous cell carcinoma of the head and neck (KEYNOTE-012): An open-label, multicentre, phase 1b trial. *Lancet Oncology, 17,* 956–965. https://doi.org/10.1016/S1470-2045(16)30066-3

Spectrum Pharmaceuticals, Inc. (2013). *Zevalin® (ibritumomab tiuxetan)* [Package insert]. Irvine, CA: Author.

van Oers, M.H.J., Klasa, R., Marcus, R.E., Wolf, M., Kimby, E., Gascoyne, R.D., ... Hagenbeek, A. (2006). Rituximab maintenance improves clinical outcome of relapsed/resistant follicular non-Hodgkin lymphoma in patients both with and without rituximab during induction: Results of a prospective randomized phase 3 intergroup trial. *Blood, 108,* 3295–3301. https://doi.org/10.1182/blood-2006-05-021113

Witzig, T.E., Gordon, L.I., Cabanillas, F., Czuczman, M.S., Emmanouilides, C., Joyce, R., ... White, C.A. (2002). Randomized controlled trial of yttrium-90–labeled ibritumomab tiuxetan radioimmunotherapy versus rituximab immunotherapy for patients with relapsed or refractory low-grade, follicular, or transformed B-cell non-Hodgkin's lymphoma. *Journal of Clinical Oncology, 20,* 2453–2463. https://doi.org/10.1200/JCO.2002.11.076

Witzig, T.E., Molina, A., Gordon, L.I., Emmanouilides, C., Schilder, R.J., Flinn, I.W., ... Wiseman, G.A. (2007). Long-term responses in patients with recurring or refractory B-cell non-Hodgkin lymphoma treated with yttrium 90 ibritumomab tiuxetan. *Cancer, 109,* 1804–1810. https://doi.org/10.1002/cncr.22617

Witzig, T.E., White, C.A., Wiseman, G.A., Gordon, L.I., Emmanouilides, C., Raubitschek, A., ... Grillo-López, A.J. (1999). Phase I/II trial of IDEC-Y2B8 radioimmunotherapy for treatment of relapsed or refractory CD20+ B-cell non-Hodgkin's lymphoma. *Journal of Clinical Oncology, 17,* 3793–3803. https://doi.org/10.1200/JCO.1999.17.12.3793

chapter ten

Biomarkers

Tracy Krause, BS, PharmD, BCOP

Introduction

Cancer is a collection of diseases that share the same characteristics of uncontrolled cellular growth and invasion. However, not all cancer cells are equal. As the understanding of cancer cell growth has expanded, patterns of pathogenesis from normal to malignant cells have been identified, including DNA mutations and changes in protein expression.

Genetic mutations, either inherited or acquired, have a significant impact on the pathogenesis of cancer. Genes that cause malignant features when mutated include proto-oncogenes and tumor suppressor genes. Proto-oncogenes code for cell growth processes and can be mutated to stay continuously active in cancer cells. Mutation of a proto-oncogene into an oncogene can lead to increased cellular growth through overexpression of specific enzymes or cellular receptors used for cell proliferation. Tumor suppressor genes help regulate cell growth, such as by DNA repair or apoptosis. Mutations in tumor suppressor genes can cause silencing of these genes, leading to unchecked cell proliferation and survival (Croce, 2008).

Knowing the characteristics of these cells is useful in assessing the risk and development of cancer and evaluating the impact of treatment beyond anatomic and morphologic assessment. Biologic markers, or biomarkers, are objectively assessed characteristics that are used as indicators of specific processes, such as pathophysiologic processes or pharmacologic responses (Biomarkers Definitions Working Group, 2001). Tumor biomarkers are quantitatively measurable molecules produced by cancer cells that can be assessed for indicators of presence, growth, or response (Chan & Schwartz, 2002).

Biomarkers can include a variety of molecules, such as genetic markers, proteins, antigens, hormones, and cell receptors. Tests for biomarkers can include many assay types and can vary depending on the molecule detected. Immunohistochemistry uses labeled molecules, such as protein- or receptor-specific antibodies, to find specific proteins in tissues; their target can include a specific receptor type, such as HER2 (Ludwig & Weinstein, 2005). Fluorescence in situ hybridization (FISH) uses fluorescent probes that detect a specific gene sequence in DNA. Because of its ability to mark parts of DNA, FISH can also be used to look for specific DNA translocations, such as the *BCR-ABL* gene in chronic myeloid leukemia. Polymerase chain reaction (PCR) can be used to detect a specific DNA sequence by generating copies of that sequence. PCR has been used in several assays to check for specific DNA mutations, such as within the genes that code for epidermal growth factor receptor (EGFR). Because of the diversity of possible markers, numerous specimen types can be used to isolate and evaluate these markers, including blood, serum, urine, and tumor tissue (Füzéry, Levin, Chan, & Chan, 2013).

History

The first oncology biomarker was recorded in 1848, when Henry Bence Jones published information on a newly discovered substance found in the urine of a patient with multiple myeloma (Jones, 1848). The light chain immunoglobulin, also called the Bence Jones protein, is still used today in the diagnosis and monitoring of patients with multiple myeloma.

In the 20th century, scientists identified alterations in other molecules in patients with cancer, including hormones and proteins. These new data led to the understanding and monitoring of markers such as the carcinoembryonic antigen (Gold, Shuster, & Freedman, 1978). In 1975, Köhler and Milstein published their experiences manufacturing specific antibodies, or monoclonal antibodies, through hybridomas. The development of monoclonal antibodies not only allowed for targeted therapies against specific proteins, but also for more sensitive, specific, and rapid testing for cancer-specific biomarkers. This led to the further development of immunoassays to target cancer-specific biomarkers, such as carbohydrate antigen 125 (Schmidt, 2011) and prostate-specific antigen (PSA) (Rao, Motiwala, & Karim, 2008). Refinement of this technology also fueled research on characteristics of and targets for chemotherapy and targeted therapies.

Research and development of genomics, the study of the function and change of a set of genes within the genome, has also expanded the use of genetic sequencing and the evaluation of gene mutations as prognostic and predictive biomarkers. Advancements in genomics, proteomics (the study of the function of cellular proteins), and cancer cell secretomics (the study of all large molecules secreted from cancer cells) have led to the identification of different types of markers (Brandi et al., 2018). As research in these fields becomes less intensive in time and resources, focus has shifted from the evaluation of disease with single-parameter assays to the evaluation of several genes and proteins via multiparametric assays, such as the Oncotype DX® assays, to evaluate the risk of cancer recurrence.

Liquid biopsy is a recent development in cancer biomarker research. Tumor cells can shed cell-free DNA into blood and urine. Analysis of a liquid sample, such as blood or serum, can detect tumor DNA in the early stages of a cancer, assess the efficacy of a cancer treatment, monitor for cancer recurrence or resistance mutations, or detect targetable driver mutations to guide treatment selection. Liquid biopsies can be completed in situations where surgical biopsy is not feasible, either because of tumor location or patient comorbidities. Blood or urine sampling for liquid biopsy screening can also be performed more often than invasive procedures, allowing for dynamic monitoring of patient response and early identification of resistance characteristics. Single-tissue samples from surgical biopsy can also miss important disease characteristics because of intertumoral and intratumoral heterogeneity; however, these may be identified in circulating free DNA. The theory of a liquid biopsy using circulating free DNA was first described in 1948 (Mandel & Metais, 1948), but it did not become practical until recent improvements in cancer pathophysiology and in the sensitivity of assays and equipment in detecting low levels of circulating tumor DNA. In 2016, the first liquid biopsy assay, the cobas® EGFR Mutation Test v2, was approved by the U.S. Food and Drug Administration (FDA). This test uses either tumor tissue or plasma samples to detect specific EGFR mutations. In patients with metastatic lung adenocarcinoma, it can detect EGFR mutations known to demonstrate efficacy or resistance with different EGFR small molecule inhibitors, allowing providers to choose the most appropriate cancer treatment (U.S. FDA, 2016). Multigene assays, such as Guardant360®, may be useful across a wide spectrum of advanced cancers.

Development

The clinical development of biomarkers into practical use is separated into five phases: clinical exploratory studies, development and validation of clinical assays, retrospective longitudinal studies of specimen repositories, prospective screening studies, and randomized controlled clinical trials (Pepe et al., 2001). Compared to clinical trials for drugs, not all biomarkers progress consecutively through phases during development and evaluation.

Clinical Uses

Biomarkers can be further defined by their impact on clinical management (see Table 10-1). Prognostic biomarkers are used to understand the qualities of a disease, including the risk of disease progression and survival. Monitoring biomarkers are used to identify disease, observe for disease progression, and evaluate therapeutic efficacy. Predictive biomarkers indicate subgroups of patients that would respond to a specific treatment. Pharmacodynamic biomarkers indicate drug effects, both efficacy and toxicity, on cells and biologic processes. Surrogate biomarkers can reliably substitute a clinically significant endpoint for outcomes (de Gramont et al., 2015). These biomarkers have become essential to clinical assessment, treatment, and drug development.

Screening, Diagnosing, and Monitoring

Some biomarkers are expressed or elevated antecedent to the development of malignant cells. Therefore, biomarker screening can be useful to evaluate patients for an increased risk of malignancy before cancer cells develop or before patients develop clinical symptoms of disease.

An example of biomarker screening is PSA for prostate cancer, as a correlation exists between increases in PSA and the incidence of prostate cancer. Normally, PSA is expressed by columnar epithelial cells, which are excreted within ejaculate and found at low levels in normal

TABLE 10-1 Clinical Questions by Biomarker Type

Biomarker Type	Questions
Screening/monitoring	Does the patient have cancer? Is the disease progressing? Is the cancer responding to treatment?
Pharmacodynamics	Is the patient at higher risk for adverse effects from a drug? Does the patient express the target for a specific medication? What is the optimal dose for a patient?
Predictive	Would the patient benefit from a specific therapy? What is the chance for response to therapy?
Prognostic	Is the patient likely to develop a specific cancer? What is the chance for survival or cure?
Surrogate	Is a clinically beneficial endpoint anticipated?

Note. Based on information from de Gramont et al., 2015.

serum. As prostate cancer develops within the glandular tissue, disruption of the basement membrane, caused by tissue invasion and luminal secretion, leads to increased secretion and diffusion of PSA into the blood. Therefore, serum PSA increases can be seen in patients with histologically proven prostate cancer. This increase can be discovered in patients before lesions are found by physical or radiologic examination. Several providers use PSA levels during assessment for prostate cancer screening (Kulasingam & Diamandis, 2008).

Histologic confirmation is usually required for a cancer diagnosis, but biomarker testing can assist in identifying appropriate patients for further assessment and biopsy (see Table 10-2). Markers for malignant mutations can be assessed through immunoassays, FISH, or PCR.

Prognostic and Predictive Tools

For patients with solid tumors, physical properties such as tumor size and lymph node involvement have been included in the standard for staging and the decision for a treatment plan, particularly when surgery is a clinical option. Physical properties and staging can roughly correlate to prognosis, in which larger and more extensive involvement correlates with poorer prognosis. However, biomarkers such as cytogenetic abnormalities and cellular molecular markers provide more information and a finer clinical assessment of prognosis (Ludwig & Weinstein, 2005). A common biomarker is lactate dehydrogenase, which is used in cancers such as lymphoma and melanoma to evaluate tumor burden and prognosis. Another biomarker includes the evaluation of acute leukemia using World Health Organization guidelines. By reviewing cytogenetic mutations, such as genetic translocations or deletions, and molecular abnormalities, such as mutated tyrosine kinases, a prognosis is more detailed than a histology review alone.

Biomarkers can also be used to predict the efficacy or toxicity of different cancer treatments (see Table 10-3). Pharmacogenomics studies the influence of genetic polymorphisms and mutations on the pharmacokinetics and pharmacodynamics of drugs. These genetic variations can be used as markers prior to therapy to assess for chance of efficacy and risk of side effects. An example of a pharmacodynamic biomarker is the evaluation of UGT1A1, an enzyme used for inactivation of SN-38 (a toxic metabolite of irinotecan). Patients with a homozygous variation of the *UGT1A1* gene, called *UGT1A1*28*, accumulate SN-38 at higher levels than patients with the normal (wild-type) enzyme, putting them at higher risk of toxicity (e.g., neutropenia) (Relling & Dervieux, 2001). The impact of *UGT1A1* is so prominent that the package insert for irinotecan includes warnings for use in this patient population and rec-

TABLE 10-2 Approved Biomarker Tests

Biomarker	Assay	Assay Type	Sample Type	Drug	Cancer Type
PD-L1	PD-L1 IHC 22C3 pharmDx™	IHC	FFPET	Pembrolizumab	Melanoma, lung
EGFR	cobas® EGFR Mutation Test	PCR	FFPET	Erlotinib	Lung
	cobas EGFR Mutation Test v2	PCR	FFPET, plasma	Erlotinib, osimertinib	Lung
	therascreen® EGFR RGQ PCR Kit	PCR	FFPET	Afatinib, gefitinib	Lung
	Dako EGFR pharmDx™ Kit	IHC	FFPET	Cetuximab, panitumumab	Colorectal
LSI TP53	Vysis CLL FISH Probe Kit	FISH	Blood	Venetoclax	CLL
KIT	KIT D816V assay	PCR	Bone marrow	Imatinib	Aggressive systemic mastocytosis
	Dako c-KIT pharmDx	IHC	FFPET	Imatinib	Gastrointestinal stromal tumors
PDGFRB	PDGFRB FISH Assay	FISH	Bone marrow	Imatinib	Myelodysplastic syndrome, myeloproliferative disease
ALK	Ventana ALK (D5F3) CDx assay	IHC	FFPET	Crizotinib	Lung

(Continued on next page)

TABLE 10-2 Approved Biomarker Tests *(Continued)*

Biomarker	Assay	Assay Type	Sample Type	Drug	Cancer Type
ALK (cont.)	Vysis ALK Break Apart FISH Probe Kit	FISH	FFPET	Crizotinib	Lung
KRAS	cobas KRAS Mutation Test	PCR	FFPET	Cetuximab, panitumumab	Colorectal
	therascreen KRAS RGQ PCR Kit	PCR	FFPET	Cetuximab, panitumumab	Colorectal
BRCA1, BRCA2	BRACAnalysis CDx™	PCR	Blood	Olaparib	Breast
HER2	INFORM HER2/NEU	FISH	FFPET	Trastuzumab	Breast
	PathVysion HER-2 DNA Probe Kit	FISH	FFPET	Trastuzumab	Breast
	PATHWAY anti-HER-2/NEU	IHC	FFPET	Trastuzumab	Breast
	InSite HER-2/NEU Kit	IHC	FFPET	Trastuzumab	Breast
	SPOT-Light® HER2 CISH Kit	CISH	FFPET	Trastuzumab	Breast
	Bond Oracle HER2 IHC System	IHC	FFPET	Trastuzumab	Breast
	HER2 CISH pharmDx Kit	CISH	FFPET	Trastuzumab	Breast
	HercepTest™	IHC	FFPET	Trastuzumab, pertuzumab, ado-trastuzumab emtan-sine	Breast

(Continued on next page)

TABLE 10-2 Approved Biomarker Tests *(Continued)*

Biomarker	Assay	Assay Type	Sample Type	Drug	Cancer Type
HER2 *(cont.)*	HER2 FISH pharmDx Kit	FISH	FFPET	Trastuzumab, pertuzumab, ado-trastuzumab emtansine	Breast
BRAF	THxID® BRAF Kit	PCR	FFPET	Trametinib, dabrafenib	Melanoma
	cobas 4800 BRAF V600 Mutation Test	PCR	FFPET	Vemurafenib	Melanoma

ALK—anaplastic lymphoma kinase; CISH—chromogenic in situ hybridization; CLL—chronic lymphocytic leukemia; EGFR—epidermal growth factor receptor; FFPET—formalin-fixed paraffin-embedded tissue; FISH—fluorescence in situ hybridization; IHC—immunohistochemistry; PCR—polymerase chain reaction; *PDGFRB*—platelet-derived growth factor receptor beta; PD-L1—programmed cell death-ligand 1

Note. From "List of Cleared of Approved Companion Diagnostic Devices (In Vitro and Imaging Tools)," by U.S. Food and Drug Administration, 2017. Retrieved from https://www.fda.gov/medicaldevices/productsandmedicalprocedures/invitrodiagnostics/ucm301431.htm.

ommends dose reductions in patients with decreased UGT1A1 activity (Pfizer Inc., 2016).

Recently, immunotherapeutic agents have increased the identification of biomarkers, improving efficacy and allowing for appropriate patient selection. In PD-1/PD-L1 (programmed cell death

TABLE 10-3 Biomarkers in Drug Labeling

Biomarker	Drugs	Impact
ALK	Alectinib, ceritinib, crizotinib	Indication
BCR-ABL1	Bosutinib, dasatinib, imatinib, nilotinib, omacetaxine, ponatinib	Indication
BRAF	Cobimetinib, dabrafenib, trametinib, vemurafenib	Indication
BRCA1/2	Olaparib	Indication
CD20 (MS4A1)	Obinutuzumab, rituximab, tositumomab	Indication
del (5q)	Lenalidomide	Indication
del (17p)	Ibrutinib	Indication
DPYD	Capecitabine, 5-fluorouracil	Safety
EGFR	Afatinib, cetuximab, erlotinib, gefitinib, osimertinib, panitumumab	Indication
ESR1	Anastrazole, exemestane, palbociclib	Indication
G6PD	Dabrafenib, rasburicase	Safety
HER2 (ERBB2)	Ado-trastuzumab emtansine, lapatinib, palbociclib, pertuzumab, trastuzumab	Indication
KIT	Imatinib	Indication
KRAS	Cetuximab, panitumumab	Indication
PD-L1 (CD274)	Nivolumab, pembrolizumab	Pharmacology
PML-RARA	Arsenic trioxide, tretinoin	Indication
PR	Anastrozole, exemestane, fulvestrant, letrozole, tamoxifen	Indication
TPMT	Cisplatin, mercaptopurine, thioguanine	Safety
UGT1A1	Belinostat, irinotecan, nilotinib, pazopanib	Safety

ALK—anaplastic lymphoma kinase; DPYD—dihydropyrimidine dehydrogenase; EGFR—epidermal growth factor receptor; PD-L1—programmed cell death-ligand 1; PR—progesterone receptor

Note. From "Table of Pharmacogenomic Biomarkers in Drug Labeling," by U.S. Food and Drug Administration, 2017. Retrieved from http://www.fda.gov/Drugs/ScienceResearch/ResearchAreas/Pharmacogenetics/ucm083378.htm.

protein 1/programmed cell death-ligand 1) immune checkpoint immunotherapy, evaluation of PD-1 expression has been correlated with improved patient response (Yuan et al., 2016). The use of immunotherapies in appropriate patients, such as those with metastatic lung cancer, can lead to durable response without the side effects of conventional chemotherapy.

Therapeutic Targets

With the increased availability of several targeted therapies, a biomarker assessment can allow for an ideal primary treatment. For example, assessment of estrogen receptor (ER), progesterone receptor (PR), and HER2 during the primary assessment of breast cancer can help prevent the use of conventional chemotherapy and its inherent toxicities in specific stages where antihormonal therapy is effective in patient treatment. Additionally, patients expressing HER2 can receive targeted therapies that increase patient response and survival. EGFR-targeting agents can also be used in patients with advanced-stage lung cancer (La Thangue & Kerr, 2011).

Surrogate Endpoints

Within clinical trials, surrogate biomarkers can be used as substitutes in the evaluation of a clinical endpoint (Biomarkers Definitions Working Group, 2001). When a biomarker is known to reliably correlate to a clinical endpoint, such as survival or response, evaluation can be cheaper, easier to measure, and faster to evaluate than clinical response (Aronson, 2005). Evaluation of laboratory responses to therapy, such as decreases in serum and urine protein, can be used as surrogate endpoints to clinical response and predict patient survival in multiple myeloma. However, finding reliable biomarkers to use as surrogate endpoints for cancer care can be complicated because of the complex mechanisms of disease and interventions and the interpatient variability of biomarker expression (Aronson, 2005).

Benefits

Compared to radiologic and physical examinations, biomarker tests can be more vigilant in finding abnormal signs related to disease. For a solid tumor to be visualized via radiologic methods, a significant number of abnormal cells are required. Specific cancer biomarkers can discover disease before the development of clinical symptoms. These markers can also find disease less than the lower limit of detection of radiologic tests.

Biomarkers can also be used as a confirmatory test prior to invasive procedures, such as a biopsy. This prevents the use of unnecessary invasive procedures and increases the yield of these procedures.

Challenges

Despite the high number of biomarkers used for cancers, not all are integrated into clinical assessment. For a biomarker to be widely used in practice, it must be practical and have an impact on clinical outcomes. Several issues may prevent the use of specific biomarkers.

An ideal tumor marker is identifiable in patients who have or will develop a specific disease. It also must have an adequate interval to intervene to improve patient outcome. Unfortunately, most biomarkers do not reach this goal (Kulasingam & Diamandis, 2008). Current biomarkers do not have perfect specificity to a type of cancer. Some biomarkers can be elevated in patients with other disease states without having cancer. An example involves the use of PSA for prostate cancer. Patients can have decreases or elevations in PSA for other reasons, such as benign prostatic hyperplasia, medication use, or age. Although biomarkers can be detected and indicate a true disease or disease recurrence, not all are found at a time when treatment can affect outcome. The U.S. Preventive Services Task Force does not currently recommend the widespread use of PSA screening, as there has not been a significant improvement in prostate cancer–related mortality to outweigh the risk of diagnostic complications (Moyer, 2012). A specific biomarker useful in the early stages of disease may lose utility in the later stages of the disease; refined understanding of the predictive power of these markers is required for effective care (Burke, 2016).

As the use of biomarkers continues to increase, standardization is necessary. In the evaluation of new biomarkers, data received from one test or one institution may not be considered equivalent to data of the same biomarker from another test or institution. Variations in specimen handling and storage, laboratory procedure and regulations for instruments and reagents needed for biomarker evaluation, and differences in study design can result in discrepancies.

Evaluation of genetic and protein biomarkers has led to the use of sophisticated instruments, including mass spectrometry, genomic microarrays, and specialized immunoassays. These instruments can be highly specialized to a specific marker and have significant monetary costs. In practice, evaluation of specific biomarkers may not be feasible at smaller institutions because of these costs. Lower utilization of specialized tests in less common diseases is also a factor. In the absence of on-site equipment, samples are usually sent to an outside facility for processing, which can lead to delays and increase the risk of mishandling by degrading or loss (de Gramont et al., 2015).

The use of biomarkers to enhance oncologic management is a promising idea, but despite rigorous research, only few have been successfully translated into practical use. Ioannidis (2013) classified failures into four separate types: clinical reversal, validation failure, nonoptimized clinical translation, and promotion despite nonpromising evidence. Clinical reversal occurs when a biomarker accepted into clinical practice is later found to not have the anticipated clinical impact. Validation failure occurs when a promising biomarker in clinical trials is later found to have exaggerated results. Nonoptimized clinical translation occurs when a promising biomarker is not followed up because of lack of support or interest. Promotion despite nonpromising evidence is the promotion of a biomarker assessment when no or little data support widespread use. In cancer research, all these failures have been seen.

Future Directions

As new biomarkers are discovered and current information regarding biomarkers increases, practical use of assessments within clinical settings continues to evolve. Currently, the American Society of Clinical Oncology recommends biomarker assessment in different malignancies only when it affects patient treatments or outcomes (Van Poznak et al., 2015). The National Comprehensive Cancer Network® (n.d.) Biomarkers Compendium can assist providers in evaluating the clinical impact of available biomarker tests. In 2010, the American Association for Cancer Research, the National Cancer Institute, and FDA collaborated to provide regulatory guidance and to find methods to speed the development and practical use of biomarker evaluation (Khleif, Doroshow, & Hait, 2010).

Nursing Implications

Knowing the impact of biomarkers on a specific disease may enhance understanding of the disease. As biomarker assessment moves from using biopsied tissue directly from the tumor to using more readily available blood samples, nurses may be called upon for appropriate drawing, handling, and delivery of these samples for evaluation. The use of targeted agents for specific biomarkers has created a multitude of FDA-approved medications and immunotherapies to treat different disease states. Nurses need to learn how to use and administer these medications, as well as how to monitor and manage their unique side effects.

Summary

Identification and evaluation of biomarkers continues to be an emerging area of clinical practice within oncology. Over recent years, several biomarkers have been identified in different disease states that have allowed for targeted therapy. As biomarkers continue to be discovered, systematic review of the utility of these biomarkers is important prior to integration into clinical practice.

References

Aronson, J.K. (2005). Biomarkers and surrogate endpoints. *British Journal of Clinical Pharmacology, 59*, 491–494. https://doi.org/10.1111/j.1365-2125.2005.02435.x

Biomarkers Definitions Working Group. (2001). Biomarkers and surrogate endpoints: Preferred definitions and conceptual framework. *Clinical Pharmacology and Therapeutics, 69*, 89–95. https://doi.org/10.1067/mcp.2001.113989

Brandi, J., Manfredi, M., Speziali, G., Gosetti, F., Marengo, E., & Cecconi, D. (2018). Proteomic approaches to decipher cancer cell secretome. *Seminars in Cell and Developmental Biology, 78*, 93–131. https://doi.org/10.1016/j.semcdb.2017.06.030

Burke, H.B. (2016). Predicting clinical outcomes using molecular biomarkers. *Biomarkers in Cancer, 8*, 89–99. https://doi.org/10.4137/BIC.S33380

Chan, D.W., & Schwartz, M.K. (2002). Tumor markers: Introduction and general principles. In E.P. Diamandis, H.A. Fritsche, H. Lilja, D.W. Chan, & M.K Schwartz (Eds.), *Tumor markers: Physiology, pathobiology, technology, and clinical applications* (pp. 9–17). Washington, DC: AACC Press.

Croce, C.M. (2008). Oncogenes and cancer. *New England Journal of Medicine, 358*, 502–511. https://doi.org/10.1056/NEJMra072367

de Gramont, A., Watson, S., Ellis, L.M., Rodón, J., Tabernero, J., de Gramont, A., & Hamilton, S.R. (2015). Pragmatic issues in biomarker evaluation for targeted therapies in cancer. *Nature Reviews Clinical Oncology, 12*, 197–212. https://doi.org/10.1038/nrclinonc.2014.202

Füzéry, A.K., Levin, J., Chan, M.M., & Chan, D.W. (2013). Translation of proteomic biomarkers into FDA approved cancer diagnostics: Issues and challenges. *Clinical Proteomics, 10*, 13. https://doi.org/10.1186/1559-0275-10-13

Gold, P., Shuster, J., & Freedman, S.O. (1978). Carcinoembryonic antigen (CEA) in clinical medicine. Historical perspectives, pitfalls and projections. *Cancer, 42*(Suppl. S3), 1399–1405.

Ioannidis, J.P.A. (2013). Biomarker failures. *Clinical Chemistry, 59*, 202–204. https://doi.org/10.1373/clinchem.2012.185801

Jones, H.B. (1848). III. On a new substance occurring in the urine of a patient with mollities ossium. *Philosophical Transactions of the Royal Society of London, 138*, 55–62. https://doi.org/10.1098/rstl.1848.0003

Khleif, S.N., Doroshow, J.H., & Hait, W.N. (2010). AACR-FDA-NCI cancer biomarkers collaborative consensus report: Advancing the use of biomarkers in cancer drug development. *Clinical Cancer Research, 16*, 3299–3318. https://doi.org/10.1158/1078-0432.CCR-10-0880

Köhler, G., & Milstein, C. (1975). Continuous cultures of fused cells secreting antibody of predefined specificity. *Nature, 256,* 495–497. https://doi.org/10.1038/256495a0

Kulasingam, V., & Diamandis, E.P. (2008). Strategies for discovering novel cancer biomarkers through utilization of emerging technologies. *Nature Reviews Clinical Oncology, 5,* 588–599. https://doi.org/10.1038/ncponc1187

La Thangue, N.B., & Kerr, D.J. (2011). Predictive biomarkers: A paradigm shift towards personalized cancer medicine. *Nature Reviews Clinical Oncology, 8,* 587–596. https://doi.org/10.1038/nrclinonc.2011.121

Ludwig, J.A., & Weinstein, J.N. (2005). Biomarkers in cancer staging, prognosis and treatment selection. *Nature Reviews Cancer, 5,* 845–856. https://doi.org/10.1038/nrc1739

Mandel, P., & Metais, P. (1948). Les acides nucleiques du plasma sanguin chez l'homme. *Comptes Rendus des Seances de la Societe de Biologie et de ses Filiales, 142,* 241–243.

Moyer, V.A. (2012). Screening for prostate cancer: U.S. Preventive Services Task Force recommendation statement. *Annals of Internal Medicine, 157,* 120–134. https://doi.org/10.7326/0003-4819-157-2-201207170-00459

National Comprehensive Cancer Network. (n.d.). About the NCCN Biomarkers Compendium®. Retrieved from https://www.nccn.org/professionals/biomarkers/default.aspx

Pepe, M.S., Etzioni, R., Feng, Z., Potter, J.D., Thompson, M.L., Thornquist, M., … Yasui, Y. (2001). Phases of biomarker development for early detection of cancer. *Journal of the National Cancer Institute, 93,* 1054–1061. https://doi.org/10.1093/jnci/93.14.1054

Pfizer Inc. (2016). *Camptosar® (irinotecan)* [Package insert]. New York, NY: Author.

Rao, A.R., Motiwala, H.G., & Karim, O.M.A. (2008). The discovery of prostate-specific antigen. *BJU International, 101,* 5–10. https://doi.org/10.1111/j.1464-410X.2007.07138.x

Relling, M.V., & Dervieux, T. (2001). Pharmacogenetics and cancer therapy. *Nature Reviews Cancer, 1,* 99–108. https://doi.org/10.1038/35101056

Schmidt, C. (2011). CA-125: A biomarker put to the test. *Journal of the National Cancer Institute, 103,* 1290–1291. https://doi.org/10.1093/jnci/djr344

U.S. Food and Drug Administration. (2016). Cobas EGFR Mutation Test v2. Retrieved from https://www.fda.gov/Drugs/InformationOnDrugs/ApprovedDrugs/ucm504540.htm

Van Poznak, C., Somerfield, M.R., Bast, R.C., Cristofanilli, M., Goetz, M.P., Gonzalez-Angulo, A.M., … Harris, L.N. (2015). Use of biomarkers to guide decisions on systemic therapy for women with metastatic breast cancer: American Society of Clinical Oncology Clinical practice guideline. *Journal of Clinical Oncology, 33,* 2695–2704. https://doi.org/10.1200/JCO.2015.61.1459

Yuan, J., Hegde, P.S., Clynes, R., Foukas, P.G., Harari, A., Kleen, T.O., … Fox, B.A. (2016). Novel technologies and emerging biomarkers for personalized cancer immunotherapy. *Journal for Immunotherapy of Cancer, 4,* 3. https://doi.org/10.1186/s40425-016-0107-3

chapter eleven

Case-Based Management Strategies and Patient Education

Susan J. McCall, MSN, ANP-BC, AOCNP®

Introduction

In an era of evolutionary cancer therapeutics, the ability to harness and manipulate the power of the human immune system has led to the ability to target, control, and—in several cases—cure deleterious malignant diagnoses. The advent of immunomodulatory drugs (IMiDs), cellular therapies, and checkpoint inhibitors has changed the landscape of available treatment options for patients with cancer. As these immune-based therapies make their way through the clinical trial pipeline and into practice, nurses and clinicians will begin to care for a greater number of patients receiving immunotherapy agents.

It is imperative for oncology nurses to have a firm understanding of the toxicity profiles of these drugs, as a sound knowledge base will optimize patient outcomes by enabling nurses to provide education to patients and family members, anticipate potential adverse reactions, and implement prompt intervention in the event of an adverse reaction.

Immune-Related Adverse Events From Checkpoint Inhibitors

Although immunotherapy and immunomodulatory agents have demonstrated significant benefits to patients with various malignancies, this class of drugs carries a unique side effect profile. Immunotherapy agents, specifically those that block checkpoint pathways, can incite a generalized inflammatory state and cause immune-related adverse events (irAEs) (Postow, 2015). These events mimic autoimmune disorders and can disrupt normal cellular function. A major driver for irAEs is activation of CD4 and CD8 T cells, which infiltrate normal tissue. This can lead to increased production of inflammatory cytokines (Kaehler et al., 2010), which can affect any organ system. No current prognostic markers can predict a patient's propensity to develop these irAEs.

The most common irAEs involve the skin, gastrointestinal tract, liver, and endocrine system. Less commonly, irAEs can also afflict the pulmonary, neurologic, ocular, renal, and hematologic systems. Of note, the term *immune-related adverse event* has not been consistently described in clinical trials and the literature (Maughan, Bailey, Gill, & Agarwal, 2017); however, for purposes of this discussion, it is any toxicity with a potential immune-mediated etiology that may or may not require use of an immune-modulating therapy (e.g., steroids) after other diagnoses have been ruled out.

No prospective randomized clinical trials have been conducted that investigate irAE treatments. Instead, expert recommendations for management of irAEs have been published based on retrospective data and analyses. The American Society of Clinical Oncology (ASCO) and the National Comprehensive Cancer Network® (NCCN®) have recently collaborated to develop formal clinical practice guidelines for the management of irAEs (Brahmer et al., 2018; NCCN & ASCO, 2018). For more current formal published guidelines on this topic, see AstraZeneca Pharmaceuticals LP, 2018; Bristol-Myers Squibb Co., n.d., 2018a, 2018b; Genentech, Inc., 2017b; Haanen et al., 2017; and Merck and Co., Inc., 2017a.

The nomenclature for organs afflicted with inflammation usually includes the suffix "-itis": thyroiditis (inflammation of the thyroid), pneumonitis (inflammation of the lungs), colitis (inflammation of the colon), pancreatitis (inflammation of the pancreas), and more. Patients should receive education regarding these potential "-itis" conditions prior to the start of therapy and for the duration of treatment, ideally at every encounter. They should also be informed of the risks of infusion-related reactions and fatigue; these adverse events have been reported with checkpoint inhibitors as well. When appropriate, education should also include family members and caregivers.

NCCN (n.d.) has developed an Immunotherapy Teaching/Monitoring Tool to help clinicians provide education to patients regarding immunotherapy and irAEs. This tool provides information for each agent, including indications, mechanisms of action, and dosing relevant to a disease. It also details toxicity information, including signs, symptoms, and monitoring parameters, organized by organ system, as well as monitoring questionnaires to be provided to patients prior to each dose. Toxicity management recommendations are also included for the healthcare team. Additionally, recently published NCCN guidelines for management of immune-related toxicities include principles of immunotherapy patient education (NCCN & ASCO, 2018). These educational concepts are a useful guide for providing education regarding immunotherapy mechanisms of action, side effects, and monitoring frequencies.

Another useful resource for patients is a wallet card, a small leaflet that includes the treatment name, physician contact information, and signs and symptoms of adverse events to report to the healthcare team. These wallet cards are intended to serve as a guide for patients and are also pertinent for other healthcare providers, such as primary care physicians or other specialists (McGettigan & Rubin, 2017). In addition to carrying a list of active home medications, patients should be encouraged to always carry a wallet card while receiving immunotherapy agents. Wallet cards have been published by various pharmaceutical companies for various medications, including IV and oral agents.

The management of adverse events varies depending on the grade (severity) of the event. The Common Terminology Criteria for Adverse Events (CTCAE) is an excellent tool for grading the severity of toxicities related to immunotherapy agents. It primarily defines symptom severity to guide clinicians on when and how to intervene (National Cancer Institute Cancer Therapy Evaluation Program, 2017). In general, grade 1 events are mild, grade 2 events are moderate, grade 3 events are severe, grade 4 events are life threatening, and grade 5 events are death. For many toxicities, treatment interruption is recommended for grade 2 or 3 events. Dose discontinuation is indicated for some grade 3 events and a majority of grade 4 events. Treatment is typically resumed when a symptom or toxicity improves to grade 1 or less (Postow & Wolchok, 2017).

The onset of adverse events varies by organ and can be seen as early as one week after first infusion to as late as several months after treatment discontinuation. Nurses must assess patients regularly, perhaps between office visits, to screen for signs and symptoms of irAEs. NCCN and ASCO (2018) recommend monitoring for irAEs for at least one year following the conclusion of immunotherapy. Patients should be reminded that irAEs are treatable, but they need to report symptoms early for prompt treatment.

For mild toxicities, monitoring may be appropriate, and immunotherapy treatment can continue. If a patient is having mild symptoms, topical or localized intervention (e.g., topical steroid cream for localized rash) is appropriate. For moderate or severe toxicities requiring treatment interruption, systemic corticosteroids (prednisone or equivalent) are indicated in most cases. The use of corticosteroids temporarily suppresses immune response, and symptoms are often improved and reversed in a short period of time. Depending on the type and severity of the toxicity, the dosage of steroids usually ranges 0.5–2 mg (of prednisone or equivalent) per kilogram of body weight per day (Brahmer et al., 2018; Postow & Wolchok, 2017). Other supportive medications and interventions may also be necessary. It is important to consider infectious disease prophylaxis for any patient with cancer receiving a prolonged taper course (NCCN, 2017), as well as blood sugar monitoring, especially in patients with a diabetic comorbidity. Referral to a specialist should be considered.

If a patient experiences a severe toxicity or if toxicity is not manageable with systemic steroids alone, referral to a specialist is compulsory, and permanent treatment discontinuation may be indicated. Other agents, such as tumor necrosis factor-alpha antagonists (infliximab [Remicade®]), cyclophosphamide, or mycophenolate mofetil, can be effective in steroid-refractory cases (Brahmer et al., 2018; Marrone, Ying, & Naidoo, 2016; Postow & Wolchok, 2017). Although no formal on-label indication for use exists, the dose of infliximab generally used to treat steroid-refractory irAEs is 5 mg/kg IV every two weeks (Janssen Biotech, Inc., 2017; Postow, 2015).

The incidence of all-grade adverse events with checkpoint inhibitors varies in the literature, ranging 30%–90% in single-agent clinical trials (Bertrand, Kostine, Barnetche, Truchetet, & Schaeverbeke, 2015; Chuzi et al., 2017; Marrone et al., 2016; Michot et al., 2016; Weber, Dummer, de Pril, Lebbé, & Hodi, 2013). Combination therapy, specifically the use of a cytotoxic T-lymphocyte antigen 4 (CTLA-4) inhibitor (ipilimumab) and a programmed cell death protein 1 (PD-1) inhibitor, has been reported to elicit a greater number of adverse events (Bristol-Myers Squibb Co., 2018b; Larkin et al., 2015). Combination immunotherapy with radiation, chemotherapy, or other targeted agents may also increase the severity of adverse events (NCCN & ASCO, 2018). In addition, higher doses of ipilimumab are associated with a higher frequency of irAEs (Wolchok et al., 2010). As new combination therapies that include checkpoint inhibitors are given to patients with cancer, it is likely adverse events incidence will increase. Table 11-1 summarizes the frequency of common adverse events, including irAEs, according to formal prescribing information for each checkpoint inhibitor.

Death has been reported in a very small number of patients receiving immunotherapy agents. In a systematic review of 1,265 patients from 22 clinical trials receiving a CTLA-4 inhibitor, death was reported in 11 patients (0.86%) (Bertrand et al., 2015). Most deaths were related to bowel perforation in the setting of colitis, but some were associated with hepatic failure. Other grade 5 (death) events related to checkpoint inhibitors include fatal pneumonitis and renal failure (EMD Serono, Inc., 2017; Genentech, Inc., 2017b; Topalian et al., 2012).

TABLE 11-1 Frequency of Immune-Related Adverse Events

All-Grade Immune-Related Adverse Events (%)	CTLA-4 Inhibitors	PD-1 Inhibitors		Combination CTLA-4 and PD-1 Inhibitors	PD-L1 Inhibitors		
	Ipilimumab (Yervoy®)	Nivolumab (Opdivo®)	Pembrolizumab (Keytruda®)	Ipilimumab and Nivolumab	Durvalumab (Imfinzi®)	Atezolizumab (Tecentriq®)	Avelumab (Bavencio®)
Rash	14.5–25	9	17–24	22.6	15.6	13–15	22
Colitis/diarrhea	13–30	2.9	1.7	26	1.3	19.7	1.5
Hepatitis	4.5–16	1.8	0.7	13	2.8–4.3	1.6–2.5	0.9
Pneumonitis	0.2	3.1	3.4	6	2.3	2.6	1.2
Endocrine	28	–	–	–	–	–	–
Thyroid dysfunction	–	11.7	12.5	30	15.3	4.9	6
Adrenal insufficiency	–	1	–	5	0.9	0.4	0.5
Hypophysitis	–	0.6	0.6	9	< 0.1	0.2	–
Type 1 DM	–	0.9	0.2	1.5	< 0.1	0.3	0.1

(Continued on next page)

TABLE 11-1 Frequency of Immune-Related Adverse Events *(Continued)*

All-Grade Immune-Related Adverse Events (%)	CTLA-4 Inhibitors	PD-1 Inhibitors		Combination CTLA-4 and PD-1 Inhibitors	PD-L1 Inhibitors		
	Ipilimumab (Yervoy®)	Nivolumab (Opdivo®)	Pembrolizumab (Keytruda®)	Ipilimumab and Nivolumab	Durvalumab (Imfinzi®)	Atezolizumab (Tecentriq®)	Avelumab (Bavencio®)
Nephritis/renal dysfunction	< 1	1.2	0.3	2.2	–	–	0.1
Infusion-related reactions	< 1	6.4	0.2	2.5	1.8	1.3–1.7	25
Fatigue	41–46	39–59	26–38	–	39	46–52	41–50

CTLA-4—cytotoxic T-lymphocyte antigen 4; DM—diabetes mellitus; PD-1—programmed cell death protein 1; PD-L1—programmed cell death-ligand 1

Note. Based on information from AstraZeneca Pharmaceuticals LP, 2018; Bristol-Myers Squibb Co, 2018a, 2018b; EMD Serono, Inc., 2017; Genentech, Inc., 2017b; Merck and Co., Inc., 2017a, 2017b.

Case-Based Management of Toxicities Related to Therapy

Dermatologic

Case 1

G.M., a 78-year-old male lawyer with a past medical history of hyperlipidemia and hypertension, was recently diagnosed with stage IV lung adenocarcinoma with metastatic disease to the brain. He received frontline therapy in a clinical trial with a PD-1 inhibitor. One month after initiating treatment, he developed a pruritic, macular rash to his upper chest that progressed to his abdomen. Complete blood count was notable for elevated eosinophils (13%). He was referred to a dermatologist for consultation, and his examination was remarkable for blanching pink macules over the anterior and posterior trunk and extremities. A biopsy of the rash demonstrated mild superficial spongiotic and perivascular dermatitis with scattered eosinophils and neutrophils, most consistent with a hypersensitivity reaction (see Figure 11-1). He was treated with topical steroids (clobetasol), and his rash improved over the next three days. He continued immunotherapy without any recurrence of rash and was able to achieve a complete remission. He is currently without any evidence of disease and is working full time as a law professor at a local university.

Case 2

C.T. is a 35-year-old male graphic design artist with a past medical history of osteosarcoma and a below-the-knee left leg amputation during childhood. He was diagnosed with renal cell carcinoma and underwent a partial nephrectomy; however, five months later, C.T. was found to have metastatic disease. He received antiangiogenic therapy but had progression of disease. C.T. initiated treatment with a PD-1 inhibitor on a clinical trial. Two months after starting therapy, he developed ill-defined pruritic eczematous plaques on his upper legs and trunk. He was referred to a dermatologist, who biopsied one of the plaques. Results demonstrated psoriasiform and spongiotic dermatitis consistent with eczema. C.T. was given a prescription for a topical steroid cream, which he used as needed with good relief. His plaques stabilized, and he continued therapy for six more months. Eventually, his plaques slowly increased in size and his pruritus became more intense. The dermatologist described the findings as a severe exacerbation of previously diagnosed psoriasis, and therapy was interrupted (see Figure 11-2). Phototherapy was recommended, but C.T. preferred other treatment. He was prescribed a course of systemic prednisone 1 mg/kg and mycophenolate mofetil, after which his plaques and pruritus resolved. Given the severity of his symptoms, he did not restart therapy.

FIGURE 11-1 Diffuse Erythematous Rash Related to a Checkpoint Inhibitor

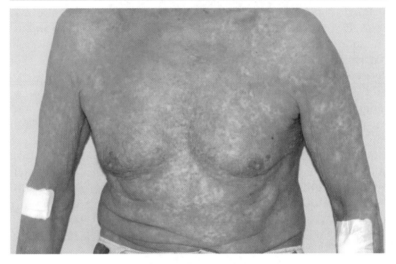

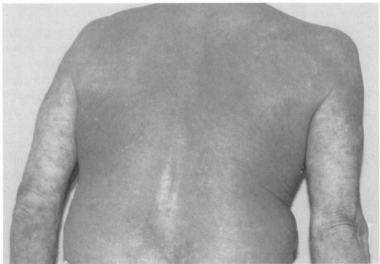

Note. Images courtesy of Meenal Khetherpal, MD. Used with permission.

FIGURE 11-2 Psoriatic Rash Related to a Checkpoint Inhibitor

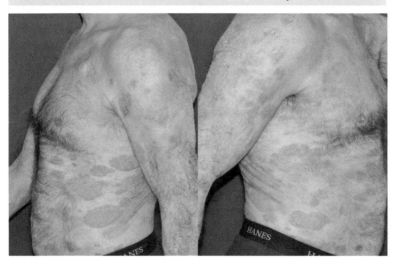

Note. Images courtesy of Mario Lacouture, MD. Used with permission.

Dermatologic toxicity is the most common irAE associated with checkpoint inhibitors and has an incidence of 18%–68% (Marrone et al., 2016; Naidoo et al., 2015; Weber, Postow, Lao, & Schadendorf, 2016). The most common presenting symptoms are a nonspecific maculopapular rash and/or pruritus on the trunk or extremities (Friedman, Proverbs-Singh, & Postow, 2016; Rapoport et al., 2017; Sibaud et al., 2016). Rash can also manifest as generalized erythema or look reticular/morbilliform in appearance. The onset of dermatologic symptoms typically occurs early in the treatment course, with an average onset of two to three weeks (Postow & Wolchok, 2017).

Other reported symptoms include Sweet's syndrome, follicular rash, urticarial dermatitis, alopecia, photosensitivity reaction, and vitiligo (Belum et al., 2016; Naidoo et al., 2015). Lichenoid dermatitis or psoriasis may also develop (Joseph et al., 2015; Murata, Kaneko, Harada, Aoi, & Morita, 2017; Ruiz-Bañobre et al., 2017). Mucosal involvement can occur, including xerostomia, stomatitis, and lichenoid reactions (Belum et al., 2016; Naidoo et al., 2015). Drug reaction with eosinophilia and systemic symptoms (known as DRESS), a potentially lethal and very rare hypersensitivity reaction with skin and possible organ involvement, can also occur. Symptoms include generalized skin eruption, typically of morbillosus/erythrodermic presentation, and may be associated with elevated eosinophils and enlarged lymph nodes (Bocquet, Bagot, & Roujeau,

1996). Other rare reactions, Stevens-Johnson syndrome and toxic epidermal necrolysis, are life threatening and require emergent treatment (Bristol-Myers Squibb Co., 2018b; Goldinger et al., 2016; Liniker et al., 2016; Nayar, Briscoe, & Fernandez Penas, 2016; Saw, Lee, & Ng, 2017). A survival analysis performed in patients receiving pembrolizumab (Keytruda®) found patients who developed cutaneous adverse events had significantly longer progression-free survival compared to those who did not (Sanlorenzo et al., 2015). It remains unclear if adverse events correlate with progression-free survival in patients using checkpoint inhibitors or immune-modulating therapy.

For patients who present with dermatologic complaints, onset and severity of symptoms should be assessed. Pruritus, rash, lesions, oral lesions, nodules, skin thickening, and erythema warrant examination. Although the development of skin rash or skin changes may be related to immunotherapy, consideration of other diagnoses, such as contact dermatitis (including contact with poison ivy/poison oak), allergy to concomitant medication, insect bites, fungal infection, and disseminated herpes zoster (shingles), is important.

Patients should be educated on proper skin care, including avoidance of irritating topical lotions, creams, and perfumes; use of sunscreen prior to sun exposure; and use of hypoallergenic moisturizers. For patients with pruritus, the goal of therapy includes relief of symptoms. Addressing the underlying cause (i.e., a rash) is the primary treatment of pruritic symptoms. Localized symptoms typically can be managed with topical steroids (medium to high potency) (Lacouture, 2015; Lacouture et al., 2014). Patients reporting more intense, generalized pruritus that may or may not be associated with a rash can benefit from other systemic pharmacologic interventions, including corticosteroids, antihistamines, gabapentin, pregabalin, mirtazapine, or aprepitant (Belum et al., 2016; Ito et al., 2017; Lacouture et al., 2014; Santini et al., 2012). Table 11-2 provides dermatologic grading and management strategies.

TABLE 11-2 Dermatologic Grading and Management Strategies*

	Grade 1	Grade 2	Grade 3	Grade 4
Symptoms	Possible mild or localized symptoms (pruritus, burning)	Possible intense/widespread symptoms (pruritus, burning), limiting instrumental ADLs	Intense/widespread pruritus, interfering with sleep and/or ADLs	Life-threatening consequences

(Continued on next page)

TABLE 11-2   Dermatologic Grading and Management Strategies*
(Continued)

	Grade 1	Grade 2	Grade 3	Grade 4
Examination findings	Rash/macules/ papules/ plaques < 10% BSA[†]	Rash/mac- ules/papules/ plaques 10%– 30% BSA[†]	Rash/macules/ papules/ plaques > 30% BSA[†]	Skin break- down with associated fluid or electrolyte abnormal- ities Life-threaten- ing conse- quences
Manage- ment for toxicity/ symptoms	Topical ste- roids (inter- mediate or high potency) Oral antihista- mines	Topical ste- roids (high potency) Oral predni- sone 0.5–1 mg/kg/day (or equiva- lent) Consider der- matology referral and skin biopsy. Oral antihista- mines	Topical ste- roids (high potency) Oral predni- sone 0.5–1 mg/kg/day (or equiv- alent); increase if no improve- ment. May require ste- roid taper. Consider der- matology referral and skin biopsy. Oral antihista- mines	Interven- tions as per grade 3 Hospitaliza- tion/critical care unit if severe skin breakdown
Manage- ment for immuno- therapy	Continue.	Consider hold- ing. If improves to ≤ grade 1, resume ther- apy.	Hold. If improves to ≤ grade 1, resume ther- apy after ste- roid taper complete. If no improve- ment, con- sider addi- tional immu- nosuppres- sion (inflix- imab, myco- phenolate).	Permanently discontinue.

(Continued on next page)

TABLE 11-2 Dermatologic Grading and Management Strategies*
(Continued)

Patient Education and Symptoms to Report
• New skin rash/lesions, dryness, or other changes in skin
• Pruritus (itching)
• Ulcers of the mouth
• History of contact with allergic triggers
• New medications
• Any other systemic symptoms

Nursing Interventions
• Perform total body skin examination and oral mucosa examination.
• Assess for infection.
• Assess severity of symptoms.
• Assess patient quality of life.
• Assess ability to perform ADLs.
• Consider dermatology referral.
• Obtain laboratory tests for blood counts and organ function, along with possible serologic studies for other autoimmune disorders.

---

* Grading of symptoms and examination findings can be found in Common Terminology Criteria for Adverse Events 5.0.

† Patients with skin changes involving blistering or ulceration should be assessed, preferably by dermatology, to rule out Stevens-Johnson syndrome.

ADLs—activities of daily living; BSA—body surface area

Note. Based on information from AstraZeneca Pharmaceuticals LP, 2018; Brahmer et al., 2018; Bristol-Myers Squibb Co., n.d., 2018a, 2018b; EMD Serono, Inc., 2017; Genentech, Inc., 2017b; Merck and Co., Inc., 2017a, 2017b; National Cancer Institute Cancer Therapy Evaluation Program, 2017; National Comprehensive Cancer Network & American Society of Clinical Oncology, 2018.

Gastrointestinal

Case 1

M.H. is a 59-year-old retired police officer. He was diagnosed with locally advanced urothelial carcinoma at age 56. Shortly after diagnosis, he underwent surgical resection and received adjuvant platinum-containing chemotherapy; however, M.H. had disease progression five months after initiating therapy. After this progression, he started treatment with a programmed cell death-ligand 1 (PD-L1) inhibitor. M.H. received this therapy for 12 months but voluntarily withdrew because of poor social and financial support.

Approximately two months after discontinuing the clinical trial therapy, M.H. developed progressive diarrhea and mild abdominal pain. He was evaluated in clinic for a routine follow-up visit and stated he had a two-week history of very loose stools without blood or mucus. His appetite was decreased and he had lower abdominal pain: a 6 out of 10 on the pain rating scale. M.H. had not had any-

thing to eat or drink for three days. His vitals were notable for orthostatic blood pressure and tachycardia. On examination, he had dry
mucous membranes, poor skin turgor, and moderate abdominal tenderness in his lower abdomen. He was admitted to the hospital for IV
fluids, pain control, and a workup.

A computed tomography scan of his abdomen and pelvis revealed
new colonic wall thickening and surrounding fat stranding involving the splenic flexure to the level of the mid transverse colon (see
Figure 11-3). Stool studies were obtained to rule out infection, and
the patient was started on prophylactic antibiotics. Colonoscopy with
blind biopsies revealed colonic mucosa with focal active colitis. When
stool studies did not reveal infection, high-dose IV steroids (methylprednisolone 1 mg/kg every 12 hours) were initiated. The patient
also received oral budesonide 9 mg daily. Within 48 hours, the
patient was feeling better, his diarrhea had significantly improved (to
grade 1), and he was discharged. M.H.'s steroids were tapered gradually over six weeks.

FIGURE 11-3 Colonic Wall Thickening Observed in a Patient With Colitis

Computed tomography scan of the abdomen (with contrast). Arrow indicates colonic wall thickening in a patient with colitis.

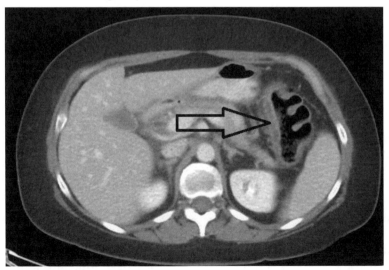

Note. Image courtesy of Susan J. McCall, MSN, ANP-BC, AOCNP®. Used with permission.

Diarrhea is a common complaint in patients receiving immunotherapy. The onset of diarrhea is approximately six to eight weeks after initiation of therapy (Weber, Yang, Atkins, & Disis, 2015). The incidence of diarrhea is higher with CTLA-4 inhibitors (30%) than with PD-1 inhibitors (8%–19%) (Garon et al., 2015; Hodi et al., 2010; Robert, Long, et al., 2015; Robert, Schachter, et al., 2015; Weber et al., 2015). Colitis, an inflammatory condition of the colon, is related to diarrhea but separate from this symptom. Patients can have diarrhea with or without colitis. Patients with colitis usually present with abdominal pain and have radiographic or endoscopic findings of inflammation (Postow, 2015). The incidence of colitis is less frequent with PD-1 blockade than with CTLA-4 blockade, with grade 3 or 4 events seen in about 1%–2% of cases (Postow & Wolchok, 2017).

Early reporting of symptoms by patients and early intervention by clinicians are critical; delayed reporting and noncompliance with management strategies can be fatal, as bowel perforation has been observed in immunotherapy-induced colitis (Eggermont et al., 2016; Mitchell, Kluger, Sznol, & Hartman, 2013). Patients should report any change in bowel patterns, abdominal pain, appetite changes, or other systemic symptoms (e.g., fever, malaise). For patients with diarrhea and possible colitis, bacterial (specifically, *Clostridium difficile*), viral, or parasitic infections; irritable bowel syndrome; dietary allergies; and medication-induced appendicitis, pancreatitis, or thyroid dysfunction should be excluded.

Treatment of immune-related diarrhea or colitis depends on the grade of the toxicity. Patients with mild (grade 1) diarrhea should be closely monitored. Antimotility agents and dietary modifications can be implemented. For patients with moderate (grade 2) symptoms, steroids are recommended, especially within five days of symptom onset (Pernot, Ramtohul, & Taieb, 2016). A systemic steroid dose of 0.5–1 mg/kg/day prednisone (or equivalent) can be used (Pernot et al., 2016; Postow & Wolchok, 2017). In cases of severe colitis (grade 3–4), 1–2 mg/kg/day prednisone (or equivalent) IV is recommended; however, patients will likely have to be admitted for additional supportive care (Pernot et al., 2016). Prophylactic use of budesonide is not recommended (Weber et al., 2009), but budesonide (9 mg daily) is often used in moderate to severe cases of diarrhea and colitis, despite a lack of prospective evidence.

It is vital for nurses and clinicians to perform frequent assessments of patient symptoms to determine the efficacy of intervention and need for additional therapy. Initiation of steroids should lead to a rapid reversal in symptoms, but in the event diarrhea/colitis are not improved with steroids, early initiation of infliximab is recommended (Merrill et al., 2014; Prieux-Klotz et al., 2017). In severe situations, or in situations in which symptoms are refractory to steroid use, a colonoscopy should be considered; however, this is only indicated if the diagnosis is unclear and should not be used in every situation (Postow, 2015). Table 11-3 provides diarrhea and colitis grading and management strategies.

TABLE 11-3 Diarrhea and Colitis Grading and Management Strategies*

	Grade 1	Grade 2	Grade 3	Grade 4
Symptoms	Increase of < 4 stools per day over baseline without abdominal pain	Increase of 4–6 stools per day over baseline with moderate abdominal pain	Increase of ≥ 7 stools per day over baseline Limiting self-care ADLs Severe abdominal pain Medical intervention indicated	Life-threatening consequences Urgent intervention indicated
Examination findings	Likely benign examination	Possible mucus or blood in stool Possible abdominal tenderness	Abdominal tenderness/peritoneal signs Ileus Fever	Abdominal tenderness/peritoneal signs Ileus Fever Failure to thrive
Management for toxicity/symptoms	Close monitoring Dietary modifications (BRAT diet) Antidiarrheal agent if infection has been ruled out	Oral prednisone 0.5–1 mg/kg (or equivalent) followed by taper Consider referral to gastroenterologist and lower gastrointestinal endoscopy.	Consider hospitalization. Oral prednisone 1–2 mg/kg/day (or equivalent) followed by taper, or IV methylprednisolone 1–2 mg/kg/day Consider referral to gastroenterologist and lower gastrointestinal endoscopy. If no improvement in 2 days, consider additional immunosuppression (infliximab 5 mg/kg, mycophenolate).	Hospitalization/critical care unit

(Continued on next page)

TABLE 11-3 Diarrhea and Colitis Grading and Management Strategies* *(Continued)*

	Grade 1	Grade 2	Grade 3	Grade 4
Management for immuno-therapy	Consider holding.	Hold. If improves to ≤ grade 1, resume therapy.	Hold PD-1 and PD-L1 agent. If improves to ≤ grade 1, resume therapy after steroid taper complete. If recurrent colitis, discontinue.	Permanently discontinue.

Patient Education and Symptoms to Report
- Change in bowel pattern or stool consistency
- Increased frequency or urgency of bowel movements
- Blood or mucus in stool; black, tar-like, or sticky stools
- Abdominal pain, nausea, vomiting, decreased appetite
- Fever
- Any other systemic symptoms
- Ongoing or worsening symptoms despite use of antidiarrheal agents or steroids

Nursing Interventions
- Obtain vital signs.
- Perform abdominal examination to assess for abdominal tenderness.
- Assess for infection.
- Assess for dehydration.
- Assess severity of symptoms.
- Assess patient quality of life.
- Assess ability to perform ADLs.
- Obtain stool sample for evaluation infection (e.g., *Clostridium difficile*).
- Administer IV fluids, if indicated.
- Consider referral to gastroenterologist.
- Consider imaging with x-ray or computed tomography scan.
- Obtain laboratory tests for blood counts and organ function.

* Grading of symptoms and examination findings can be found in Common Terminology Criteria for Adverse Events 5.0.

ADLs—activities of daily living; BRAT—bananas, rice, applesauce, and toast; PD-1—programmed cell death protein 1; PD-L1—programmed cell death-ligand 1

Note. Based on information from AstraZeneca Pharmaceuticals LP, 2018; Brahmer et al., 2018; Bristol-Myers Squibb Co., n.d., 2018a, 2018b; EMD Serono, Inc., 2017; Genentech, Inc., 2017b; Merck and Co., Inc., 2017a, 2017b; National Cancer Institute Cancer Therapy Evaluation Program, 2017; National Comprehensive Cancer Network & American Society of Clinical Oncology, 2018.

Hepatic

Case 1

L.O. is a 73-year-old nonsmoker who was recently diagnosed with metastatic non-small cell lung cancer. He enrolled in a clinical trial and received a CTLA-4 plus PD-1 inhibitor combination treatment. When L.O. returned to clinic two weeks after his treatment cycle, he was found to have elevated aspartate aminotransferase (AST) 19 times the upper limit of normal (ULN) and elevated alanine aminotransferase (ALT) 10 times ULN. L.O.'s bilirubin level was normal. He did not have any abdominal pain, changes in bowel pattern, jaundice, or changes in appetite. Treatment was held for grade 3 transaminitis, and L.O. was referred for a liver biopsy.

Results demonstrated liver tissue with modest mononuclear cell dominant inflammatory infiltrate with occasional neutrophils. L.O. initiated oral prednisone 1 mg/kg/day. Repeat hepatic function testing four days later showed AST and ALT improved to six times ULN, and L.O. remained asymptomatic. Over the next three weeks, his AST and ALT levels returned to normal. L.O. continued an oral prednisone taper over four weeks. The clinical trial was not restarted, but he did receive other therapy for his lung cancer.

The most frequently observed hepatic adverse events in patients receiving checkpoint inhibitors are elevations in AST and ALT, known as transaminitis (also synonymous with hepatitis for purposes of this discussion). Onset is typically 6–14 weeks after initiation of therapy (Spain, Diem, & Larkin, 2016). Most patients present without symptoms, although some have had associated fever (Postow, 2015). In cases of progressive hepatitis, patients may develop jaundice, hyperbilirubinemia, and fatigue. The incidence of transaminitis is less than 10% with single-agent ipilimumab, approximately 5% with single-agent PD-1 inhibitors, and 20%–30% with combination CTLA-4 and PD-1 inhibitors (Marrone et al., 2016; Naidoo et al., 2015; Spain et al., 2016; Wolchok et al., 2010).

Management of transaminitis includes systemic steroids (Cramer & Bresalier, 2017); however, prior to initiation, other etiologies for elevated transaminases must be ruled out, such as alcohol use, acetaminophen use, viral hepatitis, other medications, and metastatic liver disease. Liver function tests should be monitored at regular intervals (no less than once per week) to assess for improvement. If steroids are not effective, referral to a specialist is recommended, and mycophenolate should be given. Infliximab cannot be used because of contraindications in patients with hepatitis (Reuben, 2013). In certain cases, especially in steroid-refractory and mycophenolate-refractory instances, a liver biopsy may be helpful in establishing etiology of hepatitis

(Abdel-Wahab, Alshawa, & Suarez-Almazor, 2017). Table 11-4 provides hepatic grading and management strategies.

TABLE 11-4 Hepatic Grading and Management Strategies*

	Grade 1	Grade 2	Grade 3	Grade 4
Symptoms	Asymptomatic	Possible mild abdominal pain Patient may not be symptomatic despite grade of transaminitis.	Possible moderate to severe abdominal pain Patient may not be symptomatic despite grade of transaminitis.	Life-threatening consequences Patient may not be symptomatic despite grade of transaminitis.
Examination findings	AST or ALT > ULN–3 × ULN Bilirubin > ULN– 1.5 × ULN	AST or ALT 3–5 × ULN Bilirubin > 1.5–3 × ULN	AST or ALT > 5–20 × ULN Bilirubin > 3–10 × ULN	AST or ALT > 20 × ULN Bilirubin > 10 × ULN
Management for toxicity/ symptoms	Close monitoring	If liver function tests worsen with holding immunotherapy, start oral prednisone 0.5–1 mg/kg (or equivalent) followed by taper. Consider referral to gastroenterologist.	Oral prednisone 1–2 mg/kg/day (or equivalent) followed by taper Consider referral to gastroenterologist. If no improvement, consider additional immunosuppression (mycophenolate).	Oral prednisone 1–2 mg/kg/day (or equivalent) followed by taper Consider referral to gastroenterologist. If no improvement, consider mycophenolate.
Management for immunotherapy	Continue.	Hold. If improves to ≤ grade 1, resume therapy.	Hold. If improves to ≤ grade 1, resume therapy after steroid taper complete.	Permanently discontinue.

(Continued on next page)

TABLE 11-4 Hepatic Grading and Management Strategies*
(Continued)

Patient Education and Symptoms to Report
• Yellowing of the skin or the whites of the eyes
• Change in color of urine
• Nausea, vomiting, and decreased appetite
• Abdominal pain, abdominal bloating
• Increased lethargy and fatigue
• Bleeding or bruising
• Recent acetaminophen use
• Recent alcohol intake
• New medications
• Any other systemic symptoms

Nursing Interventions
• Obtain vital signs.
• Obtain laboratory tests for blood counts and liver function and coagulation studies.
• Perform abdominal examination to assess for abdominal tenderness.
• Perform skin and eye examinations to assess for jaundice.
• Screen for acetaminophen or alcohol use.
• Assess for infection.
• Assess for dehydration.
• Assess severity of symptoms.
• Assess patient quality of life.
• Assess ability to perform ADLs.
• Consider referral to gastroenterologist.

* Grading of symptoms and examination findings can be found in Common Terminology Criteria for Adverse Events 5.0.

ADLs—activities of daily living; ALT—alanine aminotransferase; AST—aspartate aminotransferase; ULN—upper limit of normal

Note. Based on information from AstraZeneca Pharmaceuticals LP, 2018; Brahmer et al., 2018; Bristol-Myers Squibb Co., n.d., 2018a, 2018b; EMD Serono, Inc., 2017; Genentech, Inc., 2017b; Merck and Co., Inc., 2017a, 2017b; National Cancer Institute Cancer Therapy Evaluation Program, 2017; National Comprehensive Cancer Network & American Society of Clinical Oncology, 2018.

Pulmonary

Case 1

M.J. is a 45-year-old woman who is very active and enjoys running marathons. She recently was diagnosed with unresectable *BRAF* wild-type melanoma. Approximately 11 days after receiving a PD-1 inhibitor, M.J. developed increased exertional dyspnea, which she noted when she attempted her regular morning exercise routine. She would become short of breath within seconds of starting her run. M.J. denied fevers and contact with sick people. She did have a dry cough with attempts at deep inspiration. On examination, decreased

breath sounds without wheezing in the bilateral bases on ausculta-
tion was noted. Her pulse oximetry was 98% at rest on room air
but dropped to 89% with exertion. M.J. was referred for pulmonary
consultation.

Pulmonary function testing revealed a 40% decrease in the diffusing capacity of her lungs for carbon dioxide. A computed tomography scan of her chest was performed demonstrating new diffuse bilateral pulmonary ground glass changes; no pulmonary embolus was
found (see Figure 11-4). M.J. received prednisone 0.5 mg/kg with
slow taper as per pulmonary recommendations. She was able to be
retreated and went back to running. She continues therapy without
difficulty.

Compared to other irAEs, pneumonitis is an uncommon toxicity of checkpoint inhibitors; however, it can be severe and frightening
for patients and clinicians. The incidence of pneumonitis is 5%–10%,
including rates with combination therapy (Chuzi et al., 2017; Spain et
al., 2016). An increased incidence of pneumonitis is present in patients
with prior thoracic radiation (Merck and Co., Inc., 2017b).

FIGURE 11-4 Pneumonitis

Computed tomography scan of the chest (without contrast). Arrows indicate
ground glass opacities in a patient with pneumonitis.

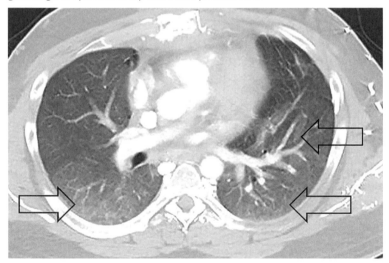

Note. Image courtesy of Susan J. McCall, MSN, ANP-BC, AOCNP®. Used with permission.

Patients should report any symptoms of acute exertional dyspnea, shortness of breath, cough, hypoxia (if able to measure this at home), feeling "easily winded," or chest pain. It may be difficult for patients to recognize symptoms, especially if they have an underlying disease for which they are symptomatic. It may be equally challenging for the clinical team; other diagnoses must be excluded, including infection (e.g., bacterial, fungal, viral), exacerbation of chronic obstructive pulmonary disease, malignant disease progression, pulmonary embolus, pulmonary effusion, atelectasis, sarcoidosis, pericardial effusion, or myocardial infarction. Drug-induced pneumonitis is a diagnosis of exclusion; after all other possibilities have been ruled out, treatment can be initiated (Postow & Wolchok, 2017). Evaluation should include physical examination, including resting and exertional pulse oximetry and radiographic imaging (e.g., chest x-ray, computed tomography scan, pulmonary function testing). It is helpful to obtain baseline pulmonary function testing prior to the start of therapy, as changes can be quantified when compared to baseline values.

Treatment with systemic steroids is indicated for symptomatic patients. It is helpful to have patients evaluated by a pulmonologist, as this professional can exclude other etiologies. Patients with previous radiation to the chest or exposure to bleomycin may be at risk of pulmonary complications. Table 11-5 provides pneumonitis grading and management strategies.

TABLE 11-5 Pneumonitis Grading and Management Strategies*

	Grade 1	Grade 2	Grade 3	Grade 4
Symptoms	Asymptomatic	Symptomatic Shortness of breath with minimal exertion, limiting ADLs	Severe symptoms Shortness of breath at rest, limiting self-care ADLs Oxygen indicated	Life-threatening consequences Urgent respiratory intervention indicated
Examination findings	Radiographic findings	Possible hypoxia with exertion Radiographic findings, decrease in DLCO	Visibly in distress Hypoxia at rest and/or with exertion Radiographic findings, decrease in DLCO	Extreme respiratory distress

(Continued on next page)

TABLE 11-5 Pneumonitis Grading and Management Strategies*
(Continued)

	Grade 1	Grade 2	Grade 3	Grade 4
Management for toxicity/ symptoms	Close monitoring	Oral prednisone 1–2 mg/kg (or equivalent) followed by taper Consider referral to pulmonologist and bronchoscopy/lung biopsy. If no improvement, consider additional immunosuppression (infliximab/ mycophenolate).	Hospitalize. Methylprednisolone IV 1–2 mg/kg/day followed by taper Consider referral to pulmonologist and bronchoscopy/lung biopsy. If no improvement, consider additional immunosuppression (infliximab/ mycophenolate).	Hospitalize. Consider intubation. Methylprednisolone IV 1–2 mg/kg/day followed by taper Consider referral to pulmonologist and bronchoscopy/lung biopsy. If no improvement, consider additional immunosuppression (infliximab/ mycophenolate).
Management for immunotherapy	Continue with close monitoring. Hold at clinician discretion.	Hold. If improves to ≤ grade 1, resume therapy at clinician discretion.	Permanently discontinue.	Permanently discontinue.

Patient Education and Symptoms to Report
• Cough
• Shortness of breath, especially with exertion
• Chest pain
• New medications
• Any other systemic symptoms

Nursing Interventions
• Obtain vital signs, including resting and ambulating pulse oximetry.
• Provide oxygen, if necessary.
• Auscultate lungs.
• Assess for infection and fever.
• Assess severity of symptoms.
• Assess patient quality of life.
• Assess ability to perform ADLs.
• Consider chest x-ray or computed tomography scan.
• Consider referral to pulmonologist.

* Grading of symptoms and examination findings can be found in Common Terminology Criteria for Adverse Events 5.0.

ADLs—activities of daily living; DLCO—diffusing capacity of the lungs for carbon dioxide

Note. Based on information from AstraZeneca Pharmaceuticals LP, 2018; Brahmer et al., 2018; Bristol-Myers Squibb Co., n.d., 2018a, 2018b; EMD Serono, Inc., 2017; Genentech, Inc., 2017b; Merck and Co., Inc., 2017a, 2017b; National Cancer Institute Cancer Therapy Evaluation Program, 2017; National Comprehensive Cancer Network, 2018.

Endocrine

Case 1

A.T. is a 31-year-old travel agent without a significant past medical history. He was recently diagnosed with refractory classical Hodgkin lymphoma. After A.T. had received three prior therapies and was not able to achieve remission, he initiated treatment with a PD-1 inhibitor, which he tolerated well. Approximately 12 weeks after starting treatment, A.T. underwent positron-emission tomography with 2-deoxy-2-[fluorine-18] fluoro-D-glucose (FDG-PET) for disease assessment. An incidental finding of acute thyroiditis was found manifested by the significant bilateral diffuse uptake of his thyroid gland (see Figure 11-5). Laboratory examination was remarkable for thyroid-stimulating hormone (TSH) of 0.32 mcU/ml (low) and normal free T4 (thyroxine), which was consistent with subclinical hyperthyroidism. A.T. underwent ultrasound of the thyroid gland, which demonstrated markedly heterogeneous thyroid consistent with thyroiditis. He was asymptomatic and continued to receive therapy with the checkpoint inhibitor.

Three weeks later, A.T.'s thyroid function tests revealed a very low TSH (0.03 mcU/ml) and normal free T4, consistent with worsening hyperthyroidism. Ten days later, his TSH was 2.45 mcU/ml (normal) with a low free T4. After another 10 days, his TSH was 85.3 mcU/ml with low free T4, consistent with hypothyroidism. The patient remained asymptomatic but was prescribed levothyroxine 75 mcg daily for the management of hypothyroidism.

FIGURE 11-5 Thyroiditis

FDG-avidity (fluoro-D-glucose) on positron-emission tomography scan of acute thyroiditis

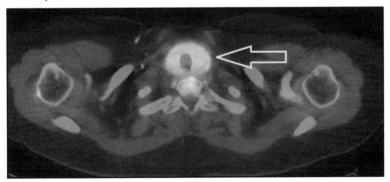

Note. Image courtesy of Susan J. McCall, MSN, ANP-BC, AOCNP®. Used with permission.

Case 2

M.Y. is a 51-year-old male insurance agent. He was recently diagnosed with head and neck squamous cell carcinoma and received combination radiation and platinum-based chemotherapy on a clinical trial. Unfortunately, M.Y. developed metastatic disease to the lung. He initiated treatment with a PD-1 inhibitor. Approximately three months later, M.Y. developed progressive fatigue and "decreased stamina." Thyroid function tests were normal, and conservative interventions were recommended. Three weeks later, he presented to clinic with increased fatigue, generalized weakness, decreased appetite, and nausea. His vital signs were within normal limits (mild tachycardia; 110 heart rate), and no evidence of extreme dehydration was present. Infectious workup did not reveal any acute infection. A magnetic resonance imaging (MRI) of the brain did not reveal an enlarged pituitary; however, M.Y. was found to have low adrenocorticotropic hormone (ACTH) and cortisol. He was started on prednisone 10 mg daily, and immunotherapy was temporarily held.

After prednisone, his symptoms improved, and he was switched to hydrocortisone and fludrocortisone. M.Y. eventually discontinued fludrocortisone but was able to continue hydrocortisone daily. He was also able to continue immunotherapy.

Case 3

R.J. is a 79-year-old retired gynecologist with a past medical history of hypertension and hyperlipidemia. She was diagnosed with locally advanced urothelial carcinoma and enrolled on a clinical trial with a PD-L1 inhibitor. During a follow-up visit approximately eight months later, R.J. noted a mild headache and nausea. She rated the headache as 3 out of 10 and indicated the nausea was not preventing her from eating. Both symptoms were intermittent and did not happen every day. She was given antiemetics for as-needed use and was monitored. Two weeks later, her daughter called the office to report her mother had been feeling dizzy and "was not her usual self." The patient was evaluated in the office shortly thereafter, where she reported increased fatigue, had a worsening headache, and appeared uncomfortable. Laboratory work demonstrated a low cortisol level, a low ACTH level, a low prolactin level, and normal thyroid levels. Given these results, a diagnosis of hypophysitis was suspected. A brain MRI was ordered, which showed an enlarged pituitary gland (see Figure 11-6A). R.J. was treated with IV methylprednisolone 1.5 mg/kg, and her symptoms improved within three days. Repeat brain MRI demonstrated a reduction in the size of the

pituitary gland (see Figure 11-6*B*), and R.J. continued an oral prednisone taper over five weeks. Immunotherapy was not reinitiated.

FIGURE 11-6 Hypophysitis

Figure A: Arrow indicates an enlarged pituitary gland.

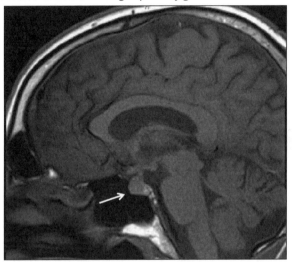

Figure B: Resolution of hypophysitis

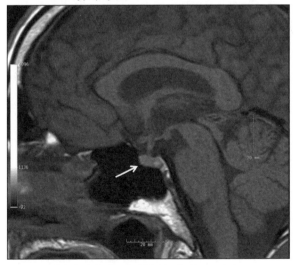

Note. Images courtesy of Kimberly D. Allman, CNP. Used with permission.

Endocrine abnormalities are perhaps the most complex group of irAEs. They are varied and include thyroid dysfunction, hypophysitis, adrenal insufficiency, and type 1 diabetes mellitus. Approximately 5%–10% of patients receiving checkpoint inhibitors develop an endocrine irAE (Michot et al., 2016). Hypophysitis (10%–15%) appears to be the most common endocrine adverse event in patients receiving ipilimumab (Faje, 2016). Other studies have found that thyroid abnormalities are more common with PD-1 inhibitors (Shang, Zhang, Li, Li, & Zhang, 2017).

The clinical presentation of endocrinopathies can be subtle and may be difficult to diagnose; frequent, thorough assessment of patients and appropriate monitoring of laboratory tests are key. Table 11-6 provides a summary of laboratory and diagnostic test findings for various endocrinopathies.

Thyroid Dysfunction

Hypothyroidism (underactive thyroid), hyperthyroidism (overactive thyroid), and thyroiditis (inflammation of the thyroid) have been observed in patients receiving checkpoint inhibitors. Hypothyroidism is more common with PD-1 inhibitors (4%–10%) than with CTLA-4 inhibitors (2%–4%) (Spain et al., 2016). Thyroid dysfunction is usually seen early—within the first few doses of a drug—and may be transient (Di Giacomo, Biagioli, & Maio, 2010; Postow, 2015). Thyroid function tests should be drawn at baseline prior to start of therapy and periodically during therapy. Most patients are asymptomatic, and diagnosis is often made through laboratory assessment. Thyroid hormone replacement with levothyroxine can be instituted without immunotherapy interruption. The patient should be made aware that thyroid replacement therapy may be lifelong.

Subclinical hyperthyroidism often precedes overt hypothyroidism (Corsello et al., 2013). For patients with labs consistent with hyperthyroidism, close monitoring will usually demonstrate resolution of abnormal labs (to euthyroid) followed by overt hypothyroidism.

Hyperthyroidism is less common (1%–7%) and is often subclinical (Postow & Wolchok, 2017). Symptomatic patients (e.g., tachycardia, tremor) should be referred to a specialist for treatment, and immunotherapy interruption should be considered.

Adrenal Insufficiency

Adrenal insufficiency is the most critical endocrinopathy. If found to be in adrenal crisis (e.g., dehydration, hypotension, shock), a patient should be hospitalized immediately and referred to an endocrinologist. Treatment with IV corticosteroids and aggressive hydration should be initiated (Postow & Wolchok, 2017). Prolonged treatment, perhaps lifelong, with glucocorticoids is indicated.

TABLE 11-6 Laboratory and Diagnostic Test Findings for Immune-Related Endocrinopathies

Endocrinopathy	Thyroid (TSH, T3, and Free T4)	Adrenal (ACTH and Cortisol)	Gonadal (LH and FSH)	Hypothalamic (Prolactin)	Other Diagnostic Findings
Hypothyroidism	Elevated TSH, normal or low free T4	Normal	Normal	Normal	Possible symptoms: fatigue/weakness, weight gain, dry skin, constipation, edema, cold intolerance
Hyperthyroidism	Low TSH, possibly normal or high T3, normal or high free T4	Normal	Normal	Normal	Possible symptoms: weight loss, tachycardia, fatigue, hair loss, protrusion of eyes, menstrual irregularity
Adrenal insufficiency	Normal	Low ACTH and cortisol	Normal	Normal	Possible electrolyte abnormalities (hyponatremia, hyperkalemia), anemia, fatigue, weight loss, arthralgias/myalgias, nausea/vomiting, hypotension
Hypophysitis	Possibly low TSH, decreased T3 and free T4	Low ACTH and cortisol	Possibly low FSH and LH	Usually low	Enlargement/enhancement of pituitary gland; possible symptoms: headache, visual changes, mental status changes
Type 1 diabetes mellitus	Normal TSH, T3, and free T4	Normal	Normal	Normal	Hyperglycemia (severe), possible diabetic ketoacidosis

ACTH—adrenocorticotropic hormone; FSH—follicle-stimulating hormone; LH—luteinizing hormone; T3—triiodothyronine; T4—thyroxine; TSH—thyroid-stimulating hormone

Note. Based on information from Jameson, 2015.

Hypophysitis

Hypophysitis is inflammation of the pituitary gland. It has a 1%–6% incidence with single-agent therapy and a 2%–10% incidence with combination therapy (Naidoo et al., 2015). Onset occurs within two to three months but can present later (Corsello et al., 2013). Symptoms include fatigue, behavioral change, loss of libido, headache, nausea, dizziness, and visual changes (Spain et al., 2016). Evaluation of the pituitary-hypothalamic, pituitary-thyroid, pituitary-gonadal, and pituitary-adrenal axes with blood tests (e.g., TSH, free T4, free T3 [triiodothyronine], luteinizing hormone, follicle-stimulating hormone, ACTH, cortisol, prolactin) will guide diagnosis; often, thyroid hormones, cortisol, ACTH, and gonadal hormone levels will be decreased (although a decrease in all levels does not confirm diagnosis). An MRI of the brain will reveal pituitary enlargement and help exclude possible brain metastases, which should be considered whenever a patient presents with mental status changes (Naidoo et al., 2015; Postow, 2015). Immediate initiation of high-dose steroids (prednisone 1 mg/kg/ day) may reverse inflammatory processes (Postow & Wolchok, 2017). Some patients may need long-term hormone replacement with hydrocortisone 20 mg in the morning and 10 mg in the evening.

Type 1 Diabetes Mellitus

The development of acute type 1 diabetes mellitus has been reported in rare cases (Hughes et al., 2015; Okamoto et al., 2016). It is diagnosed with evaluation of blood glucose, which is often significantly elevated. Referral to an endocrinologist for management is indicated. For patients who present with diabetic ketoacidosis, hospitalization is strongly recommended. Table 11-7 provides endocrinopathy grading and management strategies.

TABLE 11-7 Endocrinopathy Grading and Management Strategies*

	Grade 1	Grade 2[†]	Grade 3[†]	Grade 4[†]
Symptoms	Asymptomatic Laboratory or radiographic findings only	Hyperthyroidism: tachycardia, tremor Hypothyroidism: lethargy, weight gain Adrenal insufficiency: lethargy, dizziness Hypophysitis: headache, fatigue	Severe symptoms	Life-threatening consequences Urgent respiratory intervention indicated

(Continued on next page)

TABLE 11-7 Endocrinopathy Grading and Management Strategies*
(Continued)

	Grade 1	Grade 2[†]	Grade 3[†]	Grade 4[†]
Examination findings	–	Hypothyroidism: elevated TSH (with normal or low free T4) Hyperthyroidism: low TSH (with normal or high free T4) Adrenal insufficiency: low cortisol, possible hyperkalemia, and hyponatremia	Same as grade 2, but also with severe electrolyte imbalance and abnormal vital signs	Same as grade 3, but also with life-threatening consequences
Management for toxicity/ symptoms	Close monitoring	Consider referral to endocrinologist. Hypothyroidism: Initiate levothyroxine. Hyperthyroidism: Initiate thyroid suppressive medication and treat symptoms.	Hospitalize. Refer to endocrinologist. Initiate IV steroids and IV fluid. Rule out sepsis.	Same as grade 3
Management for immunotherapy	Continue with close monitoring. Hold at clinician discretion.	Hold. If improves to ≤ grade 1, resume therapy after completion of steroid taper.	Permanently discontinue.	Permanently discontinue.

Patient Education and Symptoms to Report
- Fatigue/lethargy
- Muscle aches
- Headaches
- Confusion
- Weight gain or loss
- Heart palpitations
- Vision changes
- Postural hypotension/dizziness
- Changes in mood or behavior/irritability
- Temperature intolerance (feeling cold)
- Excessive thirst, hunger, or frequent urination
- Nausea or vomiting
- Hair loss
- Hoarseness or deepening of voice
- New medications
- Any other systemic symptoms

(Continued on next page)

TABLE 11-7 Endocrinopathy Grading and Management Strategies*
(Continued)

Nursing Interventions
- Obtain vital signs, including orthostatic blood pressure.
- Obtain laboratory studies to examine thyroid, pituitary, adrenal function, and blood glucose.
- Assess for dehydration/orthostatic hypotension.
- Assess for mental status changes; perform mini-mental status examination.
- Anticipate order for brain MRI.
- Assess severity of symptoms.
- Assess patient quality of life.
- Assess ability to perform ADLs.
- Consider referral to endocrinologist.

* Grading of symptoms and examination findings can be found in Common Terminology Criteria for Adverse Events 5.0.

† Patients with hyperthyroidism or hypothyroidism may not be symptomatic, and findings may be limited to laboratory findings only.

ADLs—activities of daily living; MRI—magnetic resonance imaging; T4—thyroxine; TSH—thyroid-stimulating hormone

Note. Based on information from AstraZeneca Pharmaceuticals LP, 2018; Brahmer et al., 2018; Bristol-Myers Squibb Co., n.d., 2018a, 2018b; EMD Serono, Inc., 2017; Genentech, Inc., 2017b; Merck and Co., Inc., 2017a, 2017b; National Cancer Institute Cancer Therapy Evaluation Program, 2017; National Comprehensive Cancer Network & American Society of Clinical Oncology, 2018.

Neurologic

Case 1

K.B. is a 42-year-old electrical engineer. He was diagnosed with metastatic melanoma and began treatment with a PD-1 inhibitor one year ago. He experienced a complete remission after five months and continued therapy without any adverse events.

Recently, he traveled to Europe for vacation. When he returned, he reported mild lower back pain with dull achiness bilaterally, rating as 4 out of 10 on the pain scale. K.B. attributed this to increased activity while traveling and discomfort from flying; however, his symptoms worsened over the next five days, at which time he presented to clinic for evaluation. He reported lower extremity weakness, lower back pain rating as 7 out of 10, constipation, and difficulty urinating. On examination, K.B. had decreased strength in his bilateral lower extremities, tenderness of his lower lumbar spine, and required assistance to stand up from the examination table. He was admitted for immediate workup of these symptoms.

An array of examinations were performed under the guidance of a neurologist, including an electromyogram, an MRI of the spine and brain, blood tests to evaluate autoimmune markers, heavy metal screening, and a paraneoplastic panel.

The blood tests were negative, the electromyogram demonstrated decreased motor nerve conduction velocity, and the MRI of the brain was negative; however, the MRI of the spine revealed fairly diffuse leptomeningeal enhancement along the cauda equina nerve roots. A lumbar puncture was recommended for further evaluation, but the patient refused.

K.B.'s symptoms were thought to be immune mediated (diagnosis not defined), and he was treated with IV methylprednisolone 1 g for four days, then with oral prednisone, which was tapered over four weeks. His symptoms improved within a week, and K.B. was discharged. He made a full recovery but did not continue treatment with immunotherapy.

Neurologic irAEs are rare compared to previously discussed events. Eltobgy et al. (2017) performed a systematic review of immune-related neurologic toxicities and found an incidence of 1%–15% for all grades with single-agent therapy. Events were more frequent with ipilimumab and in combination studies that included chemotherapy plus a checkpoint inhibitor. The most common reported events include peripheral neuropathy, radiculopathy, Guillain-Barré syndrome, transverse myelitis, aseptic meningitis, myasthenia gravis, and posterior reversible encephalopathy syndrome (Eltobgy et al., 2017; Makarious, Horwood, & Coward, 2017; Marrone et al., 2016; Michot et al., 2016; Postow & Wolchok, 2017).

Expert consultation and workup is warranted for any patient experiencing neurologic symptoms or deficits, even if symptoms are subtle. Regardless of grade, these patients should hold therapy if neurologic symptoms are thought to be related to immunotherapy (Spain et al., 2016). Corticosteroids should be given to treat symptoms. If necessary, additional treatment is administered, such as plasmapheresis and IV immunoglobulin (Postow & Wolchok, 2017).

Fatigue

Although toxicities of immunotherapy treatments include those of autoimmune etiology, fatigue is also common (Larkin et al., 2015; Michot et al., 2016; Naidoo et al., 2015; Spain et al., 2016). Abdel-Rahman et al. (2016) found CTLA-4 inhibitors were associated with a higher risk of fatigue compared to control regimens, whereas PD-1 inhibitors were associated with a lower risk. It is important to evaluate fatigue, specifically with functional capacity (independent activities of daily living) and quality of life. Patients may have baseline fatigue from underlying disease/cancer, stress, depression, pain, poor nutrition, or other factors. Worsening fatigue, especially fatigue not relieved by rest, while receiving immunotherapy suggests drug-related etiology. However, other etiologies, such as anemia, hypothyroidism, poor sleep, or disease progression, should be considered and excluded in cases where the underlying cause of fatigue is not clear. Autoimmune toxicities may also contribute to fatigue, such as hypothyroidism, hemolytic anemia, hypophysitis, or neurologic toxicity. These should be ruled out for patients requiring evaluation of progressive fatigue.

The nurse should assess severity of symptoms and interventions to help improve fatigue. Exercise is the only level 1 intervention for fatigue currently recommended (American Cancer Society, 2016; National Cancer Institute, 2017). This can include walking or more rigorous activities depending on patient fitness and energy level. Additional interventions to treat fatigue include napping, prioritizing daily tasks, and avoiding caffeine at night (American Cancer Society, 2016).

Rare Adverse Events

Case 1

M.M. is a 62-year-old venture capitalist. He was diagnosed with classical Hodgkin lymphoma and treated with a PD-1 inhibitor on a clinical trial. M.M. tolerated this therapy very well for nearly 15 months.

He was scheduled for tumor assessment and underwent an FDG-PET scan per protocol procedure. M.M. presented to clinic for examination, review of his scan, and consideration for therapy. During this interview, he stated he had developed mild upper abdominal pain five days prior, which was 7 out of 10 on the pain rating scale. M.M. associated this pain with a decreased appetite. He attributed these symptoms to something he ate and stress, as he had been traveling frequently for work. He denied nausea, vomiting, dyspepsia, fevers, diarrhea, or constipation.

Review of his FDG-PET scan demonstrated an incidental finding of a diffusely FDG-avid enlarged pancreas (see Figure 11-7). Laboratory evaluation revealed an elevated lipase 5.5 times ULN and an elevated amylase 3 times ULN. His blood sugar was elevated three times ULN. Because of the grade of his pancreatic enzyme elevation (grade 4) and symptoms, M.M. was admitted to the hospital for management of immune-related pancreatitis.

A gastroenterologist was consulted, and M.M. was given IV systemic steroids, IV fluids, and a clear liquid diet. His pancreatic enzymes improved the following day, remarkable for an elevated lipase four times ULN, amylase at ULN, and normal blood glucose. His symptoms were significantly improved, and M.M. was discharged the next day. He did not resume treatment with the PD-1 inhibitor.

FIGURE 11-7 Pancreatitis

The central organ with FDG-avid (fluoro-D-glucose) uptake on positron-emission tomography scan represents acute pancreatitis.

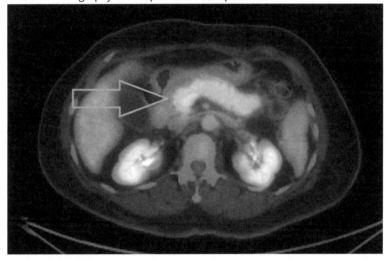

Note. Image courtesy of Susan J. McCall, MSN, ANP-BC, AOCNP®. Used with permission.

Pancreatic

Pancreatitis, defined as the presence of abdominal pain, elevation of serum lipase or amylase, and radiographic findings, has been reported in less than 1%–2% of patients receiving checkpoint inhibitors (Alabed, Aghayev, Sakellis, & Van den Abbeele, 2015; Banks et al., 2013; Blasig et al., 2017; Hofmann et al., 2016; Wachsmann, Ganti, & Peng, 2017). Elevations of amylase and lipase without symptoms have been reported in 10%–15% of patients receiving checkpoint inhibitors on clinical trials (Postow & Wolchok, 2017). In patients who have elevations in lipase or amylase without clinical or radiographic evidence of pancreatitis, the significance of and implications for therapy interruption remain unclear. It is not recommended to routinely monitor pancreatic enzymes in an asymptomatic patient, as elevations may result in unnecessary therapy interruption. No indications exist for steroids in asymptomatic patients outside of the clinical trial setting (Postow, 2015).

For patients with acute pancreatitis, other etiologies should be excluded, including alcohol-induced pancreatitis, gallstones, insult from medications, infection, or malignancy. Referral to a specialist is indicated. Patients who have immune-related pancreatitis should receive systemic corticosteroids and supportive care.

Renal

Interstitial nephritis and renal failure have been reported in less than 1%–5% of cases, more with combination therapy (Cortazar et al., 2016; Forde, Rock, Wilson, & O'Byrne, 2012; Postow & Wolchok, 2017; Rassy et al., 2016). The onset of toxicity occurs about three months after therapy initiation (Postow & Wolchok, 2017).

Manifestations of renal toxicity are usually asymptomatic and observed in rising creatinine levels in the blood. For patients with rising creatinine, therapy should be interrupted, and a consultation with specialist is warranted (Postow & Wolchok, 2017). Treatment includes systemic corticosteroids, supportive IV fluids, supportive electrolyte replacement, and/or hospitalization depending on the severity of the toxicity.

Rheumatologic

Various presentations of immune-related rheumatologic toxicities have been reported with varying incidences, including inflammatory arthritis, salivary gland dysfunction (sicca syndrome), inflammatory myositis, generalized arthralgias, tenosynovitis polymyalgia rheumatica/giant cell arteritis, celiac disease, lupus nephritis, dermatomyositis, autoimmune inflammatory myopathy, and Vogt-Koyanagi–like syndrome (Abdel-Wahab, Shah, & Suarez-Almazor, 2016; Cappelli, Gutierrez, Baer, et al., 2017; Cappelli, Gutierrez, O'Bingham, & Shah, 2017; Chan, Kefford, Carlino, Clements, & Manolios, 2015; Law-Ping-Man, Martin, Briens, Tisseau, & Safa, 2016; Naidoo et al., 2017; Postow & Wolchok, 2017). The incidence of these events ranges from 1%–7%. Generalized arthralgias were reported in 4%–22% of patients receiving checkpoint inhibitors on clinical trials (Naidoo et al., 2017).

Providers should ask patients about any new joint pain (any joint), swelling, warmth, erythema, and stiffness (especially if worse in the morning) since initiating treatment with a checkpoint inhibitor. Nonsteroidal anti-inflammatory drugs (NSAIDs) will likely provide relief of these symptoms but may also be suggestive of a rheumatologic process. Referral to a specialist is warranted if the suspicion exists of an immune-related rheumatologic toxicity. Early referral, diagnosis, and treatment are important to prevent severe psoriatic arthritis and possible erosive joint damage (Cappelli, Naidoo, O'Bingham, & Shah, 2016).

Naidoo et al. (2017) proposed guidelines for management of patients with immune-related rheumatologic toxicities. They recommend initiating treatment with systemic corticosteroids for any symptoms or toxicity greater than grade 2. If patients do not experience relief, methotrexate should be administered at a starting dose of 15 mg weekly, which can be titrated if necessary.

Cardiac

Myocarditis, heart failure, pericarditis, pericardial tamponade, heart block, and cardiomyopathy have been reported (Kushnir & Wolf, 2017). An increased likelihood of severe myocarditis was found with an ipilimumab plus nivolumab combination compared to nivolumab alone (0.27% vs. 0.06%) (Jain, Bahia, Mohebtash, & Barac, 2017). Patients presented with various symptoms, including shortness of breath, fatigue, edema, chest pain, and syncope. Most patients were found to have electrocardiogram (ECG) abnormalities on presentation.

Symptoms may be subtle, but for any patient with suspicion of cardiac dysfunction, immediate intervention should be provided. Whether cardiac symptoms are related to immunotherapy or not, immediate intervention will improve patient outcomes, as there have been reports of patients experiencing fatal immune-related cardiotoxicities (Jain et al., 2017; Kushnir & Wolf, 2017). Patients should be probed about increasing shortness of breath (also needs to be differentiated from symptoms of pneumonitis), chest pain, dizziness, acute weight gain, increasing edema, or cough. If possible in the practice setting, an ECG and troponin level should be obtained. Early specialist intervention is also warranted. Unstable patients should be hospitalized, ideally in a cardiac care unit, if troponin levels are increased or ECG abnormalities are found (Postow & Wolchok, 2017). Similar to other irAEs, cardiotoxicity should be treated with systemic corticosteroids (Jain et al., 2017).

Hematologic

Red cell aplasia, neutropenia, acquired hemophilia, autoimmune hemolytic anemia (AIHA), and thrombocytopenia/immune thrombocytopenia purpura (ITP) have been observed in less than 1% of patients receiving checkpoint inhibitors (Cooling, Sherbeck, Mowers, & Hugan, 2017; Palla, Kennedy, Mosharraf, & Doll, 2016; Postow, 2015; Shiuan et al., 2017). Spain et al. (2016) observed that most of these toxicities occurred in patients with underlying hematologic malignancy, specifically lymphoma. Shiuan et al. (2017) noted two severe cases of ITP in which steroids, IV immunoglobulin, and rituximab were required; both patients made a full recovery.

Patients may be asymptomatic, pending the degree of anemia. Patients who are found to have a low platelet count should be counseled regarding bleeding precautions and avoidance of trauma.

Mild cases of thrombocytopenia and anemia may warrant only close observation; however, severe cases of ITP and AIHA require treatment with systemic corticosteroids and should be referred to a hematologist. For patients with significant anemia or very profound thrombocytopenia with high risk of spontaneous bleeding, transfusions are indicated. If necessary, a bone marrow biopsy should be performed (Postow, 2015). In cases where patients may be refractory to steroids, rituximab or IV immunoglobulin are possible treatment options (Palla et al., 2016; Shiuan et al., 2017).

Ocular

In addition to rare organ toxicities, ocular symptoms and inflammation have also been observed with checkpoint inhibitors. Diagnoses of episcleritis, conjunctivitis, intraocular inflammation (uveitis), optic neuropathy, retinopathy, and keratitis occur in less than 1% of patients receiving CTLA-4 and PD-1 inhibitors (Papavasileiou, Prasad, Freitag, Sobrin, & Lobo, 2015; Postow & Wolchok, 2017). Ocular symptoms include vision changes (acute), dry eye, photophobia, and moderate to severe pain. Patients may assume these symptoms are allergic in etiology; this is certainly a differential diagnosis, but acute ocular changes warrant prompt ophthalmology consultation. Herpes zoster of the eye must be excluded. If a diagnosis of an immune-related ocular event is made, treatment with topical steroids (1% prednisolone or equivalent) is recommended (Postow & Wolchok, 2017). In more severe cases (grade 3 or 4 events), systemic steroids may be used, and treatment should be discontinued (Weber et al., 2016).

Infusion Reactions

The CTLA-4, PD-1, and PD-L1 inhibitors are immunomodulatory monoclonal antibodies derived from biologic sources. As such, infusion-related reactions have been reported in up to 25% of patients, most of which are mild (Postow & Wolchok, 2017).

Avelumab (Bavencio®), a PD-L1 inhibitor indicated for the treatment of Merkel cell carcinoma, requires premedication with acetaminophen and antihistamine prior to the first four infusions (EMD Serono, Inc., 2017).

Symptoms of infusion-related reactions include chills, urticaria, fever, shortness of breath, myalgia, and hypotension. The infusion should be stopped, and the patient should be assessed for suspected infusion reactions. Supportive medications should be given as per clinician or institutional guidelines, preferably with an antihistamine and/or corticosteroid.

Immune-Related Adverse Events From Other Agents

Cytokine Therapy

Although newer agents have been developed to treat metastatic melanoma, cytokine therapy continues to be the mainstay for the adjuvant treatment of surgically resected malignancies with a high risk of recurrence. Three medications—interferon alfa-2b, peginterferon alfa-2b, and aldesleukin—work by activating immune cells to elicit an inflammatory response, specifically against tumor cells. This mechanism of action is not dissimilar to that of contracting a viral infection; the body mounts an immune system response to overwhelm a foreign pathogen. During this response, symptoms of fatigue, pyrexia, and chills (typical flu-like symptoms) are very common. Approximately 94% of patients receiving peginterferon alfa-2b experience some degree of fatigue, 75% experience pyrexia, and 63% experience chills. Additional common adverse events include increased AST and ALT (77%), headache (70%), anorexia (69%), myalgia (68%), and nausea (64%) (Merck and Co., Inc., 2015). This constellation of symptoms presents challenges to patients and providers. With a majority of patients experiencing adverse events, a high risk of failure to comply with treatments exists. These symptoms also can contribute to the development of major depressive disorder, which has been observed in 59% of patients (Merck and Co., Inc., 2015).

Assessment and management of side effects is crucial. Premedication with antipyretics and increased oral hydration can reduce the intensity of flu-like symptoms. Administration of acetaminophen or NSAIDs prior to therapy may also help alleviate symptoms (Abdel-Wahab et al., 2017). Patients must have regular laboratory monitoring to assess for any organ toxicities. They should also be assessed at regular intervals for any neuropsychiatric disorders (Hauschild et al., 2008). Providing emotional support to patients and encouraging them to continue with therapy will ensure compliance with therapy. For patients experiencing increased depressive symptoms, pretreatment with paroxetine appears to be an effective strategy (Musselman et al., 2001). Referral to a psychiatrist or psychologist is also appropriate.

Oral Immune Modulators

Case 1

R.B. is a 61-year-old widowed accountant with a past medical history of chronic obstructive pulmonary disease and type 2 diabetes mellitus. She was recently diagnosed with stage I immunoglobulin G kappa multiple myeloma. She initiated treatment with lenalidomide 25 mg daily in combination with dexamethasone. Aspirin 81 mg daily was also initiated for prevention of deep vein thrombosis.

During a follow-up visit two weeks later, R.B. was found to have a platelet count of 28,000/mm³ on her complete blood count. She did not have any bleeding. R.B. was instructed to hold her lenalidomide dose and aspirin until she returned to the clinic in five days for an additional lab assessment.

R.B.'s repeat complete blood count testing demonstrated a platelet count of 44,000/mm³. She was instructed to restart lenalidomide therapy at a reduced dosage of 20 mg daily. Aspirin was not restarted until platelets improved to greater than 50,000/mm³.

The use of oral IMiDs, such as thalidomide (Thalomid®), lenalidomide (Revlimid®), and pomalidomide (Pomalyst®), for treatment of multiple myeloma and other malignancies has increased. Growing evidence suggests that continuous treatment is associated with better overall survival (Palumbo et al., 2015). Often, modification of dose and schedule are effective in managing common toxicities associated with this class of drugs (Colson, 2015). As with other therapies, management of adverse events related to this therapy will ensure patient adherence with the treatment regimen and improve outcomes (Kumar et al., 2017).

The most common adverse event associated with oral IMiDs is myelosuppression, primarily thrombocytopenia and neutropenia. For patients receiving these agents, complete blood counts should be monitored frequently, perhaps as often as once per week at the start of therapy. For patients with grade 4 thrombocytopenia, some instances of grade 3 thrombocytopenia, or grade 4 neutropenia, treatment should be interrupted (Celgene Corp., 2017a, 2017b). Patients should be advised to monitor for any signs of bleeding, bruising, or fever. Treatment can resume when the absolute neutrophil count and platelet count improve; the threshold for resuming treatment varies on the diagnosis and the patient's baseline status. When treatment is resumed, it should be given at a lower dose, usually 5 mg lower than baseline. Patients who experience neutropenia during therapy are at risk for febrile neutropenia. Prophylactic use of granulocyte macrophage–colony-stimulating factor, antibiotics (especially against *Pneumocystis jiroveci* pneumonia), and vaccines (e.g., influenza, pneumococcus, *Haemophilus*) is recommended (González Rodriguez, 2011).

Rash is seen in 27.2% of patients on lenalidomide therapy (Nardone et al., 2013). Many rashes present in a morbilliform fashion and are associated with pruritus. These cutaneous reactions are likely related to the immunomodulatory properties of these agents (Nardone et al., 2013). For localized rash or pruritus, topical corticosteroids and antihistamines are recommended (González Rodríguez, 2011; Tinsley, Kurtin, & Ridgeway, 2015). Treatment interruption or discontinuation should be considered for grade 2 rashes (10%–30% of body surface area). For more severe rashes (grade 3 or 4), treatment interruption or discontinuation should be considered (Kumar et al., 2017). Severe reactions, such as angioedema or skin exfoliation, warrant permanent discontinuation of drug (Celgene Corp., 2017a; Nardone et al., 2013).

Gastrointestinal side effects, such as diarrhea or constipation, are also associated with IMiDs (60%–70% incidence) (Celgene Corp., 2017a, 2017b). Mild and moderate diarrhea (grade 1 or 2) can be managed with antimotility agents and dietary modifications (e.g., BRAT [bananas, rice, applesauce, and toast] diet) (Colson, 2015; González Rodríguez, 2011). For grade 3 or 4 diarrhea, the IMiD should be held at clinician discretion until diarrhea improves. Dose reduction should be considered after diarrhea improves (Celgene Corp., 2017a, 2017b). It is important to manage and treat gastrointestinal side effects as soon as possible to prevent worsening toxicity and maintain adherence to the treatment regimen. Montefusco and Capecchi (2017) effectively managed IMiD-related diarrhea with cholestyramine (Questran®). In patients receiving dexamethasone, medication to reduce acid production, such as a proton pump inhibitor, may be beneficial (Kumar et al., 2017). For patients experiencing constipation, mild stimulants, stool softeners, and dietary modifications are recommended. If a patient develops symptoms of severe constipation or bowel obstruction, the IMiD should be held, and the patient should be referred for evaluation.

Venous and arterial thrombotic events, such as deep vein thrombosis and pulmonary embolus, have been reported in 7%–8% of patients receiving thalidomide or lenalidomide, especially in combination with dexamethasone (Celgene Corp., 2017a, 2017b; Palumbo et al., 2008). A 3% risk of arterial thromboembolic events, such as myocardial infarction and cerebral vascular accidents, also exists (Celgene Corp., 2017a, 2017b; Maharaj, Chang, Seegobin, Serrano-Santiago, & Zuberi, 2017). Patients with a history of thrombosis may be at greater risk; it is important to screen patients and obtain a thorough history. Education on monitoring symptoms (e.g., leg swelling, calf pain, shortness of breath) should be provided to patients. Thromboprophylaxis with aspirin 81 mg daily is recommended (Lyman et al., 2015; Palumbo et al., 2008; Zonder et al., 2006). If a patient sustains a thrombosis, treatment with anticoagulation therapy (e.g., low-molecular-weight heparin, rivaroxaban, inferior vena cava filter, thrombectomy) is required (Scarvelis & Wells, 2006).

Peripheral sensory and motor neuropathy are also associated with these agents. Autonomic symptoms, such as orthostatic hypotension, bradycardia, and constipation, can occur. Neuropathy incidence is between 15%–21% and appears to be a cumulative, dose-dependent toxicity (Celgene Corp., 2017a, 2017b). Unfortunately, no standard of care exists for treatment of IMiD-related neuropathy, and no preventive medications are available. Dose delays or reductions are indicated in patients with progressive neuropathy (greater than grade 1) (Delforge et al., 2010). Pharmacologic interventions used to treat neuropathy include gabapentin, pregabalin, tricyclic antidepressants, or dual serotonin/noradrenaline reuptake inhibitors. If these interventions are unsuccessful, extended-release opioids may be used (Koeppen, 2014).

Engineered T-Cell Therapy

Case 1

F.P. is a 50-year-old elementary school teacher without any significant medical comorbidities. She was recently diagnosed with aggressive non-Hodgkin lymphoma. Her lymphoma relapsed after receiving standard chemotherapy, and she enrolled in a clinical trial for anti-CD19 chimeric antigen receptor (CAR) T-cell therapy. F.P. was admitted to the hospital, where she received chemotherapy over four days. The next day, F.P. received day 1 of CAR T-cell therapy.

On day 2, she developed a fever of 39.3°C (102.7°F) associated with rigors and malaise. F.P. was also neutropenic ($300/mm^3$ absolute neutrophil count). Blood cultures, urine cultures, and fungal markers performed on serum samples did not demonstrate any infectious source. She was given empiric antibiotics and antiviral therapy.

On day 3, F.P.'s fever did not abate, and supportive measures continued to be implemented.

On day 4, the RN reported changes in F.P.'s mental status. She was confused (alert and oriented to place only) and intermittently noncommunicative. No seizure activity was witnessed. Vital signs were remarkable for hypotension (blood pressure 85/50), tachycardia (heart rate 130), and fever (39°C [102.2°F]). Infectious workup was again negative. F.P. was transferred to the intensive care unit, where she was consulted by a neurologist. A computed tomography of the head did not reveal any acute changes/infarcts, and an electroencephalogram did not demonstrate seizure activity. C-reactive protein (CRP) levels detected in the blood were elevated at 30.1 mg/L.

On day 5, a lumbar puncture revealed high protein levels. Tocilizumab 4 mg/kg IV was given to treat cytokine release syndrome (CRS). Later that day, CRP levels decreased to 15.2 mg/L.

On day 6, CRP levels decreased to 7.8 mg/L. F.P.'s cognition improved, and her fever abated.

On day 7, she was transferred out of the intensive care unit.

Currently, two CAR T-cell therapies are approved by the U.S. Food and Drug Administration (FDA): tisagenlecleucel (Kymriah®), for the treatment of relapsed or refractory pediatric acute lymphoblastic leukemia, and axicabtagene ciloleucel (Yescarta®), for the treatment of relapsed or refractory diffuse large B-cell lymphoma. These therapies can induce durable clinical responses; however, they can also produce serious toxicities, such as CRS (Lee et al., 2014; Maude et al., 2018; Neelapu, Locke, et al., 2017). Other sequelae of CAR T-cell therapies include neurotoxicity, myelosuppression, B-cell aplasia, hypogammaglobulinemia, and hypersensitivity reactions.

CRS is the most prevalent side effect of CAR T-cell therapy (Lee et al., 2014). CRS is a cascade of events that initially manifests clinically with mild symptoms, such as fever, rigor, flu-like symptoms, myalgia, arthralgia, and malaise, but can progress to more severe symptoms, such as high fever, hypotension, tachycardia, capillary leak, and possibly disseminated intravascular coagulation. Its underlying mechanism is related to immune activation by the infiltration of T cells, which causes vascular endothelial cells and other non–T cells to produce interleukin (IL)-6 (Obstfeld et al., 2017). Elevated inflammatory cytokine levels, specifically of IL-6, can be detected in the blood; however, this assessment method is costly. Ferritin, IL-10, and CRP levels have been used as surrogate markers, as ferritin is sensitive and specific for macrophage activation and hemophagocytic lymphohistiocytosis (Teachey et al., 2016), and CRP is made by hepatocytes in response to IL-6 (Davila et al., 2014).

Two pivotal phase 2 trials for tisagenlecleucel and axicabtagene ciloleucel reported a CRS incidence (any grade) of 77% and 93%, respectively (Maude et al., 2018; Neelapu, Locke, et al., 2017). Most cases were grade 1 or 2, but 13% of axicabtagene ciloleucel recipients and 46% of tisagenlecleucel recipients experienced CRS events classified as grade 3 or higher. CRS onset occurs within the first week after cell infusion but typically presents within two to three days and persists for a median duration of eight days (Maude et al., 2018; Neelapu, Locke, et al., 2017; Neelapu, Tummala, et al., 2017).

In patients receiving CAR T-cell therapy, CRS severity corresponds to disease burden at the time of cell infusion (Bonifant, Jackson, Brentjens, & Curran, 2016; Maude, Barrett, Teachey, & Grupp, 2014). For patients with acute lymphoblastic leukemia and a high number of circulating blasts, an increased risk of severe CRS exists. The correlation between CRS and therapy outcomes is not yet established (Maude et al., 2014).

Management of CRS can be challenging, as presenting symptoms can mimic allergic response, anaphylaxis, infection or sepsis, shock, or other underlying processes. The initial workup and care of a patient with pyrexia following CAR T-cell infusion should include blood cultures, antibiotics, IV fluids, and close vital sign and clinical monitoring. Because CRS is an inflammatory process, it is reversible with appropriate intervention. The primary goal is maintenance of hemodynamic status, as hypotension can lead to shock and organ failure. Tocilizumab, a humanized monoclonal antibody targeting the IL-6 receptor, is now FDA approved for the treatment of CRS; it is recommended for grade 2 or higher CRS or hypotension refractory to fluid boluses (Neelapu, Tummala, et al., 2017). Tocilizumab is given intravenously at doses of 4 or 8 mg/kg over one hour and tends to resolve CRS symptoms within 24–48 hours. Up to three subsequent doses can be given at least eight hours apart (Genentech, Inc., 2017a). Studies using tocilizumab in cases of grade 3 and 4 CRS have not demonstrated a negative effect on efficacy of CAR T cells (Fitzgerald et al., 2017; Neelapu, Tummala, et al., 2017). Corticosteroids are also effective in management of CRS but should only be given in cases refractory to IL-6 blockade or in patients with severe neurotoxicity (Neelapu, Tummala, et al., 2017).

Patients receiving CAR T cells can also experience neurologic toxicity, as manifested by confusion, headaches, nausea, ataxia, dysmetria, aphasia, delirium, hallucinations, somnolence, and seizures. These events often occur concurrently with CRS. Neurologic events occurred in 40% of patients receiving tisagenlecleucel (Maude et al., 2018) and 64% of patients receiving axicabtagene ciloleucel (Neelapu, Tummala, et al., 2017), with 13% and 28% reported as grade 3 or higher, respectively. The reported median onset of neurologic symptoms was 3–5 days, with median resolution occurring in 10–17 days. Neelapu, Locke, et al. (2017) described neurotoxicity as CAR-T-cell–related encephalopathy syndrome, or CRES, and developed a grading tool (CARTOX-10) for neurologic assessment of patients with symptoms after CAR T-cell infusion. For patients exhibiting neurologic changes, the authors recommended vigilant neurologic monitoring, electroencephalogram, neurology consult, and transfer to intensive care, if indicated (Neelapu, Locke, et al., 2017). CRES can be managed with corticosteroids; dexamethasone is preferred because of its high central nervous system penetrance (Czock, Keller, Rasche, & Häussler, 2005), but many study patients also received tocilizumab.

Prompt recognition of neurologic symptoms and close monitoring of hemodynamic and neurologic status are vital. Supportive care measures with IV fluids, antibiotics, antipyretics, antiemetics, and antiepileptics, as well as frequent monitoring of organ function and electrolytes, are imperative. Patients should be educated on the risk of toxicities. Education and psychological support for family members and caregivers are also essential (Smith & Venella, 2017).

Vaccine Therapy

Sipuleucel-T (Provenge®) is a unique treatment, as it is an autologous cellular immunotherapy. As such, its safety profile includes (usually) mild events and well-tolerated therapy. The primary adverse event observed with sipuleucel-T is acute infusion reaction, which includes symptoms of nausea and vomiting, fatigue, fever, chills, hypotension, hypertension, tachycardia, and dyspnea/hypoxia. The incidence of chills is 53% (Dendreon Corp., 2014; Gomella, Gelpi-Hammerschmidt, & Kundavram, 2014). In most cases, these symptoms occur during or shortly after infusion and resolve within 48 hours (Kantoff et al., 2010). A small number of patients (3.5%) have experienced cerebrovascular accidents (hemorrhagic and ischemic strokes). Overall, therapy was discontinued in less than 2% of cases (Dendreon Corp., 2014).

To minimize infusion reactions, a patient should receive premedication acetaminophen and antihistamine at least 30 minutes prior to infusion (Abdel-Wahab et al., 2017; Dendreon Corp., 2014). In the event of an acute infusion reaction, the infusion should be stopped, and the patient should be assessed. Additional supportive medications include another antihistamine, low-dose meperidine, and a slowed infusion time (Gomella et al., 2014; Hall et al., 2011). Patients with preexisting cardiopulmonary disease should be monitored closely during and after infusion (Abdel-Wahab et al., 2017). Concomitant use of immunosuppressive agents, such as systemic corticosteroids, is not recommended, as they may affect drug efficacy (Dendreon Corp., 2014). However, they may be given at clinician discretion in cases where adverse events warrant steroid use.

Oncolytic Viral Therapy

Although the previously discussed therapies are administered in a systemic fashion, talimogene laherparepvec (Imlygic®) is administered directly into melanoma lesions. The side effect profile is similar to interferon therapy, as up to 50% of patients experience flu-like symptoms (e.g., fatigue, chills, pyrexia, nausea, malaise, myalgia, arthralgia) (Amgen Inc., 2017). These symptoms are more common in the first three months of treatment. An increased risk of herpetic infection also exists after administration. Cellulitis and immune-mediated events (e.g., glomerulonephritis, vasculitis, pneumonitis, psoriasis, vitiligo) have been reported (Amgen Inc., 2017; Andtbacka et al., 2015).

Management of these adverse reactions includes supportive care measures. As with management of cytokine therapy, increased hydration and antipyretics may alleviate symptom severity. Prophylactic antiviral therapy is not recommended, as it may interfere with effectiveness of this therapy type; however, antivirals are indicated in the setting of an active disseminated herpetic infection (Amgen Inc., 2017).

Special Populations

Although a tremendous amount is known about the side effect profiles of various immunotherapy agents, a knowledge deficit or absolute contraindication for therapy exists in some special populations.

Pregnant Women and Women of Childbearing Potential

Women who are pregnant or breastfeeding have been excluded from clinical trials using immunotherapy agents (and from most cancer clinical trials in general). Antibodies are known to cross the placental barrier; therefore, FDA does not recommended that pregnant women receive any checkpoint (category D) or CTLA-4 (category C) inhibitors. The use of these agents in women who are breastfeeding has not been studied.

Immunodulatory agent use in pregnant women leads to deleterious birth defects, spontaneous abortion, and premature infant death. Pregnancy is contraindicated (category X), and women must agree to use two different forms of birth control. Women of childbearing potential should be educated on methods of highly effective birth control, including intrauterine devices, oral contraceptive pills, tubal ligations, and male vasectomies, and provided counseling on adequate contraceptive techniques. Other effective forms of birth control are barrier devices, such as male condoms and diaphragms. Natural family planning (rhythm method), progesterone-only "minipills," and female condoms are not effective methods of birth control and should not be used as a solitary means of contraception (Celgene Corp., 2017b).

Patients With Comorbidities and Preexisting Autoimmune Disorders

Patients with organ dysfunction and autoimmune conditions have largely been excluded from participation in clinical trials using checkpoint inhibitors. Consequently, data regarding safety and efficacy of checkpoint inhibitors in this patient population are lacking.

In a retrospective analysis, Kanz et al. (2016) identified 27 patients with solid tumors who had baseline organ dysfunction (renal, hepatic, or cardiac) prior to receiving anti–PD-1 agents. After exposure to drug, only 7% experienced grade 3 irAEs (three total events). Only one patient had to discontinue therapy because of worsening organ function. Moreover, efficacy of therapy was observed in nearly half (48%) of patients.

When considering the mechanism of action of CTLA-4 and PD-1 inhibitors, a theoretical concern exists that these agents could intensify an underlying autoimmune condition. Therefore, a general reluctance exists to prescribe these agents to patients with conditions such as lupus,

Crohn disease, and rheumatoid arthritis. Many of these patients may also be receiving systemic steroids and/or tumor necrosis factor–blocking agents (e.g., adalimumab, etanercept, infliximab), which have been historically contraindicated with use of checkpoint inhibitors. However, emerging evidence suggests that patients with underlying autoimmune conditions can tolerate therapy. Gutzmer et al. (2017) observed a flare of preexisting autoimmune disorder in 42% of patients treated with a checkpoint inhibitor. Approximately 35% of patients treated were receiving ongoing immunosuppression at the time of PD-L1 initiation. These patients were treated without the need to discontinue therapy. Menzies et al. (2017) found similar rates of flare in underlying autoimmune disorders (38%) that required immunosuppressive therapy. Only two patients (4%) had to discontinue therapy. Johnson et al. (2016) also found ipilimumab-induced exacerbation of underlying autoimmune conditions in 27% of study patients. The irAEs in this study did not exceed the number observed in large clinical trials.

These studies demonstrate that patients with underlying autoimmune conditions, with appropriate monitoring, may be candidates for immunotherapy. Additional prospective studies are needed to establish safety guidelines for patients with baseline autoimmune diagnoses. For patients with an underlying disorder or baseline organ dysfunction, frequent follow-up with close monitoring of symptoms, organ function, and physical examination is crucial.

Older Adults and Pediatrics

Older adult patients are frequently underrepresented in clinical trials (Lewis et al., 2003). This is often because of comorbid diagnoses, poor performance status, or poor organ function. The impact of age on the response of immunotherapy has not been described (Daste et al., 2017), and no identifiable differences were found in response rates in patients older than 65 years in clinical trials (Johnson, Sullivan, & Menzies, 2017). Friedman et al. (2017) reviewed the rates of adverse events in patients aged 80 years and older with melanoma and found that they did not differ from data in previously reported phase 3 clinical trials of all age groups. In 429 patients treated with atezolizumab (Tecentriq®) for urothelial carcinoma and non-small cell lung cancer, no differences were found in safety or efficacy in patients older than 75 years of age when compared to younger patients (Genentech, Inc., 2017b).

Little data exist for efficacy and safety in pediatric patients receiving immunotherapy agents. Merchant et al. (2016) described results of a phase 1 trial of ipilimumab, noting 55% of patients developed irAEs with a predominance of gastrointestinal and liver toxicities. Ipilimumab was tolerated at similar toxicities and pharmacokinetics as reported in adult trials. A theoretical concern of efficacy remains, as immune checkpoint inhibitors are known to be more effective in highly mutated cancers; pediatric solid tumors typically have a low mutation threshold (Park & Cheung, 2017). Clinical trials are using more of these agents for pediatric patients. One trial, NCT00586391, includes pediatric patients for assessment of combination CD19 CAR T cells and ipilimumab in B-cell lymphoid malignancies.

Patients Who Have Received Solid Organ or Allogeneic Transplantation

Nivolumab and pembrolizumab are FDA approved for use in patients with Hodgkin lymphoma (Bristol-Myers Squibb Co., 2018a). Ongoing clinical trials are also using these agents in patients with non-Hodgkin lymphoma. Many patients with relapsed/refractory lymphoma may receive an allogeneic hematopoietic stem cell transplantation (HSCT). Merryman et al. (2017) conducted a retrospective review of 39 patients with lymphoma who received prior treatment with a PD-1 inhibitor before HSCT. The incidences of acute graft-versus-host disease were 44% for grades 1 and 2 and 23% for grades 3 and 4 (median follow-up time of 12 months). This suggests an increased risk of early immune-related toxicity in this population. Haverkos et al. (2017) also found graft-versus-host disease to have a rapid and severe onset in patients treated with a PD-1 inhibitor who subsequently underwent HSCT.

Kittai, Oldham, Cetnar, and Taylor (2017) reviewed case studies of 12 patients who received a checkpoint inhibitor after solid organ transplantation. Four patients (33%) experienced organ rejection. Unfortunately, no guidelines exist for treatment with checkpoint inhibitors in patients who have received a bone marrow or solid organ transplant; however, some patients have been able to tolerate therapy after transplantation. Further prospective studies are warranted.

Pseudoprogression

Pseudoprogression is an interesting phenomenon observed with immunomodulating agents, checkpoint inhibitors, and CAR T cells. It is characterized by a measurable increase in size of the primary tumor after initiation of treatment followed by subsequent tumor regression. An analysis of tumor tissue biopsied in events of pseudoprogression (tumor flare) has found the initial increase in tumor size is actually caused by migration of T cells into the tumor, which causes inflammation (Di Giacomo et al., 2009). The subsequent reduction of tumor size is related to a decrease in inflammatory cells and tumor cell burden (see Figure 11-8).

FIGURE 11-8 Melanoma Pseudoprogression

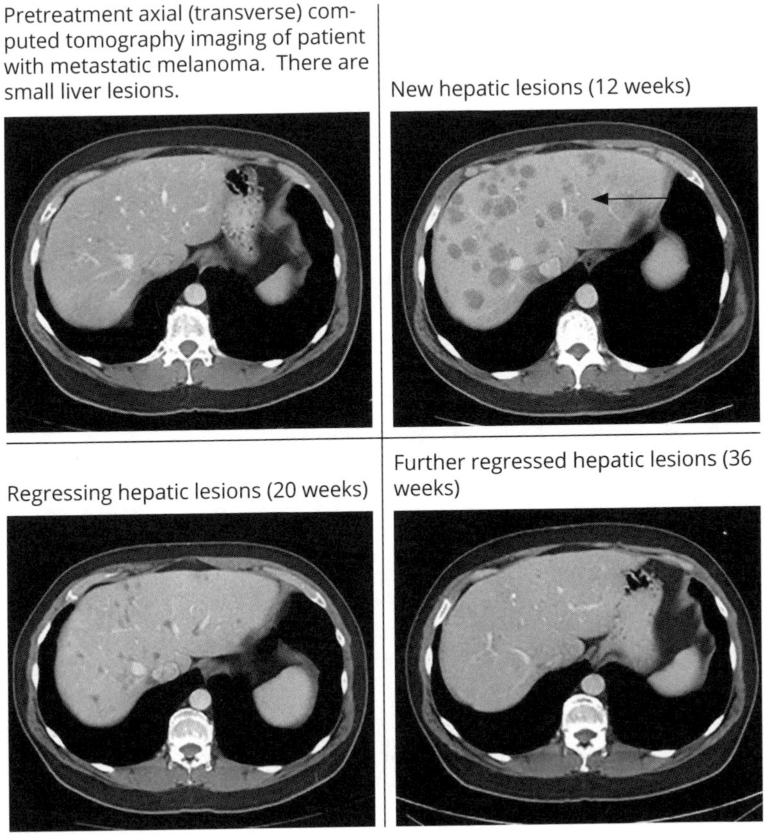

Pretreatment axial (transverse) computed tomography imaging of patient with metastatic melanoma. There are small liver lesions.

New hepatic lesions (12 weeks)

Regressing hepatic lesions (20 weeks)

Further regressed hepatic lesions (36 weeks)

Note. Images courtesy of Michael Postow, MD, and Jedd Wolchok, MD. Used with permission.

Pseudoprogression represents a challenging issue in current practice. Initial assessment of patients receiving this therapy shows a lack of patient response to therapy, manifested by enlarged tumor size. Historically, these patients would have been labeled as "progression of disease" by World Health Organization or Response Evaluation Criteria In Solid Tumors (RECIST) criteria, which dictate strict cutoffs for definitions of progression, stable disease, partial remission, and complete response (Chiou & Burotto, 2015). However, these findings have prompted recommendations for the development of immune-related response criteria (Wolchok et al., 2009). In 2017, the RECIST working group developed guidelines (iRECIST) for response criteria for patients receiving immunotherapy agents in clinical trials (Seymour et al., 2017). In the event a patient experiences a mixed response or has an equivocal finding, continuation of treatment and reassessment at a future time to rule out or confirm pseudoprogression are recommended. New criteria for evaluation of response of clinical trial therapy in patients with lymphoma have been developed as well. The LYRIC criteria include the category of "indeterminate response," an identifier for lesions until confirmed as flare/pseudoprogression or true progression of disease by either biopsy or subsequent imaging (Cheson et al., 2016).

Patients and caregivers should be educated about the potential for pseudoprogression; the appearance of worsening disease early in treatment may elicit feelings of fear, hopelessness, and anxiety. Acknowledging that not every patient who experiences progression is a pseudoprogressor, the healthcare team must provide support and reinforce the importance of continuing therapy, especially if the patient is gaining clinical benefit. Early responses (or appearance of lack of a response) can be misleading, and patients should be encouraged to adhere to therapy and primary team recommendations.

Adherence to Oral Therapy

The number of novel agents used for antineoplastic purposes is increasing. Although many of these agents are given intravenously, more than 80 oral anticancer medications (OACs) have been approved, and many more are in clinical trial development for patients with various cancers. In addition to providing efficacious, less invasive therapy, most patients prefer oral medications because of their convenience and perceived sense of autonomy (Liu, Franssen, Fitch, & Warner, 1997; Twelves, Gollins, Grieve, & Samuel, 2006).

Many reports have assessed adherence to antineoplastic agents. In a large systematic review, Greer et al. (2016) observed adherence rates of 46%–100%. These rates were dependent on patient population, medication, duration of follow-up, assessment tool, and calculation of adherence.

To help facilitate proper administration and ensure patient compliance, the healthcare team must assess barriers to compliance and provide education and support to patients and caregivers. It is vital for patients to understand their treatment regimen and the importance of taking oral medications as prescribed. Patient adherence to therapy is directly related to survival rate and risk of recurrence; poor adherence to therapy negatively affects patient outcomes.

The International Society for Pharmacoeconomics and Outcomes Research defines *medication compliance* (also referred to as *adherence*) as "the act of conforming to the recommendations made by the provider with respect to the timing, dosage, and frequency of medication taking" (Cramer et al., 2008, p. 46). It defines *medication persistence* as "the duration of time from initiation to discontinuation of therapy" (Cramer et al., 2008, p. 46). In most circumstances, patients will underadhere (e.g., taking fewer tablets per day than prescribed, not starting a cycled drug on the day prescribed). Alternatively, some patients may overadhere (e.g., doubling doses, taking more pills than prescribed).

Many factors and barriers contribute to patient compliance with OACs. Understanding and acknowledging these potential barriers allows clinicians, as part of an interprofessional team approach, to design a treatment plan to improve patient compliance and safety. Demographic and clinical factors are often not modifiable (e.g., age, comorbidities), but understanding psychological factors (e.g., patient perception of illness) may be beneficial when considering interventions to increase adherence (Lin, Clark, Tu, Bosworth, & Zullig, 2017). Patients who do not understand the rationale for treatment are less likely to be compliant with therapy (Kurtin, Colson, Tariman, Faiman, & Finley-Oliver, 2016).

In addition to the Oncology Nursing Society's (2016) Oral Adherence Toolkit, the Multinational Association of Supportive Care in Cancer (n.d.) Oral Agent Teaching Tool was developed for patients receiving OACs. This tool includes generic education points for all OACs, resources, and an evaluation to assess education effectiveness. Table 11-8 details some of the most common barriers one may encounter when caring for patients taking OACs.

Evidence for therapeutic patient education interventions is lacking for patients treated in an ambulatory setting (Arthurs et al., 2015). Additional research is needed in this arena.

Financial Considerations

Although positive strides have been made in developing new agents to treat cancer, the cost of these therapeutic drugs has set a different, higher bar on the economics of today's cancer care. Whereas traditional, off-patent chemotherapy agents may cost several hundred dollars (or in some cases, just several dollars) per dose, the cost of a checkpoint inhibitor for a 70 kg patient is between $6,000 and $11,000 per dose. This amount increases to nearly $35,000 for CTLA-4 inhibitors (Wolters Kluwer, n.d.). Oral agents for multiple myeloma, such as lenalidomide and pomalidomide, can cost $15,000–$17,000 per month (Wolters Kluwer, n.d.). CAR T-cell therapy also falls into this category. An infusion of tisagenlecleucel costs $475,000, and an infusion of axicabtagene ciloleucel costs $373,000 (Wolters Kluwer, n.d.).

TABLE 11-8 Barriers to Oral Cancer Therapy

Factors	Barrier	Intervention
Patient related	Age	For young patients, engage parents. For older adults, engage family members.
	Polypharmacy	Review with clinical pharmacist to screen for drug–drug interactions. Change drug class in the event of an interaction if possible.
	Emotional and mental status	Assess for depression/poor coping. Refer to specialist if needed.
	Socioeconomic status	Assess for lack of financial support. Engage social work or other philanthropic organizations if needed.
	Social support	Identify caregiver support. If lack of support, engage social work.
	Comorbid conditions (including dysphagia)	Screen for uncontrolled conditions. Refer to specialist if needed.
	Language and health literacy	Provide information in format easiest for patient to understand.
	Lifestyle	Assess patient schedule and tailor treatment regimen to fit schedule.
	Perceived benefit of treatment/expectations about medication efficacy	Provide education to patient and family continuously; ensure entire clinical team reinforces. Provide motivational interviewing and counseling.
	Lack of understanding of side effects	Provide education to patient and family continuously; ensure entire clinical team reinforces.
	Substance abuse	Screen for drug or alcohol abuse. Refer to specialist if needed.
Treatment related	Side effect profile	Provide education prior to start of therapy. Assess symptoms regularly. Encourage patient to call.
	Complexity of regimen/frequency of dosing	Use pill diary/calendar, pill box (AM and PM compartments), and reminders (phone, alarm clock, phone call). Assess and monitor adherence at each visit.

(Continued on next page)

TABLE 11-8 Barriers to Oral Cancer Therapy *(Continued)*

Factors	Barrier	Intervention
Treatment related *(cont.)*	Cost	Assess patient insurance coverage and financial ability/willingness to pay (for drug or co-payment). Seek financial support programs if needed.
Healthcare team related	Relationship/trust with providers	Identify methods to improve communication between patient and team. Assess patient comfort with team members.
	Poor communication	Consider implementing communication training sessions for staff members.
	Access to healthcare team (geographic and communication)	Discuss with social work or case management. Assess patient means of communication.

Note. Based on information from Burhenn & Smuddle, 2015; Hartigan, 2003; Kurtin et al., 2016; Mislang et al., 2017; Zolnierek & DiMatteo, 2009.

From "Oral Adherence Toolkit," by Oncology Nursing Society. Copyright 2016 by Oncology Nursing Society. Adapted with permission.

Several publications have discussed the financial implications of immunotherapy cancer care on a macrolevel (Oh et al., 2017; Vivot et al., 2017; Wang et al., 2017), but patients will incur some degree of financial burden for these agents on a microlevel, depending on insurance coverage, co-payment requirements, and deductibles. Indirect costs are also incurred through transportation, time off work, family burden, and treatment-related decisions. Davidoff et al. (2013) found that patients with cancer had an average out-of-pocket cost for care of nearly $5,000 per year. Bestvina, Zullig, and Zafar (2014) reviewed the impact of these costs on the patient experience and found that they may add to the burden of the cancer diagnosis itself.

Fortunately, patients can receive financial support through many means (see Table 11-9). Discussing financial concerns and burdens with patients and caregivers will help the clinical team to individualize a treatment plan. If available, social workers and case managers may have recommendations for additional resources. Many pharmaceutical companies and philanthropic organizations have programs for reimbursement and drug coverage. Local and community organizations may also provide support for patients receiving anticancer therapies. The patient and clinical team may have to fill out applications for financial support.

TABLE 11-9 Financial Resources

Type	Resources
Pharmaceutical companies	AstraZeneca Access 360™ (durvalumab)
	Bristol-Myers Squibb Access Support® (nivolumab and ipilimumab)
	Celgene Patient Support (lenalidomide and pomalidomide)
	CoverOne® from EMD Serono, Inc. (avelumab)
	Genentech Access to Care Foundation
	Kite Konnect™ (axicabtagene ciloleucel)
	Kymriah Cares™ (tisagenlecleucel)
	Merck Access Program (pembrolizumab)
Philanthropic organizations	American Cancer Society
	Cancer*Care* Co-Payment Assistance Foundation
	Good Days from Chronic Disease Fund
	HealthWell Foundation
	The Leukemia and Lymphoma Society's Co-Pay Assistance Program
	Livestrong Foundation
	National Cancer Institute support and resources
	Partnership for Prescription Assistance
	Patient Access Network Foundation
	Patient Advocate Foundation's Co-Pay Relief Program
	Patient Services, Inc.

Note. This list is not comprehensive.

Summary

Immune-based therapy to treat cancer is not a new concept; however, newer agents are becoming more mainstream for the treatment of melanoma, non-small cell lung cancer, renal cell carcinoma, bladder cancer, Hodgkin lymphoma, and multiple myeloma. Although monitoring of adverse events is a collaborative effort, the oncology nurse is often the most frequent contact for patients. It is important for the nurse to provide education, in both written form and orally, to patients and caregivers regarding the mechanism of action and potential side effects of immunotherapy agents. This education should start before therapy onset and continue at every contact point during active treatment. As with other antineoplastic agents, immediate intervention to manage side effects of therapy will minimize treatment delays, thus maximizing efficacy of the treatment regimen and optimizing patient care and quality of life.

All identifying information for case studies presented in this work (such as pseudonyms used) has been changed for privacy.

References

Abdel-Rahman, O., Helbling, D., Schmidt, J., Petrausch, U., Giryes, A., Mehrabi, A., ... Oweira, H. (2016). Treatment-associated fatigue in cancer patients treated with immune checkpoint inhibitors; A systematic review and meta-analysis. *Clinical Oncology, 28,* e127–e138. https://doi.org/10.1016/j.clon.2016.06.008

Abdel-Wahab, N., Alshawa, A., & Suarez-Almazor, M.E. (2017). Adverse events in cancer immunotherapy. In A. Naing & J. Hajjar (Eds.), *Immunotherapy: Advances in experimental medicine and biology* (pp. 155–174). New York, NY: Springer.

Abdel-Wahab, N., Shah, M., & Suarez-Almazor, M.E. (2016). Adverse events associated with immune checkpoint blockade in patients with cancer: A systematic review of case reports. *PLOS ONE, 11,* e0160221. https://doi.org/10.1371/journal.pone.0160221

Alabed, Y.Z., Aghayev, A., Sakellis, C., & Van den Abbeele, A.D. (2015). Pancreatitis secondary to anti–programmed death receptor 1 immunotherapy diagnosed by FDG PET/CT. *Clinical Nuclear Medicine, 40,* e528–e529. https://doi.org/10.1097/RLU.0000000000000940

American Cancer Society. (2016). Managing cancer-related fatigue. Retrieved from https://www.cancer.org/treatment/treatments-and-side-effects/physical-side-effects/fatigue/managing-cancer-related-fatigue.html

Amgen Inc. (2017). *Imlygic® (talimogene laherparepvec)* [Package insert]. Thousand Oaks, CA: Author.

Andtbacka, R.H., Kaufman, H.L., Collichio, F., Amatruda, T., Senzer, N., Chesney, J., ... Coffin, R.S. (2015). Talimogene laherparepvec improves durable response rate in patients with advanced melanoma. *Journal of Clinical Oncology, 33,* 2780–2788. https://doi.org/10.1200/JCO.2014.58.3377

Arthurs, G., Simpson, J., Brown, A., Kyaw, O., Shyrier, S., & Concert, C.M. (2015). The effectiveness of therapeutic patient education on adherence to oral anti-cancer medicines in adult cancer patients in ambulatory care settings: A systematic review. *JBI Database of Systematic Reviews and Implementation Reports, 13,* 244–292. https://doi.org/10.11124/jbisrir-2015-2057

AstraZeneca Pharmaceuticals LP. (2018). *Imfinzi® (durvalumab)* [Package insert]. Wilmington, DE: Author.

Banks, P.A., Bollen, T.L., Dervenis, C., Gooszen, H.G., Johnson, C.D., Sarr, M.G., ... Vege, S.S. (2013). Classification of acute pancreatitis—2012: Revision of the Atlanta classification and definitions by international consensus. *Gut, 62,* 102–111. https://doi.org/10.1136/gutjnl-2012-302779

Belum, V.R., Benhuri, B., Postow, M.A., Hellmann, M.D., Lesokhin, A.M., Segal, N.H., ... Lacouture, M.E. (2016). Characterisation and management of dermatologic adverse events to agents targeting the PD-1 receptor. *European Journal of Cancer, 60,* 12–25. https://doi.org/10.1016/j.ejca.2016.02.010

Bertrand, A., Kostine, M., Barnetche, T., Truchetet, M.-E., & Schaeverbeke, T. (2015). Immune related adverse events associated with anti-CTLA-4 antibodies: Systematic review and meta-analysis. *BMC Medicine, 13,* 211. https://doi.org/10.1186/s12916-015-0455-8

Bestvina, C.M., Zullig, L.L., & Zafar, S.Y. (2014). The implications of out-of-pocket cost of cancer treatment in the USA: A critical appraisal of the literature. *Future Oncology, 10,* 2189–2199. https://doi.org/10.2217/fon.14.130

Blasig, H., Bender, C., Hassel, J.C., Eigentler, T.K., Sachse, M.M., Hiernickel, J., ... Gutzmer, R. (2017). Reinduction of PD1-inhibitor therapy: First experience in eight patients with metastatic melanoma. *Melanoma Research, 27,* 321–325. https://doi.org/10.1097/CMR.0000000000000341

Bocquet, H., Bagot, M., & Roujeau, J.C. (1996). Drug-induced pseudolymphoma and drug hypersensitivity syndrome (drug rash with eosinophilia and systemic symptoms: DRESS). *Seminars in Cutaneous Medicine and Surgery, 15,* 250–257. https://doi.org/10.1016/S1085-5629(96)80038-1

Bonifant, C.L., Jackson, H.J., Brentjens, R.J., & Curran, K.J. (2016). Toxicity and management in CAR T-cell therapy. *Molecular Therapy Oncolytics, 3,* 16011. https://doi.org/10.1038/mto.2016.11

Brahmer, J.R., Lacchetti, C., Schneider, B.J., Atkins, M.B., Brassil, K.J., Caterino, J.M., ... Thompson, J.A. (2018). Management of immune-related adverse events in patients treated with checkpoint inhibitor therapy: American Society of Clinical Oncology clinical practice guideline. *Journal of Clinical Oncology, 36*, 1714–1768. https://doi.org/10.1200/JCO.2017.77.6385

Bristol-Myers Squibb Co. (n.d.). Opdivo® safety tool. Retrieved from https://www.opdivosafetytool.com/#/superhome

Bristol-Myers Squibb Co. (2018a). *Opdivo® (nivolumab)* [Package insert]. Princeton, NJ: Author.

Bristol-Myers Squibb Co. (2018b). *Yervoy® (ipilimumab)* [Package insert]. Princeton, NJ: Author.

Burhenn, P.S., & Smuddle, J. (2015). Using tools and technology to promote education and adherence to oral agents for cancer. *Clinical Journal of Oncology Nursing, 19*(Suppl. 3), 53–59. https://doi.org/10.1188/15.S1.CJON.53-59

Cappelli, L.C., Gutierrez, A.K., Baer, A.N., Albayda, J., Manno, R.L., Haque, U., ... O'Bingham, C.O., III. (2017). Inflammatory arthritis and sicca syndrome induced by nivolumab and ipilimumab. *Annals of the Rheumatic Diseases, 76*, 43–50. https://doi.org/10.1136/annrheumdis-2016-209595

Cappelli, L.C., Gutierrez, A.K., O'Bingham, C.O., III, & Shah, A.A. (2017). Rheumatic and musculoskeletal immune-related adverse events due to immune checkpoint inhibitors: A systematic review of the literature. *Arthritis Care and Research, 69*, 1751–1763. https://doi.org/10.1002/acr.23177

Cappelli, L.C., Naidoo, J., O'Bingham, C.O., III., & Shah, A.A. (2016). Inflammatory arthritis due to immune checkpoint inhibitors: Challenges in diagnosis and treatment. *Immunotherapy, 9*, 5–8. https://doi.org/10.2217/imt-2016-0117

Celgene Corp. (2017a). *Pomalyst® (pomalidomide)* [Package insert]. Summit, NJ: Author.

Celgene Corp. (2017b). *Revlimid® (lenalidomide)* [Package insert]. Summit, NJ: Author.

Chan, M.M.K., Kefford, R.F., Carlino, M., Clements, A., & Manolios, N. (2015). Arthritis and tenosynovitis associated with the anti-PD1 antibody pembrolizumab in metastatic melanoma. *Journal of Immunotherapy, 38*, 37–39. https://doi.org/10.1097/CJI.0000000000000060

Cheson, B.D., Ansell, S., Schwartz, L., Gordon, L.I., Advani, R., Jacene, H.A., ... Armand, P. (2016). Refinement of the Lugano Classification lymphoma response criteria in the era of immunomodulatory therapy. *Blood, 128*, 2489–2496. https://doi.org/10.1182/blood-2016-05-718528

Chiou, V.L., & Burotto, M. (2015). Pseudoprogression and immune-related response in solid tumors. *Journal of Clinical Oncology, 33*, 3541–3543. https://doi.org/10.1200/JCO.2015.61.6870

Chuzi, S., Tavora, F., Cruz, M., Costa, R., Chae, Y.K., Carneiro, B.A., & Giles, F.J. (2017). Clinical features, diagnostic challenges, and management strategies in checkpoint inhibitor-related pneumonitis. *Cancer Management and Research, 9*, 207–213. https://doi.org/10.2147/CMAR.S136818

Colson, K. (2015). Treatment-related symptom management in patients with multiple myeloma: A review. *Supportive Care in Cancer, 23*, 1431–1445. https://doi.org/10.1007/s00520-014-2552-1

Cooling, L.L., Sherbeck, J., Mowers, J.C., & Hugan, S.L. (2017). Development of red blood cell autoantibodies following treatment with checkpoint inhibitors: A new class of anti-neoplastic, immunotherapeutic agents associated with immune dysregulation. *Immunohematology, 33*, 15–21.

Corsello, S.M., Barnabei, A., Marchetti, P., De Vecchis, L., Salvatori, R., & Torino, F. (2013). Endocrine side effects induced by immune checkpoint inhibitors. *Journal of Clinical Endocrinology and Metabolism, 98*, 1361–1375. https://doi.org/10.1210/jc.2012-4075

Cortazar, F.B., Marrone, K.A., Troxell, M.L., Ralto, K.M., Hoenig, M.P., Brahmer, J.R., ... Leaf, D.E. (2016). Clinicopathological features of acute kidney injury associated with immune checkpoint inhibitors. *Kidney International, 90*, 638–647. https://doi.org/10.1016/j.kint.2016.04.008

Cramer, J.A., Roy, A., Burrell, A., Fairchild, C.J., Fuldeore, M.J., Ollendorf, D.A., & Wong, P.K. (2008). Medication compliance and persistence: Terminology and definitions. *Value Health, 11*, 44–47. https://doi.org/10.1111/j.1524-4733.2007.00213.x

Cramer, P., & Bresalier, R.S. (2017). Gastrointestinal and hepatic complications of immune checkpoint inhibitors. *Current Gastroenterology Reports, 19*, 3. https://doi.org/10.1007/s11894-017-0540-6

Czock, D., Keller, F., Rasche, F.M., & Häussler, U. (2005). Pharmacokinetics and pharmacodynamics of systemically administered glucocorticoids. *Clinical Pharmacokinetics, 44,* 61–98. https://doi.org/10.2165/00003088-200544010-00003

Daste, A., Domblides, C., Gross-goupil, M., Chakiba, C., Quivy, A., Cochin, V., ... Ravaud, A. (2017). Immune checkpoint inhibitors and elderly people: A review. *European Journal of Cancer, 82,* 155–166. https://doi.org/10.1016/j.ejca.2017.05.044

Davidoff, A.J., Erten, M., Shaffer, T., Shoemaker, J.S., Zuckerman, I.H., Pandya, N., ... Stuart, B. (2013). Out-of-pocket health care expenditure burden for Medicare beneficiaries with cancer. *Cancer, 15,* 1257–1265. https://doi.org/10.1002/cncr.27848

Davila, M.L., Riviere, I., Wang, X., Bartido, S., Park, J., Curran, K., ... Brentjens, R. (2014). Efficacy and toxicity management of 19-28z CAR T cell therapy in B cell acute lymphoblastic leukemia. *Science Translational Medicine, 6,* 224–225. https://doi.org/10.1126/scitranslmed.3008226

Delforge, M., Bladé, J., Dimopoulos, M.A., Facon, T., Kropff, M., Ludwig, H., ... Sonneveld, P. (2010). Treatment-related peripheral neuropathy in multiple myeloma: The challenge continues. *Lancet Oncology, 11,* 1086–1095. https://doi.org/10.1016/S1470-2045(10)70068-1

Dendreon Corp. (2014). *Provenge® (sipuleucel-T)* [Package insert]. Seattle, WA: Author.

Di Giacomo, A.M., Biagioli, M., & Maio, M. (2010). The emerging toxicity profiles of anti–CTLA-4 antibodies across clinical indications. *Seminars in Oncology, 37,* 499–507. https://doi.org/10.1053/j.seminoncol.2010.09.007

Di Giacomo, A.M., Danielli, R., Guidoboni, M., Calabrò, L., Carlucci, D., Miracco, C., ... Maio, M. (2009). Therapeutic efficacy of ipilimumab, an anti-CTLA-4 monoclonal antibody, in patients with metastatic melanoma unresponsive to prior systemic treatments: Clinical and immunological evidence from three patient cases. *Cancer Immunology and Immunotherapy, 58,* 1297–1306. https://doi.org/10.1007/s00262-008-0642-y

Eggermont, A.M.M., Chiarion-Sileni, V., Grob, J.-J., Dummer, R., Wolchok, J.D., Schmidt, H., ... Testori, A. (2016). Prolonged survival in stage III melanoma with ipilimumab adjuvant therapy. *New England Journal of Medicine, 375,* 1845–1855. https://doi.org/10.1056/NEJMoa1611299

Eltobgy, M., Oweira, H., Petrausch, U., Helbling, D., Schmidt, J., Mehrabi, A., ... Abdel-Rahman, O. (2017). Immune-related neurological toxicities among solid tumor patients treated with immune checkpoint inhibitors: A systematic review. *Expert Review of Neurotherapeutics, 17,* 725–736. https://doi.org/10.1080/14737175.2017.1336088

EMD Serono, Inc. (2017). *Bavencio® (avelumab)* [Package insert]. Rockland, MA: Author.

Faje, A. (2016). Immunotherapy and hypophysitis: Clinical presentation, treatment, and biologic insights. *Pituitary, 19,* 82–92. https://doi.org/10.1007/s11102-015-0671-4

Fitzgerald, J.C., Weiss, S.L., Maude, S.L., Barrett, D.M., Lacey, S.F., Melenhorst, J., ... Teachey, D.T. (2017). Cytokine release syndrome after chimeric antigen receptor T cell therapy for acute lymphoblastic leukemia. *Critical Care Medicine, 45,* e124–e131. https://doi.org/10.1097/CCM.0000000000002053

Forde, P.M., Rock, K., Wilson, G., & O'Byrne, K.J. (2012). Ipilimumab-induced immune-related renal failure—A case report. *Anticancer Research, 32,* 4607–4608.

Friedman, C.F., Horvat, T.Z., Minehart, J., Panageas, K., Callahan, M.K., Chapman, P.H., ... Lichtman, S.M. (2017). Efficacy and safety of checkpoint blockade for treatment of advanced melanoma (mel) in patients (pts) age 80 and older (80+). *Journal of Clinical Oncology, 34*(Suppl. 15), 10009. https://doi.org/10.1200/JCO.2016.34.15_suppl.10009

Friedman, C.F., Proverbs-Singh, T.A., & Postow, M.A. (2016). Treatment of the immune-related adverse effects of immune checkpoint inhibitors: A review. *JAMA Oncology, 2,* 1346–1353. https://doi.org/10.1001/jamaoncol.2016.1051

Garon, E.B., Rizvi, N.A., Hui, R., Leighl, N., Balmanoukian, A.S., Eder, J.P., ... Gandhi, L. (2015). Pembrolizumab for the treatment of non–small-cell lung cancer. *New England Journal of Medicine, 372,* 2018–2028. https://doi.org/10.1056/NEJMoa1501824

Genentech, Inc. (2017a). *Actemra® (tocilizumab)* [Package insert]. South San Francisco, CA: Author.

Genentech, Inc. (2017b). *Tecentriq® (atezolizumab)* [Package insert]. South San Francisco, CA: Author.

Goldinger, S.M., Stieger, P., Meier, B., Micaletto, S., Contassot, E., French, L.E., & Dummer, R. (2016). Cytotoxic cutaneous adverse drug reactions during anti-PD-1 therapy. *Clinical Cancer Research, 22*, 4023–4029. https://doi.org/10.1158/1078-0432.CCR-15-2872

Gomella, L.G., Gelpi-Hammerschmidt, F., & Kundavram, C. (2014). Practical guide to immunotherapy in castration resistant prostate cancer: The use of sipuleucel-T immunotherapy. *Canadian Journal of Urology, 21*(Suppl. 1), 48–56.

González Rodríguez, A.P. (2011). Management of the adverse effects of lenalidomide in multiple myeloma. *Advances in Therapy, 28*(Suppl. 1), 1–10. https://doi.org/10.1007/s12325-010-0104-8

Greer, J.A., Amoyal, N., Nisotel, L., Fishbein, J.N., MacDonald, J., Stagl, J., ... Pirl, W.F. (2016). A systematic review of adherence to oral antineoplastic sipuleucel-T. *Oncologist, 21*, 354–376. https://doi.org/10.1634/theoncologist.2015-0405

Gutzmer, R., Koop, A., Meier, F., Hassel, J.C., Terheyden, P., Zimmer, L., ... Kähler, K.C. (2017). Programmed cell death protein-1 (PD-1) inhibitor therapy in patients with advanced melanoma and preexisting autoimmunity or ipilimumab-triggered autoimmunity. *European Journal of Cancer, 75*, 24–32. https://doi.org/10.1016/j.ejca.2016.12.038

Haanen, J.B.A.G., Carbonnel, F., Robert, C., Kerr, K.M., Peters, S., Larkin, J., & Jordan, K. (2017). Management of toxicities from immunotherapy: ESMO Clinical Practice Guidelines for diagnosis, treatment and follow up. *Annals of Oncology, 28*(Suppl. 4), iv119–iv142. https://doi.org/10.1093/annonc/mdx225

Hall, S.J., Klotz, L., Pantuck, A.J., George, D.J., Whitmore, J.B., Frohlich, M.W., & Sims, R.B. (2011). Integrated safety data from 4 randomized, double-blind, controlled trials of autologous cellular immunotherapy with sipuleucel-T in patients with prostate cancer. *Journal of Urology, 186*, 877–881. https://doi.org/10.1016/j.juro.2011.04.070

Hartigan, K. (2003). Patient education: The cornerstone of successful oral chemotherapy treatment. *Clinical Journal of Oncology Nursing, 7*(Suppl. 6), 21–24. https://doi.org/10.1188/03.CJON.S6.21-24

Hauschild, A., Gogas, H., Tarhini, A., Middleton, M.R., Testori, A., Dréno, B., & Kirkwood, J.M. (2008). Practical guidelines for the management of interferon-α-2b side effects in patients receiving adjuvant treatment for melanoma. *Cancer, 112*, 982–994. https://doi.org/10.1002/cncr.23251

Haverkos, B.M., Abbott, D., Hamadani, M., Armand, P., Flowers, M.E., Merryman, R., ... Devine, S.M. (2017). PD-1 blockade for relapsed lymphoma post-allogeneic hematopoietic cell transplant: High response rate but frequent GVHD. *Blood, 130*, 221–228. https://doi.org/10.1182/blood-2017-01-761346

Hodi, F.S., O'Day, S.J., McDermott, D.F., Weber, R.W., Sosman, J.A., Haanen, J.B., ... Urba, W.J. (2010). Improved survival with ipilimumab in patients with metastatic melanoma. *New England Journal of Medicine, 363*, 711–723. https://doi.org/10.1056/NEJMoa1003466

Hofmann, L., Forschner, A., Loquai, C., Goldinger, S.M., Zimmer, L., Ugurel, S., ... Heinzerling, I.M. (2016). Cutaneous, gastrointestinal, hepatic, endocrine, and renal side-effects of anti-PD-1 therapy. *European Journal of Cancer, 60*, 190–209. https://doi.org/10.1016/j.ejca.2016.02.025

Hughes, J., Vudattu, N., Sznol, M., Gettinger, S., Kluger, H., Lupsa, B., & Herold, K.C. (2015). Precipitation of autoimmune diabetes with anti-PD-1 immunotherapy. *Diabetes Care, 38*, e55–e57.

Ito, J., Fujimoto, D., Nakamura, A., Nagano, T., Uehara, K., Imai, Y., & Tomii, K. (2017). Aprepitant for refractory nivolumab-induced pruritus. *Lung Cancer, 109*, 58–61. https://doi.org/10.1016/j.lungcan.2017.04.020

Jain, V., Bahia, J., Mohebtash, M., & Barac, A. (2017). Cardiovascular complications associated with novel cancer immunotherapies. *Current Treatment Options in Cardiovascular Medicine, 19*, 36. https://doi.org/10.1007/s11936-017-0532-8

Jameson, J.L. (2015). Approach to the patient with endocrine disorders. In D. Kasper, A. Fauci, S. Hauser, D. Longo, J.L. Jameson, & J. Loscalzo (Eds.), *Harrison's principles of internal medicine* (19th ed.). New York, NY: McGraw-Hill.

Janssen Biotech, Inc. (2017). *Remicade® (infliximab)* [Package insert]. Horsham, PA: Author.

Johnson, D.B., Sullivan, R.J., & Menzies, A.M. (2017). Immune checkpoint inhibitors in challenging populations. *Cancer, 123,* 1904–1911. https://doi.org/10.1002/cncr.30642

Johnson, D.B., Sullivan, R.J., Ott, P.A., Carlino, M.S., Khushalani, N.I., Ye, F., … Clark, J.I. (2016). Ipilimumab therapy in patients with advanced melanoma and preexisting autoimmune disorders. *JAMA Oncology, 2,* 234–240. https://doi.org/10.1001/jamaoncol.2015.4368

Joseph, R.W., Cappel, M., Goedjen, B., Gordon, M., Kirsch, B., Gilstrap, C., … Jambusaria-Pahlajani, A. (2015). Lichenoid dermatitis in three patients with metastatic melanoma treated with anti–PD-1 therapy. *Cancer Immunology Research, 3,* 18–22. https://doi.org/10.1158/2326-6066.CIR-14-0134

Kaehler, K.C., Piel, S., Livingstone, E., Schilling, B., Hauschild, A., & Schadendorf, D. (2010). Update on immunologic therapy with anti–CTLA-4 antibodies in melanoma: Identification of clinical and biological response patterns, immune-related adverse events, and their management. *Seminars in Oncology, 37,* 485–498. https://doi.org/10.1053/j.seminoncol.2010.09.003

Kantoff, P.W., Higano, C.S., Shore, N.D., Berger, E.R., Small, E.J., Penson, D.F., … Schellhammer, P.F. (2010). Sipuleucel-T immunotherapy for castration-resistant prostate cancer. *New England Journal of Medicine, 363,* 411–422. https://doi.org/10.1056/NEJMoa1001294

Kanz, B.A., Pollack, M.H., Johnpulle, R., Puzanov, I., Horn, L., Morgans, A., … Johnson, D.B. (2016). Safety and efficacy of anti-PD-1 in patients with baseline cardiac, renal, or hepatic dysfunction. *Journal for Immunotherapy of Cancer, 4,* 60. https://doi.org/10.1186/s40425-016-0166-5

Kittai, A.S., Oldham, H., Cetnar, J., & Taylor, M. (2017). Immune checkpoint inhibitors in organ transplant patients. *Journal of Immunotherapy, 40,* 277–281. https://doi.org/10.1097/CJI.0000000000000180

Koeppen, S. (2014). Treatment of multiple myeloma: Thalidomide-, bortezomib-, and lenalidomide-induced peripheral neuropathy. *Oncology Research and Treatment, 37,* 506–513. https://doi.org/10.1159/000365534

Kumar, S.K., Vij, R., Noga, S.J., Berg, D., Brent, L., Dollar, L., & Chari, A. (2017). Treating multiple myeloma patients with oral therapies. *Clinical Lymphoma, Myeloma and Leukemia, 17,* 243–251. https://doi.org/10.1016/j.clml.2017.02.024

Kurtin, S., Colson, K., Tariman, J.D., Faiman, B., & Finley-Oliver, E. (2016). Adherence, persistence, and treatment fatigue in multiple myeloma. *Journal of the Advanced Practitioner in Oncology, 7,* 71–77. https://doi.org/10.6004/jadpro.2016.7.2.16

Kushnir, I., & Wolf, I. (2017). Nivolumab-induced pericardial tamponade: A case report and discussion. *Cardiology, 136,* 49–51. https://doi.org/10.1159/000447053

Lacouture, M.E. (2015). Management of dermatologic toxicities. *Journal of the National Comprehensive Cancer Network, 13,* 686–689. https://doi.org/10.6004/jnccn.2015.0204

Lacouture, M.E., Wolchok, J.D., Yosipovitch, G., Kähler, K.C., Busam, K.J., & Hauschild, A. (2014). Ipilimumab in patients with cancer and the management of dermatologic adverse events. *Journal of the American Academy of Dermatology, 71,* 161–169. https://doi.org/10.1016/j.jaad.2014.02.035

Larkin, J., Chiarion-Sileni, V., Gonzalez, R., Grob, J.J., Cowey, C.L., Lao, C.D., … Wolchok, J.D. (2015). Combined nivolumab and ipilimumab or monotherapy in untreated melanoma. *New England Journal of Medicine, 373,* 23–34. https://doi.org/10.1056/NEJMoa1504030

Law-Ping-Man, S., Martin, A., Briens, E., Tisseau, L., & Safa, G. (2016). Psoriasis and psoriatic arthritis induced by nivolumab in a patient with advanced lung cancer. *Rheumatology, 55,* 2087–2089. https://doi.org/10.1093/rheumatology/kew281

Lee, D.W., Gardner, R., Porter, D.L., Louis, C.U., Ahmed, N., Jensen, M., … Mackall, C.L. (2014). Current concepts in the diagnosis and management of cytokine release syndrome. *Blood, 124,* 188–195. https://doi.org/10.1182/blood-2014-05-552729

Lewis, J.H., Kilgore, M.L., Goldman, D.P., Trimble, E.L., Kaplan, R., Montello, M.J., … Escarce, J.J. (2003). Participation of patients 65 years of age or older in cancer clinical trials. *Journal of Clinical Oncology, 21,* 1383–1389. https://doi.org/10.1200/JCO.2003.08.010

Lin, C., Clark, R., Tu, P., Bosworth, H.B., & Zullig, L.L. (2017). Breast cancer oral anti-cancer medication adherence: A systematic review of psychosocial motivators and barriers.

Breast Cancer Research and Treatment, 165, 247–260. https://doi.org/10.1007/s10549-017 -4317-2

Liniker, E., Menzies, A.M., Kong, B.Y., Cooper, A., Ramanujam, S., Lo, S., ... Long, G.V. (2016). Activity and safety of radiotherapy with anti-PD-1 drug therapy in patients with metastatic melanoma. *Oncoimmunology, 5,* e1214788. https://doi.org/10.1080 /2162402X.2016.1214788

Liu, G., Franssen, E., Fitch, M.I., & Warner, E. (1997). Patient preferences for oral versus intravenous palliative chemotherapy. *Journal of Clinical Oncology, 15,* 110–115. https:// doi.org/10.1200/JCO.1997.15.1.110

Lyman, G.H., Bohlke, K., Khorana, A.A., Kuderer, N.M., Lee, A.Y., Arcelus, J.I., ... Falanga, A. (2015). Venous thromboembolism prophylaxis and treatment in patients with cancer: American Society of Clinical Oncology clinical practice guideline update 2014. *Journal of Clinical Oncology, 33,* 654–656. https://doi.org/10.1200/JCO.2014.59.7351

Maharaj, S., Chang, S., Seegobin, K., Serrano-Santiago, I., & Zuberi, L. (2017). Increased risk of arterial thromboembolic events with combination lenalidomide/dexamethasone therapy for multiple myeloma. *Expert Review of Anticancer Therapy, 17,* 585–591. https:// doi.org/10.1080/14737140.2017.133015

Makarious, D., Horwood, K., & Coward, J.I.G. (2017). Myasthenia gravis: An emerging toxicity of immune checkpoint inhibitors. *European Journal of Cancer, 82,* 128–136. https://doi .org/10.1016/j.ejca.2017.05.041

Marrone, K.A., Ying, W., & Naidoo, J. (2016). Immune-related adverse events from immune checkpoint inhibitors. *Clinical Pharmacology and Therapeutics, 100,* 242–251. https://doi .org/10.1002/cpt.394

Maude, S.L., Barrett, D., Teachey, D.T., & Grupp, S.A. (2014). Managing cytokine release syndrome associated with novel T cell-engaging therapies. *Cancer Journal, 20,* 119–122. https://doi.org/10.1097/PPO.0000000000000035

Maude, S.L., Laetsch, T.W., Buechner, J., Rives, S., Boyer, M., Bittencourt, H., ... Grupp, S.A. (2018). Tisagenlecleucel in children and young adults with B-cell lymphoblastic leukemia. *New England Journal of Medicine, 378,* 439–448. https://doi.org/10.1056/ NEJMoa1709866

Maughan, B.L., Bailey, E., Gill, D.M., & Agarwal, N. (2017). Incidence of immune-related adverse events with program death receptor-1- and program death receptor-1 ligand-directed therapies in genitourinary cancers. *Frontiers in Oncology, 7,* 56. https://doi.org /10.3389/fonc.2017.00056

McGettigan, S., & Rubin, K.M. (2017). PD-1 inhibitor therapy: Consensus statement from the faculty of the melanoma nursing initiative on managing adverse events. *Clinical Journal of Oncology Nursing, 21*(Suppl. 4), 42–51.

Menzies, A.M., Johnson, D.B., Ramanujam, S., Atkinson, V.G., Wong, A.N.M., Park, J.J., ... Long, G.V. (2017). Anti-PD-1 therapy in patients with advanced melanoma and preexisting autoimmune disorders or major toxicity with ipilimumab. *Annals of Oncology, 28,* 368–376. https://doi.org/10.1093/annonc/mdw443

Merchant, M.S., Wright, M., Baird, K., Wexler, L.H., Rodriguez-Galindo, C., Bernstein, D., ... Mackall, C.L. (2016). Phase I clinical trial of ipilimumab in pediatric patients with advanced solid tumors. *Clinical Cancer Research, 22,* 1364–1370. https://doi.org/10.1158 /1078-0432.CCR-15-0491

Merck and Co., Inc. (2015). *Sylatron® (peginterferon alfa-2b)* [Package insert]. Whitehouse Station, NJ: Author.

Merck and Co., Inc. (2017a). Guide your patients through treatment with Keytruda® (pembrolizumab). Retrieved from https://www.keytruda.com/static/pdf/adverse -reaction-management-tool.pdf

Merck and Co., Inc. (2017b). *Keytruda® (pembrolizumab)* [Package insert]. Whitehouse Station, NJ: Author.

Merrill, S.P., Reynolds, P., Kalra, A., Biehl, J., Vandivier, R.W., & Mueller, S.W. (2014). Early administration of infliximab for severe ipilimumab-related diarrhea in a critically ill patient. *Annals of Pharmacotherapy, 48,* 806–810. https://doi.org/10.1177/1060028014528152

Merryman, R.W., Kim, H.T., Zinzani, P.L., Carlo-Stella, C., Ansell, S.M., Perales, M.-A., ... Armand, P. (2017). Safety and efficacy of allogeneic hematopoietic stem cell transplant after PD-1 blockade in relapsed/refractory lymphoma. *Blood, 129,* 1380–1388. https://doi.org/10.1182/blood-2016-09-738385

Michot, J.M., Bigenwald, C., Champiat, S., Collins, M., Carbonnel, F., Postel-Vinay, S., ... Lambotte, O. (2016). Immune-related adverse events with immune checkpoint blockade: A comprehensive review. *European Journal of Cancer, 54,* 139–148. https://doi.org/10.1016/j.ejca.2015.11.016

Mislang, A.R., Wildes, T.M., Kanesvaran, R., Baldini, C., Holmes, H.M., Nightingale, G., ... Biganzoli, L. (2017). Adherence to oral cancer therapy in older adults: The International Society of Geriatric Oncology (SIOG) taskforce recommendations. *Cancer Treatment Reviews, 57,* 58–66. https://doi.org/10.1016/j.ctrv.2017.05.002

Mitchell, K.A., Kluger, H., Sznol, M., & Hartman, D.J. (2013). Ipilimumab-induced perforating colitis. *Journal of Clinical Gastroenterology, 47,* 781–785. https://doi.org/10.1097/MCG .0b013e31828f1d51

Montefusco, V., & Capecchi, M. (2017). Diarrhea incidence in multiple myeloma patients treated with lenalidomide and pomalidomide. *Clinical Lymphoma, Myeloma and Leukemia, 17*(Suppl.), e46. https://doi.org/10.1016/j.clml.2017.03.082

Multinational Association of Supportive Care in Cancer. (n.d.). MASCC Oral Agent Teaching Tool. Retrieved from http://www.mascc.org/MOATT

Murata, S., Kaneko, S., Harada, Y., Aoi, N., & Morita, E. (2017). Case of de novo psoriasis possibly triggered by nivolumab. *Journal of Dermatology, 44,* 99–100. https://doi.org/10 .1111/1346-8138.13450

Musselman, D.L., Lawson, D.H., Gumnick, J.F., Manatunga, A.K., Penna, S., Goodkin, R.S., ... Miller, A.H. (2001). Paroxetine for the prevention of depression induced by high-dose interferon alfa. *New England Journal of Medicine, 344,* 961–966. https://doi.org/10.1056 /NEJM200103293441303

Naidoo, J., Cappelli, L.C., Forde, P.M., Marrone, K.A., Lipson, E.J., Hammers, H.J., ... Brahmer, J.R. (2017). Inflammatory arthritis: A newly recognized adverse event of immune checkpoint blockade. *Oncologist, 22,* 627–630. https://doi.org/10.1634/theoncologist.2016-0390

Naidoo, J., Page, D.B., Li, B.T., Connell, L.C., Schindler, K., Lacouture, M.E., ... Wolchok, J.D. (2015). Toxicities of the anti-PD-1 and anti-PD-L1 immune checkpoint antibodies. *Annals of Oncology, 26,* 2375–2391. https://doi.org/10.1093/annonc/mdv383

Nardone, B., Wu, S., Garden, B.C., West, D.P., Reich, L.M., & Lacouture, M.E. (2013). Risk of rash associated with lenalidomide in cancer patients: A systematic review of the literature and meta-analysis. *Clinical Lymphoma, Myeloma and Leukemia, 13,* 424–429. https://doi.org /10.1016/j.clml.2013.03.006

National Cancer Institute. (2017). Fatigue (PDQ®)[Health professional version]. Retrieved from https://www.cancer.gov/about-cancer/treatment/side-effects/fatigue/fatigue-hp-pdq

National Cancer Institute Cancer Therapy Evaluation Program. (2017). *Common terminology criteria for adverse events* [v.5.0]. Retrieved from https://ctep.cancer.gov/protocoldevelop ment/electronic_applications/docs/CTCAE_v5_Quick_Reference_8.5x11.pdf

National Comprehensive Cancer Network. (n.d.). Immunotherapy teaching/monitoring tool. Retrieved from https://www.nccn.org/immunotherapy-tool/pdf/NCCN _Immunotherapy_Teaching_Monitoring_Tool.pdf

National Comprehensive Cancer Network. (2017). *NCCN Clinical Practice Guidelines in Oncology (NCCN Guidelines®): Prevention and treatment of cancer-related infections* [v.1.2018]. Retrieved from http://www.nccn.org/professionals/physician_gls/pdf/infections.pdf

National Comprehensive Cancer Network & American Society of Clinical Oncology. (2018). *NCCN Clinical Practice Guidelines in Oncology (NCCN Guidelines®): Management of immunotherapy-related toxicities* [v.1.2018]. Retrieved from http://www.nccn.org /professionals/physician_gls/pdf/immunotherapy.pdf

Nayar, N., Briscoe, K., & Fernandez Penas, P. (2016). Toxic epidermal necrolysis-like reaction with severe satellite cell necrosis associated with nivolumab in a patient with ipilimumab refractory metastatic melanoma. *Journal of Immunotherapy, 39,* 149–152. https://doi.org /10.1097/CJI.0000000000000112

Neelapu, S.S., Locke, F.L., Bartlett, N.L., Lekakis, L.J., Miklos, D.B., Jacobson, C.A., ... Go, W.Y. (2017). Axicabtagene ciloleucel CAR T-cell therapy in refractory large B-cell lymphoma. *New England Journal of Medicine, 377,* 2531–2544. https://doi.org/10.1056/ NEJMoa1707447

Neelapu, S.S., Tummala, S., Kebriaei, P., Wierda, W., Gutierrez, C., Locke, F.L., ... Shpall, E.J. (2017). Chimeric antigen receptor T-cell therapy—Assessment and management of toxicities. *Nature Reviews Clinical Oncology, 15,* 47–62. https://doi.org/10.1038/ nrclinonc.2017.148

Obstfeld, A.E., Frey, N.V., Mansfield, K., Lacey, S.F., June, C.H., Porter, D.L., ... Wasik, M.A. (2017). Cytokine release syndrome associated with chimeric-antigen receptor T-cell therapy: Clinicopathological insights [Letter]. *Blood, 130,* 2569–2572. https://doi. org/10.1182/blood-2017-08-802413

Oh, A., Tran, D.M., McDowell, L.C., Keyvani, D., Barcelon, J.A., Merino, O., & Wilson, L. (2017). Cost-effectiveness of nivolumab-ipilimumab combination therapy compared with monotherapy for first-line treatment of metastatic melanoma in the United States. *Journal of Managed Care and Specialty Pharmacy, 23,* 653–664. https://doi.org/10.18553/jmcp.2017.23.6.653

Okamoto, M., Okamoto, M., Gotoh, K., Masaki, T., Ozeki, Y., Ando, H., ... Shibata, H. (2016). Fulminant type 1 diabetes mellitus with anti-programmed cell death-1 therapy. *Journal of Diabetes Investigation, 7,* 915–918. https://doi.org/10.1111/jdi.12531

Oncology Nursing Society. (2016). Oral adherence toolkit. Retrieved from https://www.ons .org/sites/default/files/ONS_Toolkit_ONLINE.pdf

Palla, A.R., Kennedy, D., Mosharraf, H., & Doll, D. (2016). Autoimmune hemolytic anemia as a complication of nivolumab therapy. *Case Reports in Oncology, 7,* 691–697. https://doi .org/10.1159/000452296

Palumbo, A., Gay, F., Cavallo, F., Di Raimondo, F., Larocca, A., Hardan, I., ... Boccadoro, M. (2015). Continuous therapy versus fixed duration of therapy in patients with newly diagnosed multiple myeloma. *Journal of Clinical Oncology, 33,* 3459–3466. https://doi.org /10.1200/JCO.2014.60.2466

Palumbo, A., Rajkumar, S.V., Dimopoulos, M.A., Richardson, P.G., San Miguel, J., Barlogie, B., ... Hussein, M.A. (2008). Prevention of thalidomide- and lenalidomide-associated thrombosis in myeloma. *Leukemia, 22,* 414–423. https://doi.org/10.1038/sj.leu.2405062

Papavasileiou, E., Prasad, S., Freitag, S.K., Sobrin, L., & Lobo, A.-M. (2016). Ipilimumab-induced ocular and orbital inflammation—A case series and review of the literature. *Ocular Immunology and Inflammation, 24,* 140–146. https://doi.org/10.3109/09273948.2014.1001858

Park, J.A., & Cheung, N.-K.V. (2017). Limitations and opportunities for immune checkpoint inhibitors in pediatric malignancies. *Cancer Treatment Reviews, 58,* 22–33. https://doi.org /10.1016/j.ctrv.2017.05.006

Pernot, S., Ramtohul, T., & Taieb, J. (2016). Checkpoint inhibitors and gastrointestinal immune-related adverse events. *Current Opinion in Oncology, 28,* 264–268. https://doi.org /10.1097/CCO.0000000000000292

Postow, M.A. (2015). Managing immune checkpoint-blocking antibody side effects. *American Society of Clinical Oncology Educational Book, 2015,* 76–83. https://doi.org/10.14694 /EdBook_AM.2015.35.76

Postow, M.A., & Wolchok, J. (2017). Toxicities associated with checkpoint inhibitor immunotherapy. In M.E. Ross (Ed.), *UpToDate.* Retrieved February 20, 2017, from https://www .uptodate.com/contents/toxicities-associated-with-checkpoint-inhibitor-immunotherapy

Prieux-Klotz, C., Dior, M., Damotte, D., Dreanic, J., Brieau, B., Brezault, C., ... Coriat, R. (2017). Immune checkpoint inhibitor-induced colitis: Diagnosis and management. *Targeted Oncology, 12,* 301–308. https://doi.org/10.1007/s11523-017-0495-4

Rapoport, B.L., van Eeden, R., Sibaud, V., Epstein, J.B., Klastersky, J., Aapro, M., & Moodley, D. (2017). Supportive care for patients undergoing immunotherapy. *Supportive Care in Cancer, 25,* 3017–3030. https://doi.org/10.1007/s00520-017-3802-9

Rassy, E.E., Kourie, H.R., Rizkallah, J., Karak, F.E., Hanna, C., Chelala, D.N., & Ghosn, M. (2016). Immune checkpoint inhibitors renal side effects and management. *Immunotherapy, 8,* 1417–1425. https://doi.org/10.2217/imt-2016-0099

Reuben, A. (2013). Hepatotoxicity of immunosuppressive drugs. In N. Kaplowitz & L.D. DeLeve (Eds.), *Drug-induced liver disease* (3rd ed., pp. 569–591). https://doi.org/10.1016/B978-0-12-387817-5.00031-5

Robert, C., Long, G.V., Brady, B., Dutriaux, C., Maio, M., Mortier, L., ... Ascierto, P.A. (2015). Nivolumab in previously untreated melanoma without BRAF mutation. *New England Journal of Medicine, 372*, 320–330. https://doi.org/10.1056/NEJMoa1412082

Robert, C., Schachter, J., Long, G.V., Arance, A., Grob, J.J., Mortier, L., ... Ribas, A. (2015). Pembrolizumab versus ipilimumab in advanced melanoma. *New England Journal of Medicine, 372*, 2521–2532. https://doi.org/10.1056/NEJMoa1503093

Ruiz-Bañobre, J., Abdulkader, I., Anido, U., León, L., López-López, R., & García-González, J. (2017). Development of *de novo* psoriasis during nivolumab therapy for metastatic renal cell carcinoma: Immunohistochemical analyses and clinical outcome. *APMIS, 125*, 259–263. https://doi.org/10.1111/apm.12658

Sanlorenzo, M., Vujic, I., Daud, A., Algazi, A., Gubens, M., Alcántara Luna, S., ... Ortiz-Urda, S. (2015). Pembrolizumab cutaneous adverse events and their association with disease progression. *JAMA Dermatology, 151*, 1206–1212. https://doi.org/10.1001/jamadermatol.2015.1916

Santini, D., Vincenzi, B., Guida, F.M., Imperatori, M., Schiavon, G., Venditti, O., ... Tonini, G. (2012). Aprepitant for management of severe pruritus related to biological cancer treatments: A pilot study. *Lancet Oncology, 13*, 1020–1024. https://doi.org/10.1016/S1470-2045(12)70373-X

Saw, S., Lee, H.Y., & Ng, Q.S. (2017). Pembrolizumab-induced Stevens–Johnson syndrome in non-melanoma patients. *European Journal of Cancer, 81*, 237–239. https://doi.org/10.1016/j.ejca.2017.03.026

Scarvelis, D., & Wells, P.S. (2006). Diagnosis and treatment of deep-vein thrombosis. *Canadian Medical Association Journal, 175*, 1087–1092. https://doi.org/10.1503/cmaj.060366

Seymour, L., Bogaerts, J., Perrone, A., Ford, R., Schwartz, L.H., Mandrekar, S., ... de Vries, E.G.E. (2017). iRECIST: Guidelines for response criteria for use in trials testing immunotherapeutics. *Lancet Oncology, 18*, e143–e152. https://doi.org/10.1016/S1470-2045(17)30074-8

Shang, Y.H., Zhang, Y., Li, J.H., Li, P., & Zhang, X. (2017). Risk of endocrine adverse events in cancer patients treated with PD-1 inhibitors: A systematic review and meta-analysis. *Immunotherapy, 9*, 261–272. https://doi.org/10.2217/imt-2016-0147

Shiuan, E., Beckermann, K.E., Ozgun, A., Kelly, C., McKean, M., McQuade, J., ... Johnson, D. (2017). Thrombocytopenia in patients with melanoma receiving immune checkpoint inhibitor therapy. *Journal for Immunotherapy of Cancer, 5*, 8. https://doi.org/10.1186/s40425-017-0210-0

Sibaud, V., Meyer, N., Lamant, L., Vigarios, E., Mazieres, J., & Delord, J.P. (2016). Dermatologic complications of anti-PD-1/PD-L1 immune checkpoint antibodies. *Current Opinion in Oncology, 28*, 254–263. https://doi.org/10.1097/CCO.0000000000000290

Smith, L.T., & Venella, K. (2017). Cytokine release syndrome: Inpatient care for side effects of CAR T-cell therapy. *Clinical Journal of Oncology Nursing, 21*, 29–34. https://doi.org/10.1188/17.CJON.S2.29-34

Spain, L., Diem, S., & Larkin, J. (2016). Management of toxicities of immune checkpoint inhibitors. *Cancer Treatment Reviews, 44*, 51–60. https://doi.org/10.1016/j.ctrv.2016.02.001

Teachey, D.T., Lacey, S.F., Shaw, P.A., Melenhorst, J.J., Maude, S.L., Frey, N., ... Grupp, S.A. (2016). Identification of predictive biomarkers for cytokine release syndrome after chimeric antigen receptor T-cell therapy for acute lymphoblastic lymphoma. *Cancer Discovery, 6*, 664–679. https://doi.org/10.1158/2159-8290.CD-16-0040

Tinsley, S.M., Kurtin, S.E., & Ridgeway, J.A. (2015). Practical management of lenalidomide-related rash. *Clinical Lymphoma, Myeloma and Leukemia, 15*(Suppl.), S64–S69. https://doi.org/10.1016/j.clml.2015.02.008

Topalian, S.L., Hodi, F.S., Brahmer, J.R., Gettinger, S.N., Smith, D.C., McDermott, D.F., ... Sznol, M. (2012). Safety, activity, and immune correlates of anti–PD1 antibody in cancer. *New England Journal of Medicine, 366,* 2443–2454. https://doi.org/10.1056/NEJMoa1200690

Twelves, C., Gollins, S., Grieve, R., & Samuel, L. (2006). A randomised cross-over trial comparing patient preference for oral capecitabine and 5-fluorouracil/leucovorin regimens in patients with advanced colorectal cancer. *Annals of Oncology, 17,* 239–245. https://doi.org/10.1093/annonc/mdj023

Vivot, A., Jacot, J., Zeitoun, J.-D., Ravaud, P., Crequit, P., & Porcher, R. (2017). Clinical benefit, price and approval characteristics of FDA-approved new drugs for treating advanced solid cancer, 2000–2015. *Annals of Oncology, 28,* 1111–1116. https://doi.org/10.1093/annonc/mdx053

Wachsmann, J.W., Ganti, R., & Peng, F. (2017). Immune-mediated disease in ipilimumab immunotherapy of melanoma with FDG PET-CT. *Academic Radiology, 24,* 111–115. https://doi.org/10.1016/j.acra.2016.08.005

Wang, J., Chmielowski, B., Pellissier, J., Xu, R., Stevinson, K., & Liu, F.X. (2017). Cost-effectiveness of pembrolizumab versus ipilimumab in ipilimumab-naïve patients with advanced melanoma in the United States. *Journal of Managed Care and Specialty Pharmacy, 23,* 184–194. https://doi.org/10.18553/jmcp.2017.23.2.184

Weber, J.S., Dummer, R., de Pril, V., Lebbé, C., & Hodi, F.S. (2013). Patterns of onset and resolution of immune-related adverse events of special interest with ipilimumab: Detailed safety analysis from a phase 3 trial in patients with advanced melanoma. *Cancer, 119,* 1675–1682. https://doi.org/10.1002/cncr.27969

Weber, J.S., Postow, M., Lao, C.D., & Schadendorf, D. (2016). Management of adverse events following treatment with anti-programmed death-1 agents. *Oncologist, 21,* 1230–1240. https://doi.org/10.1634/theoncologist.2016-0055

Weber, J.S., Thompson, J.A., Hamid, O., Minor, D., Amin, A., Ron, I., ... O'Day, S.J. (2009). A randomized, double-blind, placebo-controlled, phase II study comparing the tolerability and efficacy of ipilimumab administered with or without prophylactic budesonide in patients with unresectable stage III or intravenous melanoma. *Clinical Cancer Research, 15,* 5591–5598. https://doi.org/10.1158/1078-0432.CCR-09-1024

Weber, J.S., Yang, J.C., Atkins, M.B., & Disis, M.L. (2015). Toxicities of immunotherapy for the practitioner. *Journal of Clinical Oncology, 33,* 2092–2099. https://doi.org/10.1200/JCO.2014.60.0379

Wolchok, J.D., Hoos, A., O'Day, S., Weber, J.S., Hamid, O., Lebbé, C., ... Hodi, F.S. (2009). Guidelines for the evaluation of immune therapy activity in solid tumors: Immune-related response criteria. *Clinical Cancer Research, 15,* 7412–7420. https://doi.org/10.1158/1078-0432.CCR-09-1624

Wolchok, J.D., Neyns, B., Linette, G., Negrier, S., Lutzky, J., Thomas, L., ... Lebbé, C. (2010). Ipilimumab monotherapy in patients with pretreated advanced melanoma: A randomised, double-blind, multicentre, phase 2, dose-ranging study. *Lancet Oncology, 11,* 155–164. https://doi.org/10.1016/S1470-2045(09)70334-1

Wolters Kluwer. (n.d.). Lexicomp online. Retrieved from http://www.wolterskluwercdi.com/lexicomp-online

Zolnierek, K.B., & DiMatteo, M.R. (2009). Physician communication and patient adherence to treatment: A meta-analysis. *Medical Care, 47,* 826–834. https://doi.org/10.1097/MLR.0b013e31819a5acc

Zonder, J.A., Barlogie, B., Durie, B.G.M., McCoy, J., Crowley, J., & Hussein, M.A. (2006). Thrombotic complications in patients with newly diagnosed multiple myeloma treated with lenalidomide and dexamethasone: Benefit of aspirin prophylaxis. *Blood, 108,* 403–404. https://doi.org/10.1182/blood-2006-01-0154

Index

The letter *f* after a page number indicates that relevant content appears in a figure; the letter *t*, in a table.

A

abatacept, 40
acquired immunity. *See* adaptive immunity
activator protein 1 (AP-1), 35–36
active immunity, defined, 119
active immuno-oncology, 49, 119, 120. *See also* vaccine therapy
active immunotherapy, 49, 119, 120. *See also* vaccine therapy
acute inflammatory response, 21–22
acute lymphoblastic leukemia (ALL)
  adoptive cell therapy for, 12
  antibody–drug conjugates for, 189–190
  bispecific T-cell engager antibodies for, 194–195
  monoclonal antibodies for, 8
acute myeloid leukemia (AML), 185, 188–189
acute-phase proteins, 21, 45*t*
adaptive immunity, 21*f*, 28–39
  cell-mediated, 29, 33–36, 35*t*
  components of, 28, 30*t*, 36–39, 38*t*

defined, 20, 28, 45*t*
  humoral, 29–33, 32*f*
  in immunotherapy, 48
adenosine A2a receptor (A2AR), 74
adherence to oral therapy, 287–289, 290*t*–291*t*
adipokines in innate immunity, 28
adjuvant in vaccine development, 123
adoptive cell transfer (ACT), 197
  defined, 197
  history of, 6, 12
  IL-2 in, 58
adoptive transfer, 45*t*
ado-trastuzumab emtansine, 148*t*, 186–188
adrenal insufficiency due to checkpoint inhibitors, 86, 245*t*, 264, 266, 267*t*
aldesleukin, 39
alemtuzumab (Campath), 148*t*, 182–183
allogeneic transplantation, adverse events with, 286
allogeneic vaccine therapy, 125–126
alopecia due to EGFR-specific monoclonal antibodies, 152–154, 154*f*
alternative pathway of complement system, 27

amino acid terminus (N-terminus), 32
AMP-224, 75*t*
anaplastic large-cell lymphoma
  antibody–drug conjugates for, 185
  monoclonal antibodies for, 8
anaplastic lymphoma kinase (ALK) as biomarker, 232*t*–233*t*, 235*t*
anemia
  due to blinatumomab, 195
  due to CD20-targeted mAbs, 175
anergy, 40
angiogenesis inhibitor
  thalidomide as, 105
  VEGFR, 161–167
antibodies
  in adaptive immunity, 37
  chimeric, 139
  in humoral immunity, 31, 32
  monoclonal. *See* monoclonal antibodies (mAbs)
  structure of, 32*f*, 139, 140*f*
antibody-dependent cellular cytotoxicity (ADCC), 45*t*
antibody–drug conjugates, 140, 142*t*, 184–191

ado-trastuzumab emtansine as, 148t, 186–188
brentuximab vedotin as, 148t, 185–186
gemtuzumab ozogamicin as, 188–189
inotuzumab ozogamicin as, 189–191
mechanism of action of, 184–185
side effects of, 148t
antibody–radiopharmaceutical conjugates, 148t, 191–194
anti–CTLA-4 agents, 70, 71, 74, 75t
dual checkpoint blockade with, 221–223
antigen, 20–21, 33, 45t
antigen–adjuvant solution in vaccine therapy, 120–121
antigen binding, 31
antigen-binding sites, 31
antigen presentation, loss or downregulation of, 48
antigen-presenting cells (APCs), 24, 25, 33, 45t
in vaccine therapy, 121, 123, 127
antigen recognition, 28
anti-OX40 mAbs, 74
anti–PD-1 agents, 71–72, 75t
combination immunotherapy with, 221
dual checkpoint blockade with, 221–223
anti–PD-L1, 71, 72–73, 75t
anti–PD-L2, 75t
antitumor immune response, 41–44, 42f
apoptosis, 37
arterial thrombotic events due to oral immunomodulators, 279
atezolizumab (Tecentriq), 72, 75t

adverse events due to, 245t–246t
autoimmune conditions, 40
adverse events with, 284–285
autoimmune hemolytic anemia (AIHA) due to checkpoint inhibitors, 275–276
autoimmune reaction in vaccine development, 124
autoimmunity, 40
autologous stem cell transplantation (ASCT), lenalidomide after, 111
autologous vaccine therapy, 125–126
avelumab (Bavencio), 72–73, 75t, 76
adverse events due to, 245t–246t

B

B1 cells, 31
B2 cells, 31
B7-1, 68
B7-2, 68
B7-DC, 68, 70
B7-H1, 67–68, 70
B7-H3, 73
B7-H4, 73
B7-S1, 73
B7x, 73
bacillus Calmette-Guérin (BCG), 95–100
history of, 4–5, 95–96
mechanism of action of, 96–97
nursing administration of, 97–99
side effects of, 99
B- and T-lymphocyte attenuator (BTLA), 73–74
basophils in innate immunity, 23t
B-cell activation, 31

B-cell lymphoma
chemoimmunotherapy for, 217
monoclonal antibodies for, 169
radioimmunotherapy for, 191, 193
B-cell proliferation, 31
B-cell receptor (BCR), 30–31, 45t
B-cell recognition, 29–30
BCR-ABL1 as biomarker, 235t
belatacept, 40
Bence Jones, Henry, 228
Bence Jones protein, 228
bendamustine, rituximab with, 218t
bevacizumab (Avastin), 161–164
dosing for, 162, 163t
efficacy of, 162–164
history of, 8
indications for, 162
side effects of, 146t, 165–167
biochemotherapy, 217–219
biologic markers. See biomarkers
biomarkers, 227–239
benefits of, 236–237
challenges with, 237–238
for checkpoint inhibitors, 70–71
clinical uses of, 230–236, 230t
for drug labeling, 231–235, 235t
for pharmacodynamics, 230t
as prognostic and predictive tools, 230t, 231–236, 235t
for screening, diagnosing, and monitoring, 230–231, 230t, 232t–234t
as surrogate endpoints, 230t, 236

as therapeutic targets, 236
defined, 227
development of, 229
evaluation of, 237–238
future directions for, 238
history of, 228–229
ideal, 237
nursing implications of, 238–239
overview of, 227–228
standardization of, 237
bispecific T-cell engager (BiTE) antibodies, 140–141, 142*t*, 148*t*, 194–196
bladder cancer, BCG for, 5, 47–48, 95–96
blinatumomab (Blincyto)
administration of, 194–195
efficacy of, 195
history of, 8
indications for, 194
mechanism of action of, 194
side effects of, 148*t*, 195–196
B lymphocytes (B cells)
in adaptive immune system, 29–33, 30*t*
defined, 45*t*
development of, 31
BMS-936559, 75*t*
BMS-986016, 75*t*
bone metastases, monoclonal antibodies for, 183–184
BRAF mutation, 222
as biomarker, 234*t*, 235*t*
BRCA1/2 as biomarker, 233*t*, 235*t*
breast cancer
antibody–drug conjugates for, 185, 187
biomarkers for, 233*t*, 236
chemoimmunotherapy for, 216
monoclonal antibodies for, 155–158

brentuximab vedotin (Adcetris), 185–186
history of, 8
side effects of, 148*t*, 186

C

Calmette, Albert, 4, 95
cancer and immune system, 40–41
cancer cell recognition, 43
cancer–immunity cycle, 41–44, 42*f*
cancer immunoediting, 40–41
cancer immunosurveillance, 6–8, 40–41
cancer symptoms, cytokines and, 61–62
carbohydrate antigen 125, 228
carboxy-terminus (C-terminus), 32
carcinoembryonic antigen, 228
cardiotoxicity
of checkpoint inhibitors, 87, 275
of HER2-targeted mAbs, 159–161
carfilzomib with lenalidomide-dexamethasone doublet, 110
CAR T-cell–related encephalopathy syndrome, 199–200
case-based management of toxicities related to therapy
with autoimmune disorders, 284–285
with checkpoint inhibitors, 247–277
dermatologic, 247–252, 248*f*, 249*f*, 250*t*–252*t*
endocrine, 263–270, 263*f*, 265*f*, 267*t*–270*t*

fatigue as, 271–272
frequency of, 245*t*–246*t*
gastrointestinal, 252–256, 253*f*, 255*t*–256*t*
hepatic, 257–259, 258*t*–259*t*
infusion reactions as, 276
neurologic, 270–271
pulmonary, 259–262, 260*f*, 261*t*–262*t*
rare, 272–276, 273*f*
with comorbidities, 284–286
with cytokine therapy, 277
with engineered T-cell therapy, 280–282
in older adults, 285
with oncolytic viral therapy, 283
with oral immune modulators, 277–280
in pediatric patients, 285–286
in pregnancy or lactation, 284
pseudoprogression as, 286–288, 287*f*
with solid organ or allogeneic transplantation, 286
in special populations, 284–286
with vaccine therapy, 283
Castleman disease, 180–181
CD20 as biomarker, 235*t*
CD20-targeted monoclonal antibodies, 168–176
obinutuzumab as, 147*t*, 172–173
ofatumumab as, 147*t*, 170–172
rituximab and hyaluronidase as, 146*t*, 169–170
rituximab as, 146*t*, 168–170

side effects of,
146t–147t, 173–176
CD28, 68
CD38-targeted monoclo-
nal antibodies, 147t,
178–180
CD52-targeted monoclonal
antibodies, 148t, 182–183
CD80, 68
CD86, 68
CD152, 38, 67, 68
CD223, 73
CD272, 73
CD273, 68, 70
CD274, 67–68, 70
as biomarker, 232t,
235t
CD276, 73
CD279, 11, 34, 35t, 38–39,
67, 69–70
cell-mediated immunity,
29, 33–36, 35t, 45t
central memory cells,
36, 37
central tolerance, 40
cereblon, 105
cervical cancer
HPV vaccine and, 11,
121–122
monoclonal antibodies
for, 162, 163t
cetuximab (Erbitux), 141,
143–144
administration of, 143
history of, 8
response to, 143–144
side effects of, 144–155,
145t, 153f–154f
checkpoint(s), 37
checkpoint inhibitors,
67–89
adverse events from,
76–88, 79f–81f, 241–
244
cardiac, 87, 275
case-based manage-
ment of, 247–277
dermatologic, 78–82,
80f, 82f, 245t, 247–
252, 248f, 249f,
250t–252t

endocrine, 81f,
85–86, 245t, 263–
270, 263f, 265f,
267t–270t
fatigue as, 246t, 271–
272
frequency of,
245t–246t
gastrointestinal,
79f, 82–83, 245t,
252–256, 253f,
255t–256t
hematologic, 87–88,
275–276
hepatic, 80f, 84–85,
245t, 257–259,
258t–259t
infusion reactions as,
76, 246t, 276
nephritis/renal dys-
function as, 246t
neurologic, 86–87,
270–271
ophthalmic/ocular,
87, 276
other toxicities as,
87–88
pancreatitis as, 272–
274, 273f
pulmonary, 79f,
83–84, 245t,
259–262, 260f,
261t–262t
rare, 272–276, 273f
renal, 246t, 274
rheumatologic, 274–
275
anti–CTLA-4 as, 70, 71,
74, 75t
anti–PD-1 as, 71–72
anti–PD-L1 as, 71,
72–73
with autoimmune dis-
eases, 77–78
biomarkers for, 70–71
in combination thera-
pies, 74–75, 128–129
defined, 45t
in dual checkpoint
blockade, 221–223
history of, 9t, 11

mechanism of action
of, 48
in metastatic setting, 76
nursing administration
of, 76
other promising, 73–74,
75t
patient education on, 78
in pregnancy and lacta-
tion, 88
in transplant recipients,
78, 286
checkpoint receptors,
67–70
A2AR as, 74
B7-H3 as, 73
B7-H4 as, 73
BTLA as, 73–74
coinhibitory, 34, 35t,
68, 69f
costimulatory, 34, 68,
69f, 74
CTLA-4 as, 67, 68
LAG-3 as, 73
PD-1 as, 67–68, 69–70
TIM-3 as, 73
chemoattractant cyto-
kines in innate immu-
nity, 22, 28
chemoimmunotherapy
(CIT), 215–219
biochemotherapy as,
217–219
common regimens for,
217, 218t
defined, 215
as immunosuppressive,
215
with R-CHOP, 216–217
side effects of, 217
chemokines, 54–55
defined, 45t, 54
and dendritic cells, 55
functions of, 54–55
in innate immunity, 27,
28, 29t
chemotaxis in innate
immunity, 22
chemotherapy as immu-
nosuppressive, 215–216
chimeric antibodies, 139

chimeric antigen receptor (CAR) T cells, 2, 198–201
adverse events with, 149t, 198–201, 280–281
defined, 198
development of, 198
indications for, 198
CHOP regimen, rituximab combined with, 216–217, 218t
chronic lymphocytic leukemia (CLL)
adoptive cell therapy for, 12
biomarkers for, 232t
monoclonal antibodies for, 8, 168, 170–173, 182–183
chronic myeloid leukemia (CML), 56
classical pathway of complement system, 27
clonal deletion in vaccine development, 122
clonal expansion, 34, 36
cluster of differentiation (CD) molecules, 45t
coinhibitor(s) in adaptive immunity, 37–39
coinhibitory receptors, 34, 35t, 68, 69f
Coley, William, 2–3, 54
Coley toxins, 3, 4
colitis
due to checkpoint inhibitors, 79f, 82–83, 245t, 253–256, 253f, 255t–256t
due to EGFR-specific monoclonal antibodies, 150
colony-stimulating factor (CSF) in innate immunity, 22
colorectal cancer
biomarkers for, 232t–233t
chemoimmunotherapy for, 216

monoclonal antibodies for, 8, 144, 162, 163t, 164
combination immunotherapy, 221–223
adverse events due to, 245t–246t
with anti–PD-1 agents, 221
with dual checkpoint blockade, 221–223
combination therapies, 215–224
checkpoint inhibitors in, 74–75
chemoimmunotherapy as, 215–219
biochemotherapy as, 217–219
common regimens for, 217, 218t
with R-CHOP, 216–217
combination immunotherapy as, 221–223
with anti–PD-1 agents, 221
with dual checkpoint blockade, 221–223
radioimmunotherapy as, 219–220
combination vaccine therapy, 128–129
common lymphoid progenitor cells, 26, 31
Common Terminology Criteria for Adverse Events (CTCAE), 243
comorbidities, adverse events with, 284–285
complement
defined, 46t
in innate immunity, 27–28
complement activation, 27
complementarity-determining regions, 31
complement cascade, 27
complement-dependent cytotoxicity, 27

compliance with oral therapy, 288–289, 290t–291t
conjugated monoclonal antibodies, 140, 142t, 184–191
ado-trastuzumab emtansine as, 148t, 186–188
brentuximab vedotin as, 148t, 185–186
gemtuzumab ozogamicin as, 188–189
inotuzumab ozogamicin as, 189–191
mechanism of action of, 184–185
side effects of, 148t
constant region, 32
corneal abnormalities due to EGFR-specific monoclonal antibodies, 149
cost considerations, 289–291, 292t
costimulatory receptors, 34, 68, 69f, 74
C-reactive proteins, 21
CRS-207 vaccine, 12
CTLA-4–specific antibody, 11
CVD regimen in biochemotherapy, 218–219
cytokine(s), 53–63
in adaptive immunity, 39
adverse events from, 277
B-cell release of, 31, 34
in cancer, 54
and cancer symptoms, 61–62
and chemokines, 54–55
defined, 46t, 53
GM-CSF as, 59–60
in history of immunotherapy, 7–8, 9t, 54
IL-2 as, 57–58
IL-6 as, 58
immuno-, 60–61
in innate immunity, 21–22, 27–28, 29t

interferon alfa as, 55–56
and natural killer cells, 26–27
nursing implications of, 62–63
production of, 54
proinflammatory, 61
in T-cell activation, 36
types of, 54, 55–60
cytokine release syndrome (CRS)
due to CD20-targeted mAbs, 174
due to chimeric antigen receptor T cells, 198–199, 280–282
cytopenias due to CD20-targeted mAbs, 175
cytotoxic T cells (CD8+)
in adaptive immune system, 30*t*, 33, 36, 37
cytotoxic T-lymphocyte antigen 4 (CTLA-4), 67, 68
as coinhibitor, 34, 35*t*, 38
history of, 6
radiation therapy and, 74–75
cytotoxic T-lymphocyte antigen 4 (CTLA-4) inhibitors, 71, 75, 75*t*
adverse events due to, 245*t*–246*t*
hepatic, 257–258
in combination immunotherapy, 11, 221
in dual checkpoint blockade, 222–223

D

dacarbazine, immunocytokine with, 61
daratumumab (Darzalex), 147*t*, 178–180
with lenalidomidedexamethasone doublet, 110
Dashiell, Bessie, 1–2

deep vein thrombosis due to oral immunomodulators, 279
defined antigen vaccine therapy, 127*t*, 128
del (5q) as biomarker, 235*t*
del (17p) as biomarker, 235*t*
delayed-onset hypogammaglobulinemia due to CD20-targeted mAbs, 176
dendritic cells (DCs), 7
antigen-presenting, 33
in cancer–immunity cycle, 42, 44
and cytokines, 55
in innate immunity, 23*t*, 25
and natural killer cells, 26
dendritic cell (DC) therapy, ex vivo, 129–130
denosumab (Xgeva, Prolia), 148*t*, 183–184
dermatologic toxicity
of checkpoint inhibitors, 78–82, 80*f*, 82*f*
assessment of, 250
case-based management of, 247–252, 248*f*, 249*f*
frequency of, 245*t*
grading of, 250*t*–252*t*
patient education on, 250
pruritus as, 79–81, 247, 249
rash as, 79–81, 82*f*, 245*t*, 247–248, 248*f*, 249, 249*f*
Stevens-Johnson syndrome and toxic epidermal necrolysis as, 81–82
treatment of, 80*f*
vitiligo as, 78–79
of EGFR-specific monoclonal antibodies, 151–155, 153*f*–154*f*

desensitization, 197
dexamethasone with lenalidomide, 110
diabetes mellitus (DM) type 1 due to checkpoint inhibitors, 85–86, 245*t*, 267*t*, 268
diagnosing, biomarkers for, 230–231, 230*t*, 232*t*–234*t*
diarrhea
due to checkpoint inhibitors, 79*f*, 82–83, 245*t*, 253–256, 253*f*, 255*t*–256*t*
due to EGFR-specific monoclonal antibodies, 150
dihydropyrimidine dehydrogenase (DPYD) as biomarker, 235*t*
disseminated intravascular coagulation due to CD20-targeted mAbs, 174
DNA-based vaccine therapy, 123, 128
docetaxel, 61
drug labeling, biomarkers for, 231–235, 235*t*
dual checkpoint blockade, combination immunotherapy with, 221–223
durvalumab (Imfinzi), 73, 75*t*
adverse events due to, 245*t*–246*t*

E

eczema due to checkpoint inhibitors, 247–248, 249*f*
effector cells, 37
in cancer–immunity cycle, 42, 44
effector memory T cells, 37
effector T cells in cancer–immunity cycle, 42

EGFR Mutation Test v2, 229
elimination phase of cancer immunoediting, 41
elotuzumab (Empliciti), 147*t*, 176–178
elotuzumab with lenalidomide-dexamethasone doublet, 110
encephalopathy, CAR T-cell–related, 199–200
endocrine toxicity of checkpoint inhibitors, 85–86, 263–270
adrenal insufficiency as, 86, 245*t*, 264, 266, 267*t*
case-based management of, 263–270, 263*f*, 265*f*
frequency of, 245*t*
grading of, 268*t*–270*t*
hypophysitis as, 85–86, 245*t*, 264–265, 265*f*, 267*t*, 268
laboratory and diagnostic test findings for, 267*t*
thyroid dysfunction due to, 85–86, 245*t*, 263, 263*f*, 266, 267*t*
treatment of, 81*f*
type 1 diabetes mellitus as, 85–86, 245*t*, 267*t*, 268
engineered T-cell therapy. *See* chimeric antigen receptor (CAR) T cells
enterocolitis due to checkpoint inhibitors, 79*f*, 83
eosinophils in innate immunity, 24*t*
epidermal growth factor receptor (EGFR) as biomarker, 232*t*, 235*t*, 236
epidermal growth factor receptor (EGFR) mutations, 229

epidermal growth factor receptor (EGFR)-specific monoclonal antibodies, 141–155
cetuximab as, 141, 143–144, 145*t*
mechanism of action of, 141–143
panitumumab as, 141, 143, 144, 145*t*
side effects of, 144–155, 145*t*, 153*f*–154*f*
equilibrium phase of cancer immunoediting, 41
erysipelas and round cell sarcoma, 2–3, 54
erythema nodosum leprosum (ENL), 104, 105, 108
escape phase of cancer immunoediting, 41
ESR1 as biomarker, 235*t*
estrogen receptor (ER) as biomarker, 236
etanercept, 62
ex vivo dendritic cell therapy, 129–130

F
fallopian tube cancer, 162, 163*t*
fatigue
due to checkpoint inhibitors, 246*t*, 271–272
cytokines and, 61–62
fever due to chimeric antigen receptor T cells, 200
financial considerations, 289–292, 292*t*
fluorescence in situ hybridization (FISH), 228
FOLFOX plus panitumumab, 144
follicular lymphoma chemoimmunotherapy for, 217
history of immunotherapy for, 8

monoclonal antibodies for, 8, 168
Forkhead box protein 3 (FOXP3) in adaptive immunity, 37
4-1BB ligand, 74
fragment antigen-binding (Fab) region, 32
fragment crystallizable (Fc) region, 32

G
gastric adenocarcinoma, 164
gastroesophageal junction adenocarcinoma, 164–165
gastrointestinal adverse effects
of checkpoint inhibitors, 82–83, 252–256
case-based management of, 252–256, 253*f*
frequency of, 245*t*
grading of, 255*t*–256*t*
treatment of, 79*f*, 254–255
of oral immunomodulators, 279
gastrointestinal perforations due to VEGF inhibitors, 165–166
gastrointestinal stromal tumors, biomarkers for, 232*t*
gemtuzumab ozogamicin (GO, Mylotarg), 188–189
genome, 46*t*
germ line, 46*t*
glioblastoma, 162, 163*t*
glucose-6-phosphate dehydrogenase (G6PD) as biomarker, 235*t*
graft-versus-host disease, 286
granulocyte macrophage–colony-stimulating factor (GM-CSF), 59–60

in vaccine therapy, 123, 127
Guérin, Camille, 4, 95
GVAX Pancreas vaccine, 11–12
GVAX vaccine, 7

H

hair changes due to EGFR-specific monoclonal antibodies, 152–154, 154f
hairy cell leukemia (HCL), 7, 56
HAVCR2, 73
heavy chains, 32, 32f
helper T cells (CD4+) in adaptive immune system, 30t, 33, 36, 37, 38t
hematologic toxicities
of CD20-targeted mAbs, 175
of checkpoint inhibitors, 87–88, 275–276
hematopoietic stem cells
in adaptive immunity, 31, 33
in innate immunity, 22, 23t
hematopoietic stem cell transplantation (HSCT)
inotuzumab ozogamicin prior to, 190
PD-1 inhibitor prior to, 286
hemophagocytic lymphohistiocytosis (HLH)/macrophage activation syndrome due to blinatumomab, 195
hemorrhagic events due to VEGF inhibitors, 165
hepatic adverse events due to checkpoint inhibitors, 84–85, 257–259
case-based management of, 257–259

frequency of, 245t
grading of, 258t–259t
treatment of, 80f
hepatitis, due to checkpoint inhibitors, 80f, 84–85, 237–238
hepatitis B virus (HBV) vaccine (Recombivax HB), 121–122
hepatocellular carcinoma (HCC), HBV vaccine and, 121–122
hepatotoxicity
of checkpoint inhibitors, 84–85, 257–259
case-based management of, 257–259
frequency of, 245t
grading of, 258t–259t
treatment of, 80f
of inotuzumab ozogamicin, 190
Hodgkin lymphoma
antibody–drug conjugates for, 185, 186
checkpoint inhibitors for, 263, 272–273
monoclonal antibodies for, 8
host immunity, escape from, 43
human epidermal growth factor receptor 2 (HER2) as biomarker, 233t–235t, 236
human epidermal growth factor receptor 2 (HER2)-targeted monoclonal antibodies, 155–161
mechanism of action of, 155
pertuzumab as, 145t, 157–158
side effects of, 145t, 158–161
trastuzumab as, 145t, 156–157
human papillomavirus (HPV) vaccine (Gardasil), 11, 121–122

humoral hypercalcemia of malignancy, 183
humoral immunity, 29–33, 32f
HVEM, 73
hybridomas, 228
hypercalcemia of malignancy
humoral, 183
monoclonal antibodies for, 183–184
hyperparathyroidism due to RANKL-targeted monoclonal antibodies, 184
hypersensitivity reactions
due to checkpoint inhibitors, 76
to monoclonal antibodies, 196–197
hyperthyroidism due to checkpoint inhibitors, 86, 263, 263f, 267t
hypervariable regions, 31
hypocalcemia due to RANKL-targeted monoclonal antibodies, 184
hypogammaglobulinemia, delayed-onset, due to CD20-targeted mAbs, 176
hypomagnesemia due to EGFR-specific monoclonal antibodies, 150–151
hypophysitis due to checkpoint inhibitors, 85–86, 245t, 264–265, 265f, 267t, 268
hypothyroidism due to checkpoint inhibitors, 85, 267t

I

ibritumomab tiuxetan (Zevalin), 148t, 191–194, 219, 220
immune checkpoint inhibitors. See checkpoint inhibitors

immune recognition, 40
immune-related adverse
events (irAEs), 241–
292
with autoimmune disor-
ders, 284–285
from checkpoint inhibi-
tors, 76–88, 79*f*–81*f*,
241–244
case-based manage-
ment of, 247–277
dermatologic, 78–82,
80*f*, 82*f*, 247–
252, 248*f*, 249*f*,
250*t*–252*t*
endocrine, 81*f*, 85–86,
263–270, 263*f*,
265*f*, 267*t*–270*t*
fatigue as, 271–272
frequency of,
245*t*–246*t*
gastrointestinal, 79*f*,
82–83, 252–256,
253*f*, 255*t*–256*t*
hematologic, 87–88
hepatic, 80*f*, 84–85,
257–259, 258*t*–259*t*
infusion reactions as,
76, 276
neurologic, 86–87,
270–271
pulmonary, 79*f*,
83–84, 259–262,
260*f*, 261*t*–262*t*
rare, 272–276, 273*f*
Common Terminology
Criteria for Adverse
Events for, 243
with comorbidities,
284–285
from cytokine therapy,
277
from engineered T-cell
therapy, 149*t*, 198–
201, 280–282
grading of, 243
Immunotherapy
Teaching/Monitoring
Tool for, 242–243
management of, 243–
244

monitoring of, 243–244
in older adults, 285
from oncolytic viral
therapy, 283
from oral immune mod-
ulators, 108, 109*t*,
112–114, 277–280
in pediatric patients,
285–286
in pregnancy or lacta-
tion, 284
pseudoprogression as,
286–288, 287*f*
with solid organ or allo-
geneic transplanta-
tion, 286
in special populations,
284–286
from vaccine therapy,
283
wallet card for, 243
immune response
adaptive (specific,
acquired), 21*f*, 28–39
cell-mediated, 29,
33–36, 35*t*
components of, 28,
30*t*, 36–39, 38*t*
defined, 20, 28
humoral, 29–33, 32*f*
components of, 21, 21*f*
innate, 21–28, 21*f*
components of, 22–27,
23*t*–24*t*
defined, 20, 21
soluble factors of,
27–28, 29*t*
immune suppression in
vaccine development,
122–123
immune system, 19–50
cancer and, 40–41
and immune tolerance,
39–40
overview of, 20–21
immune thrombocyto-
penic purpura (ITP)
due to checkpoint
inhibitors, 275–276
immune tolerance,
39–40, 46*t*

immunity
adaptive (specific,
acquired), 21*f*, 28–39
cell-mediated, 29,
33–36, 35*t*
components of, 28,
30*t*, 36–39, 38*t*
defined, 20, 28, 46*t*
humoral, 29–33, 32*f*
in cancer–immunity
cycle, 41–44, 42*f*
cell-mediated, 29,
33–36, 35*t*
defined, 19
humoral, 29–33, 32*f*
innate, 21–28, 21*f*
components of, 22–27,
23*t*–24*t*
defined, 20, 21
soluble factors of,
27–28, 29*t*
immunocytokines, 60–61
immunogen, 46*t*
immunoglobulin(s) (Igs),
31–32, 37, 46*t*
immunoglobulin A (IgA),
32
immunoglobulin D
(IgD), 32
immunoglobulin E (IgE),
33
immunoglobulin G
(IgG), 33
immunoglobulin M
(IgM), 33
immunologic memory,
28, 36
immunomodulatory drugs
(IMiDs). *See* checkpoint
inhibitors; oral immu-
nomodulatory agents
immunostimulatory fac-
tors in vaccine develop-
ment, 123–124
immunostimulatory ther-
apies, 20
immunosuppressive envi-
ronment in vaccine
development, 123
immunosurveillance,
6–8, 40–41

immunotherapy
adaptive immunity in,
48
defined, 44–47
history of, 1–13, 44–49
prior to 1900, 1–3
in 1900s–1980s, 3–5
in 1980s, 5–6
in 1990s, 6–8
in 2000s, 8–12
adoptive cell therapy
in, 6, 12
bacillus
Calmette-Guérin
in, 4–5
checkpoint inhibitors
in, 9t, 11
Coley toxins in, 3, 4
cytokines (interfer-
ons) in, 7–8, 9t
IL-2 in, 6
immunosurveillance
in, 6–8
monoclonal antibod-
ies in, 7, 8, 9t–10t
oncolytic viral thera-
pies in, 10t
targeted therapies in,
6, 8, 10t
timeline of FDA
approval in, 9t–10t
tumor necrosis factor
in, 4
vaccines in, 4–5, 7,
11–12
passive vs. active, 49
terminology for, 45t–
47t
Immunotherapy Teach-
ing/Monitoring Tool,
242–243
IMP321, 75t
indoleamine
2,3-dioxygenase
(IDO), 74, 75t
indoximod, 75t
inducible T-cell costimu-
lator protein, 74
induction phase in dual
checkpoint blockade,
222

inflammation
in cancer–immunity
cycle, 44
chronic, 22
defined, 46t
in innate immunity,
21–22
signs of, 22
infliximab, 62
infusion reactions
to CD20-targeted mAbs,
173–174
to CD38-targeted mAbs,
179–180
to checkpoint inhibi-
tors, 76, 246t, 276
desensitization for, 197
to EGFR-specific mono-
clonal antibodies, 151
to HER2-targeted
mAbs, 158
to inotuzumab ozogami-
cin, 191
to monoclonal antibod-
ies, 196–197
to vaccine therapy, 283
inhibitory checkpoints
for T cells, 34, 35t
innate immunity, 21–28,
21f
components of, 22–27,
23t–24t
defined, 20, 21, 46t
soluble factors of,
27–28, 29t
innate lymphoid cells
(ILCs), 26
inotuzumab ozogami-
cin (InO, Besponsa),
189–191
interferon(s)
in history of immuno-
therapy, 7–8, 9t
in innate immunity, 28
interferon alfa (IFN-α),
55–56
dosing schedules for, 56
in innate immunity, 29t
side effects of, 56
interferon alfa-2b (Intron
A), 7–8

interferon beta in innate
immunity, 29t
interferon gamma in
innate immunity, 29t
interleukin(s) (ILs), in
innate immunity, 28, 29t
interleukin-1 (IL-1) in
innate immunity, 28, 29t
interleukin-2 (IL-2),
57–58
in adaptive immunity,
39
in adoptive cell ther-
apy, 58
functions of, 57
in history of immuno-
therapy, 6
and interleukin-19, 61
side effects of, 57–58
structure of, 57
interleukin-6 (IL-6),
29t, 59
interleukin-6
(IL-6)-targeted mono-
clonal antibodies, 148t,
180–181
interleukin-10 (IL-10) in
innate immunity, 29t
interleukin-12 (IL-12)
in innate immunity,
26, 29t
interleukin-15 (IL-15) in
innate immunity, 29t
interleukin-18 (IL-18)
in innate immunity,
28, 29t
interleukin-19 (IL-19),
IL-2 and, 61
interstitial lung disease
due to EGFR-specific
monoclonal antibod-
ies, 151
ipilimumab (Yervoy),
71, 75t
adverse events due to,
245t–246t
as coinhibitor, 38
in combination immuno-
therapy, 11, 75, 221
in dual checkpoint
blockade, 222–223

ixazomib with
  lenalidomide-
  dexamethasone dou-
  blet, 110

J

Janus kinase(s) (JAKs)
  IL-6 and, 59
  in T-cell activation, 36
Janus kinase 3 (JAK-3), 7
JAK-STAT pathway, 7,
  36, 39

K

Kelsey, Frances Oldham,
  104
keratosis due to
  EGFR-specific mono-
  clonal antibodies, 149
KIR, 75*t*
KIT as biomarker, 232*t*,
  235*t*
KRAS mutation, 142–
  143, 144
  as biomarker, 233*t*, 235*t*

L

lactate dehydrogenase, 231
lactation
  adverse events during, 284
  checkpoint inhibitors
    and, 88
lactic acid in cancer–
  immunity cycle, 44
LAG-3, 35*t*
lectin pathway of comple-
  ment system, 27
lenalidomide (Revlimid),
  109–113
  in combination ther-
    apy, 110
  with dexamethasone, 110
  formulation of, 106*f*, 109
  indications for, 110–112
  in maintenance ther-
    apy, 111
  mechanism of action
    of, 106

side effects of, 109*t*,
  112–113, 277–280
leukemia
  acute lymphoblastic, 12
    antibody–drug conju-
      gates for, 189–190
    bispecific T-cell
      engager antibodies
      for, 194–195
    monoclonal antibod-
      ies for, 8
  acute myeloid, 185, 188–
    189
  chronic lymphocytic
    adoptive cell therapy
      for, 12
    biomarkers for, 232*t*
    monoclonal antibod-
      ies for, 8, 168, 170–
      173, 182–183
  chronic myeloid, 56
  hairy cell, 7, 56
light chains, 32, 32*f*
liquid biopsy, 229
lirilumab, 75*t*
liver function alteration
  due to EGFR-specific
    monoclonal antibod-
    ies, 150
  with elotuzumab, 178
LSI TP53 as biomarker,
  232*t*
Lübeck disaster, 4
lung cancer
  biomarkers for,
    232*t*–233*t*, 236
  checkpoint inhibitors
    for, 247
  non-small cell
    checkpoint inhibitors
      for, 73
    combination immuno-
      therapy for, 257
    monoclonal antibod-
      ies for, 162, 163*t*,
      164
lymphocyte-activation
  gene 3 (LAG-3), 35*t*,
  73, 75*t*
lymphoid progenitor
  cells, 33

lymphoma
  anaplastic large-cell
    antibody–drug conju-
      gates for, 185
    monoclonal antibod-
      ies for, 8
  B-cell
    chemoimmunother-
      apy for, 217
    monoclonal antibod-
      ies for, 169
    radioimmunotherapy
      for, 191, 193
  biomarkers for, 231
  follicular
    chemoimmunother-
      apy for, 217
    history of immuno-
      therapy for, 8
    monoclonal antibod-
      ies for, 8, 168
  Hodgkin
    antibody–drug conju-
      gates for, 185, 186
    checkpoint inhibitors
      for, 263, 272–273
    monoclonal antibod-
      ies for, 8
  mantle cell, 111
  non-Hodgkin
    adoptive cell therapy
      for, 12
    chemoimmunother-
      apy for, 217
    chimeric antigen
      receptor T-cell
      therapy for, 280
    history of immuno-
      therapy for, 7
    monoclonal antibodies
      for, 8, 168, 169, 170
    radioimmunotherapy
      for, 191–194, 219–
      220
  pseudoprogression of, 288

M

macrophages
  in cancer–immunity
    cycle, 44

in innate immunity, 22, 24
maintenance phase in dual checkpoint blockade, 222–223
major histocompatibility complex (MHC) molecules
  in cell-mediated immunity, 33–34
  defined, 46t
  and dendritic cells, 25
  in immunotherapy, 48
  in vaccine therapy, 121
mammalian target of rapamycin (mTOR) pathway, 36
mantle cell lymphoma (MCL), 111
mast cells in innate immunity, 23t
mastocytosis, biomarkers for, 232t
MEDI0680, 75t
medication persistence with oral therapy, 288–289, 290t–291t
melanoma
  adoptive cell therapy for, 12, 58
  biochemotherapy for, 217–219
  biomarkers for, 231, 232t
  checkpoint inhibitors for, 11, 71, 72, 75, 259–260, 270–271
  combination immunotherapy for, 221–223
  cytokines (interferons) for, 8, 55–56
  GM-CSF for, 60
  history of immunotherapy for, 6, 8
  IL-2 for, 57, 58
  immunocytokines for, 61
  oncolytic viral therapy for, 132–134, 133f
  pseudoprogression of, 287f
  vaccine therapy for, 12, 132

memory B cells, 31
memory cells, 36
memory T cells, 37
Merkel cell carcinoma, checkpoint inhibitors for, 72
mertansine, 186
mesenchymal growth factors in innate immunity, 28
monitoring, biomarkers for, 230–231, 230t, 232t–234t
monoclonal antibodies (mAbs), 139–197
  in antibody–drug conjugates (conjugated), 140, 142t, 184–191
    ado-trastuzumab emtansine as, 148t, 186–188
    brentuximab vedotin as, 148t, 185–186
    gemtuzumab ozogamicin as, 188–189
    inotuzumab ozogamicin as, 189–191
    mechanism of action of, 184–185
    side effects of, 148t
  in antibody–radiopharmaceutical conjugates (ibritumomab tiuxetan), 148t, 191–194
  bispecific T-cell engager (blinatumomab), 140–141, 142t, 148t, 194–196
  CD20-targeted, 168–176
    obinutuzumab as, 147t, 172–173
    ofatumumab as, 147t, 170–172
    rituximab and hyaluronidase as, 146t, 169–170
    rituximab as, 146t, 168–170
    side effects of, 146t–147t, 173–176

CD38-targeted (daratumumab), 147t, 178–180
CD52-targeted (alemtuzumab), 148t, 182–183
and chimeric antigen receptor T cells, 149t, 198–201
defined, 47t
EGFR-specific, 141–155
  cetuximab as, 141, 143–144, 145t
  mechanism of action of, 141–143
  panitumumab as, 141, 143, 144, 145t
  side effects of, 144–155, 145t, 153f–154f
HER2-targeted, 155–161
  mechanism of action of, 155
  pertuzumab as, 145t, 157–158
  side effects of, 145t, 158–161
  trastuzumab as, 145t, 156–157
in history of immunotherapy, 7, 8, 9t–10t
human, humanized, and chimeric, 142t
hypersensitivity reactions to, 196–197
IL-6–targeted (siltuximab), 148t, 180–181
with lenalidomide-dexamethasone doublet, 110
mechanism of action of, 140
naked, 140, 142t
nomenclature for, 139, 142t
PDGFR-α–targeted (olaratumab plus doxorubicin), 146t, 167–168
RANKL-targeted (denosumab), 148t, 183–184

SLAMF7-targeted (elo-
tuzumab), 147*t*, 176–
178
structure of, 139, 140*f*,
141*f*
toxicities of, 145*t*–149*t*
tumor necrosis fac-
tor–specific (tigatu-
zumab), 140
types of, 140–141, 142*t*
VEGF-targeted, 161–167
bevacizumab as, 146*t*,
161–164, 163*t*
mechanism of action
of, 161
ramucirumab as, 146*t*,
164–165
side effects of, 146*t*,
165–167
monocytes in innate
immunity, 22, 23*t*, 24
monomethyl auristatin E
(MMAE), 186
Morales, Alvaro, 5
MS4A1 as biomarker, 235*t*
multiple myeloma
biomarkers for, 228, 236
monoclonal antibodies
for, 176–180
oral immunomodula-
tory agents for, 105,
106, 108, 110–111,
113, 277–278
multivalency in vaccine
development, 127
muromonab-CD3, 8
mutation(s), 21, 41, 43,
227
mutational burden of
cancer, 41, 43
myelodysplastic syn-
drome (MDS)
biomarkers for, 232*t*
lenalidomide for, 111–
112
myeloid cells in cancer–
immunity cycle, 44
myeloma, multiple
biomarkers for, 228, 236
monoclonal antibodies
for, 176–180

oral immunomodula-
tory agents for, 105,
106, 108, 110–111,
113, 277–278
myeloproliferative dis-
ease, biomarkers for,
232*t*
myelosuppression
due to inotuzumab ozo-
gamicin, 191
due to oral immuno-
modulators, 278

N

nail changes due to
EGFR-specific mono-
clonal antibodies, 152,
154*f*
National Cancer Moon-
shot Initiative, 12
natural killer (NK) cells,
7
in cancer–immunity
cycle, 44
immune memory func-
tion of, 27
in innate immunity, 24*t*,
26–27
neoantigens, 21, 41–43,
47*t*
nephritis due to check-
point inhibitors, 246*t*
neurologic toxicities
of blinatumomab, 195–
196
of checkpoint inhibi-
tors, 86–87, 270–271
neutropenia
due to blinatumomab,
195
due to CD20-targeted
mAbs, 175
due to CD38-targeted
mAbs, 180
due to chimeric antigen
receptor T cells, 200
due to oral immuno-
modulators, 278
neutrophils in innate
immunity, 22, 24*t*

nivolumab (Opdivo),
71–72, 75*t*
adverse events due to,
245*t*–246*t*
in combination immu-
notherapy, 11, 75,
221
in dual checkpoint
blockade, 222–223
history of, 11
mechanism of action
of, 39
prior to transplanta-
tion, 286
non-Hodgkin lymphoma
(NHL)
adoptive cell therapy
for, 12
chemoimmunotherapy
for, 217
chimeric antigen recep-
tor T-cell therapy
for, 280
history of immunother-
apy for, 7
monoclonal antibodies
for, 8, 168, 169, 170
radioimmunotherapy
for, 191–194, 219–
220
non-small cell lung can-
cer (NSCLC)
checkpoint inhibitors
for, 73
combination immuno-
therapy for, 257
monoclonal antibodies
for, 162, 163*t*, 164
nuclear factor
kappa-light-chain-
enhancer of activated
B cells (NF-κB), 35
nuclear factor of acti-
vated T cells (NF-AT),
35
NY-ESO-1, 7

O

obinutuzumab (Gazyva),
172–173

• Guide to Cancer Immunotherapy

173
history of, 8
indications for, 172
results for, 173
side effects of, 147t,
173–176
ocular toxicities
of checkpoint inhibi-
tors, 87, 276
of EGFR-specific mono-
clonal antibodies,
149–150
ofatumumab (Arzerra),
170–172
administration of, 170–
171
efficacy of, 171–172
indications for, 170
side effects of, 147t,
173–176
olaratumab plus doxoru-
bicin, 146t, 167–168
Old, Lloyd, 4
older adults, adverse
events in, 285
oncogenesis, 41–43
oncolytic viral therapy
(OVT), 130
adverse events with, 283
first approved agent for,
132–134, 133f
history of, 10t
Oncotype DX assays, 229
ophthalmic toxicities
of checkpoint inhibi-
tors, 87, 276
of EGFR-specific mono-
clonal antibodies,
149–150
opsonization, 47t
Oral Agent Teaching
Tool, 289
oral anticancer medica-
tions (OACs), adherence
to, 288–289, 290t–291t
oral immunomodulatory
agents, 103–114
adverse events from,
108, 109t, 112–114,
277–280

clinical applications of,
107–114
history of, 103–104
mechanism of action of,
105–106
nursing implications
of, 114
risk evaluation and miti-
gation strategy for,
106–107
structure of, 106f
organ transplantation,
adverse events with, 286
osteonecrosis due to
RANKL-targeted
monoclonal antibod-
ies, 184
osteosarcoma, 247–248
ovarian cancer, 162, 163t
OX40 ligand (OX40L), 74

P

P2X purinoceptor 7
(P2RX7), 216
paclitaxel, 61
pain, cytokines and, 62
pancreatic cancer, 11–12
pancreatitis due to checkpoint inhibitors, 272–
274, 273f
panitumumab (Vectibix),
141, 143, 144, 145t
side effects of, 144–155,
145t, 153f–154f
parathyroid hormone–
related protein
(PTHrP), 183
passive immuno-
oncology, 49, 119, 120,
139. See also monoclo-
nal antibodies (mAbs)
passive immunotherapy,
49, 119, 120, 139. See
also monoclonal anti-
bodies (mAbs)
pathogen-associated
molecular patterns
(PAMPs), 26, 47t
pattern recognition
receptors (PRRs)

defined, 47t
in innate immunity,
25–26
pediatric patients, adverse
events in, 285–286
peginterferon alfa-2b
(PegIntron), 8
pembrolizumab (Key-
truda), 72, 75t
adverse events due to,
245t–246t
in combination immu-
notherapy, 221
history of, 11
mechanism of action
of, 39
prior to transplanta-
tion, 286
peripheral neuropathy
due to checkpoint
inhibitors, 270–271
cytokines and, 62
due to oral immuno-
modulators, 279–280
due to thalidomide, 108
peripheral tolerance, 40
peritoneal cancer, 162,
163t
pertuzumab (Perjeta),
157–158
side effects of, 145t,
158–161
phagocytic cells in innate
immunity, 22
phagocytosis, 47t
pharmacodynamics, bio-
markers for, 230t
pidilizumab, 75t
pinocytosis, 25
platelet-derived
growth factor alpha
(PDGFR-α) inhibitors,
146t, 167–168
platelet-derived growth
factor beta (PDGFRB)
as biomarker, 232t
PML-RARA as biomarker,
235t
pneumonitis due to
checkpoint inhibitors,
83–84, 260–261

case-based management of, 260–261
frequency of, 245t
grading of, 261t–262t
treatment of, 79f
polyclonal antibody, 47t
polymerase chain reaction (PCR), 228
polymorphonuclear leukocytes in innate immunity, 22, 24t
pomalidomide (Pomalyst), 113–114
formulation of, 106f, 113
indication for, 113
mechanism of action of, 106
side effects of, 109t, 113–114, 278–280
predictive tools, biomarkers as, 230t, 231–236, 235t
pregnancy
adverse events in, 284
checkpoint inhibitors in, 88
thalidomide and, 106–107
primitive pattern recognition receptors in innate immunity, 25–26
progesterone receptor (PR) as biomarker, 235t, 236
prognostic tools, biomarkers as, 230t, 231–236
programmed cell death-ligand 1 (PD-L1), 67–68, 69, 70
as biomarker, 232t, 235–236, 235t
radiation therapy and, 74–75
in vaccine development, 122
programmed cell death-ligand 1 (PD-L1) inhibitors, 72–73, 75t, 76

adverse events due to, 245t–246t
dermatologic, 247–249, 248f, 249f
endocrine, 263–266, 263f, 265f
gastrointestinal, 252–253, 253f
hepatic, 257–258
pancreatitis as, 272–273, 273f
pulmonary, 259–261, 260f
programmed cell death-ligand 2 (PD-L2), 68, 69, 70
in vaccine development, 122
programmed cell death protein 1 (PD-1), 11, 34, 35t, 38–39, 67, 69–70
in vaccine development, 122
programmed cell death protein 1 (PD-1) inhibitors, 71–72, 75, 75t
adverse events due to, 245t–246t
in combination immunotherapy, 11, 221
in dual checkpoint blockade, 222–223
history of, 11
mechanism of action of, 39
progressive multifocal leukoencephalopathy (PML) due to CD20-targeted mAbs, 176
prostate cancer
biomarkers for, 230–231, 237
checkpoint inhibitors for, 11
vaccine therapy for, 130–131
prostate-specific antigen (PSA), 228, 230–231, 237

prostatic acid phosphatase (PAP) and vaccine therapy, 131
proteasome inhibitors (PIs) with lenalidomide-dexamethasone doublet, 110
proteinuria due to VEGF inhibitors, 166–167
proto-oncogenes, 227
pruritus
due to checkpoint inhibitors, 79–81, 247, 249
due to EGFR-specific monoclonal antibodies, 154f
pseudoprogression, 286–288, 287f
psoriasis due to checkpoint inhibitors, 247–248, 249f
pulmonary embolism due to oral immunomodulators, 279
pulmonary toxicity
of CD20-targeted mAbs, 175–176
of checkpoint inhibitors, 83–84, 259–262
case-based management of, 259–262, 260f
frequency of, 245t
grading of, 261t–262t
treatment of, 79f
of HER2-targeted mAbs, 159, 161

R

radiation therapy
combination, 148t, 191–194, 219–220
with checkpoint inhibitors, 74–75
and cytokine release, 61
radioimmunotherapy (RIT), 148t, 191–194, 219–220

with checkpoint inhibitors, 74–75
ramucirumab, 164–165
side effects of, 146t, 165–167
rash
due to checkpoint inhibitors, 79–81, 82f, 245t, 247–248, 248f, 249, 249f
due to EGFR-specific monoclonal antibodies, 151–152, 153f
due to oral immunomodulators, 278–279
R-CHOP regimen, 216–217, 218t
R-CVP regimen, 218t
receptor activator of nuclear factor kappa-B ligand (RANKL)-targeted (denosumab) monoclonal antibodies, 148t, 183–184
regulatory B cells, 31
regulatory T cells (Tregs)
in adaptive immune system, 30t, 37
in immunotherapy, 49
renal cell carcinoma (RCC)
checkpoint inhibitors for, 11
IL-2 for, 57
immunocytokines for, 61
monoclonal antibodies for, 162, 163t
renal dysfunction due to checkpoint inhibitors, 246t, 274
rheumatologic toxicities due to checkpoint inhibitors, 274–275
Risk Evaluation and Mitigation Strategy (REMS) program, 104, 106–107
rituximab (Rituxan), 168–170

with bendamustine, 218t
dosing schedule for, 168–169
history of, 7, 8
and hyaluronidase, 146t, 169–170
in R-CHOP regimen, 216–217, 218t
results for, 170
side effects of, 146t, 173–176
Rockefeller, John D., Jr., 2
round cell sarcoma, 1–3

S

sarcoma
checkpoint inhibitors for, 247–248
history of immunotherapy for, 1–3
monoclonal antibodies for, 167–168
screening, biomarkers for, 230–231, 230t, 232t–234t
secondary lymphoid tissue, 25
secondary primary malignancies (SPMs)
with elotuzumab, 177–178
with lenalidomide, 112–113
self-antigens in vaccine development, 122
self-tolerance, 40
in vaccine development, 122
serum sickness due to CD20-targeted mAbs, 174
signaling lymphocytic activation molecule F7 (SLAMF7)-targeted monoclonal antibodies, 147t, 176–178
signal transducer and activator of transcription (STAT), 7, 36, 39
IL-6 and, 56

siltuximab (Sylvant), 148t, 180–181
sipuleucel-T (Provenge), 130–131
adverse effects with, 283
skeletal-related events, monoclonal antibodies for, 183–184
skin infection due to EGFR-specific monoclonal antibodies, 152
solid organ transplantation, adverse events with, 286
specific immunity. See adaptive immunity
squamous cell carcinoma
checkpoint inhibitors for, 264
monoclonal antibodies for, 143
Stevens-Johnson syndrome due to checkpoint inhibitors, 81–82
stomatitis due to EGFR-specific monoclonal antibodies, 150
Streptococcus pyogenes and round cell sarcoma, 2–3, 54
stress level, cytokines and, 62
surrogate endpoints, biomarkers as, 230t, 236
System for Thalidomide Education and Prescribing Safety (S.T.E.P.S.), 104
systemic inflammatory response syndrome (SIRS) due to CD20-targeted mAbs, 174

T

talimogene laherparepvec (Imlygic, T-VEC), 132–134
administration of, 132, 133f

adverse events with,
132–134, 283
approval of, 60
history of, 12
indications for, 132
response to, 134
targeted therapies
in combination with
anti–CTLA-4, 74
history of, 6, 8, 10*t*
T-cell activation, 34, 36
T-cell exclusion, 44
T-cell expansion, 43
T-cell immunity, 7
T-cell membrane protein
3 (TIM-3), 35*t*, 73
T-cell metabolism
in immunotherapy, 49
regulation of, 43
T-cell precursors, 33
T-cell proliferation, 34
T-cell receptor (TCR),
33, 47*t*
T-cell recognition, 34
T-cell tolerance, 7
thalidomide (Thalomid)
clinical applications of,
107–108
formulation of, 106*f*, 107
history of, 103–104
indications for, 108
mechanism of action of,
105–106
nursing implications
of, 114
risk evaluation and miti-
gation strategy for,
106–107
side effects of, 108, 109*t*,
278–280
Theracys (BCG live intra-
vesical), 97, 98
therapeutic targets, bio-
markers as, 236
thrombocytopenia
due to CD20-targeted
mAbs, 175
due to CD38-targeted
mAbs, 180
due to oral immuno-
modulators, 278

thromboembolic events
due to immunomodula-
tory drugs, 106, 107
due to oral immuno-
modulators, 279
due to VEGF inhibi-
tors, 166
thromboprophylaxis
with immunomodula-
tory drugs, 107
with oral immunomod-
ulators, 279
thrombotic events due to
oral immunomodula-
tors, 279
thymocytes, 33
thyroid dysfunction due
to checkpoint inhibi-
tors, 85–86, 245*t*, 263,
263*f*, 266, 267*t*
thyroiditis due to check-
point inhibitors, 263,
263*f*
TICE BCG, 97, 98
TIGIT, 35*t*
TIM-3, 35*t*, 73
tisagenlecleucel (Kym-
riah), 12
tissue-resident memory
cells, 36
T lymphocytes (T cells).
See also under T-cell
in adaptive immune sys-
tem, 29, 30*t*, 33–36,
35*t*, 37, 38*t*
in adoptive cell trans-
fer, 197
in cancer–immunity
cycle, 42–44
chimeric antigen recep-
tor (CAR), 2, 149*t*,
198–201
inhibitory checkpoints
for, 34, 35*t*
tocilizumab (Actemra), 199
tolerance in vaccine
development, 123
Toll-like receptor(s)
(TLRs), 25, 47*t*
Toll-like receptor 4 (TLR-
4), 216

tositumomab (Bexxar), 8,
191, 219
toxic epidermal necrol-
ysis (TEN) due to
checkpoint inhibitors,
81–82
TPMT as biomarker, 235*t*
transaminitis due to
checkpoint inhibitors,
80*f*, 84–85, 237–238
transforming growth
factor beta in innate
immunity, 29*t*
trastuzumab (Her-
ceptin), 156–157
administration of, 156
in combination with
chemotherapy, 157
history of, 8
mechanism of action
of, 156
response to, 156
side effects of, 145*t*,
158–161
tuberculosis (TB) vac-
cine, 4–5, 95
tumor antigens, unde-
tectable, 43
tumor-associated anti-
gen (TAA) in vaccine
therapy, 120–121, 124–
125, 128
tumor cell recognition,
43
tumor flare, 286–288,
287*f*
tumor heterogeneity in
vaccine development,
124, 126
tumor-infiltrating lym-
phocytes (TILs) in
adoptive cell trans-
fer, 197
tumor lysis syndrome
(TLS)
due to CD20-targeted
mAbs, 174–175
due to chimeric anti-
gen receptor T cells,
200–201
tumor marker, ideal, 237

tumor microenviron-
ment (TME), 22, 24,
25, 43–44
tumor necrosis factor
(TNF)
in adaptive immunity,
39
in history of immuno-
therapy, 4
in innate immunity,
28, 29t
tumor suppressor genes,
227
tumor-targeting mono-
clonal antibodies. *See*
monoclonal antibodies
(mAbs)

U

UGT1A1 as biomarker,
231–235, 235t
urothelial carcinoma, 72,
73, 252–253, 264–265
U.S. Food and Drug
Administration (FDA)
approval, timeline of,
9t–10t

V

vaccine(s), prophylactic
vs. therapeutic, 121–
122
vaccine therapy, 119–134
adverse events with, 283
approved agents for,
130–134
sipuleucel-T as, 130–
131

talimogene laher-
parepvec as, 132–
134, 133f
combination, 128–129
defined antigen, 127t,
128
development of, 122–
129
autologous vs. alloge-
neic tumor sources
in, 125–126
inducing immunos-
timulatory factors
in, 123–124
overcoming immune
suppression in,
122–123
selection of
tumor-associated
antigen in, 124–
125
DNA-based, 123, 128
ex vivo dendritic cell,
129–130
history of, 4–5, 7, 11–12
mechanism of action of,
120–122
oncolytic viral therapy
as, 130
first approved agent
for, 132–134, 133f
whole-cell, 126–127,
127t
vascular endothelial
growth factor recep-
tor (VEGF)-targeted
monoclonal antibod-
ies, 161–167
bevacizumab as, 146t,
161–164, 163t

mechanism of action
of, 161
ramucirumab as, 146t,
164–165
side effects of, 146t,
165–167
vasculitis due to CD20-t
argeted mAbs, 175
VCTN1, 73
veno-occlusive disease
(VOD)
due to gemtuzumab
ozogamicin, 189
due to inotuzumab ozo-
gamicin, 190
venous thromboembo-
lism (VTE) due to
VEGF inhibitors, 166
venous thrombotic events
due to oral immuno-
modulators, 279
viral vector therapy, 130
VISTA, 35t
vitiligo due to checkpoint
inhibitors, 78–79

W

wallet card, 243
white blood cell growth
factor in innate immu-
nity, 22
whole-cell vaccine ther-
apy, 126–127, 127t

X

xerosis due to EGFR-
specific monoclonal
antibodies, 152, 153f